RADIANT HEALTH AGELESS BEAUTY

Dr. Christine Horner's **30-Day Program** to Extraordinary Health, Beauty, and Longevity

CHRISTINE HORNER, M.D., F.A.C.S.

D0029477

Elgea Publishing
San Diego, CA

The information contained in this book is based upon the research and personal and professional experiences of the author. It is not intended as a substitute for consulting with your physician or other healthcare provider. Any attempt to diagnose and treat an illness should be done under the direction of a healthcare professional.

The author does not advocate the use of any particular healthcare protocol but believes the information in this book should be available to the public. The author is not responsible for any adverse effects or consequences resulting from the use of the suggestions, preparations, or procedures discussed in this book. Should the reader have any questions concerning the appropriateness of any procedures or preparation mentioned, the author strongly suggests consulting a professional healthcare advisor.

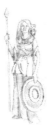

Published by:
Elgea Publishing
San Diego, CA

Copyright © 2016 Christine Horner

ISBN-13   Hardcover: 978-0-9972884-1-4
              Softcover: 978-0-9972884-0-7

The image on page 19 is reprinted by permission of Jai Shree Krishn
    www.haribhakt.com
The images on page 35 and 36 are reprinted by permission of Dr. Masaru Emoto.
The image on page 38 is reprinted by permission of Global Good News
    Administration, http://globalgoodnews.com/
The image on page 198 is reprinted by permission of Jacqueline Rizk,
    www.thedetoxdiva.com
The image on page 209 is reprinted by permission of Todd Strane, Life Vessel
    Advanced Wellness, www.lifevessel.com
The image on page 245 is reprinted by the permission of Barbara Litchfield,
    HTCP, MA, CCA, www.HealingTouchCincinnati.com

Edited by Carol Killman Rosenberg • www.CarolKillmanRosenberg.com
Cover and interior design by Gary A. Rosenberg • www.thebookcouple.com
Cover photo by Dorie Hagler

Printed in the United States of America.

Contents

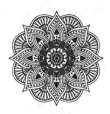

Laying Down the Scalpel
for the Secrets to Radiant Health

*D*o you fear growing older because you think your mind and body will start to falter? Do you imagine that one by one your organs will begin to fail—first your eyesight will go, then your joints, your mind, your skin tone, and ultimately your heart? But what if there was another option—a way to age gracefully and beautifully, and stay radiantly healthy, vibrant, limber, and strong?

You might think preventing the stereotypical decline in old age requires an austere life with hours of meditation every day, along with juice fasts and yoga; or hours of rigorous exercise and a diet of lettuce, carrots, and wheat grass, along with expensive spa treatments and plastic surgery. Or you may believe that your health and longevity are programmed in your genes and there's nothing you can do about it. After all, Jeanne Calmet from France, who had the longest recorded lifespan, died in 1997 at the age of 122 years old and smoked cigarettes, drank port wine, and ate chocolate every day. She must have been blessed with longevity genes, right? Not so fast.

What if I were to tell you that no matter what you were dealt in the genetic lottery, you could enjoy a long life of radiant health and ageless beauty—and achieving it could be simple, fun, and adventurous? That's what this book is all about.

As a board-certified plastic surgeon, I know all too well how you can spend thousands of dollars on topical treatments and surgery in an attempt to turn back the clock. Streams of women, regardless of their income, along with an ever-growing percentage of men, continuously came to my office seeking the latest techniques to help them look younger.

But one week in 1997 changed my entire concept of health and rejuvenation, and ultimately, my career and my life. I was at a spa in Fairfield, Iowa. It was an unusual spa that specialized in a technique called *panchakarma*, a detoxification and rejuvenation program based on *Ayurveda*. After forty-eight hours of receiving the unique individualized treatments—which were not uncomfortable, but rather luxurious and relaxing—I looked in the mirror and was amazed to see that I looked a decade younger, and I had never felt better in my life!

At that moment I realized that most of my patients, although they couldn't articulate it, actually desired the youthful, healthy glow I saw staring back at me in the mirror—a look that could never be achieved with surgery and topical chemicals.

My plastic surgery training had only taught me how to anatomically reposition skin and underlying tissue to a more youthful contour, and use chemicals and other materials to artificially enhance appearance. I was taught nothing about how to naturally create youthful beauty from the inside out, as this ancient system of medicine understands, not to mention its side benefits of extraordinary health, vitality, and longevity. After all, how great is it to artificially look good after surgery, when inside you feel rundown, tired, depressed, and unhealthy? It was clear to me that *Ayurveda* held the answers to many of the mysteries of the fountain of youth. So, I dove in eagerly, learning the timeless truths and wisdom from this incredible system of medicine.

Ayur means life and *veda* means knowledge, so *Ayurveda* literally means the "knowledge of life or lifespan." It teaches the "natural laws" that govern human beings. If you follow these fundamental principles and guidelines, you create balance in your physiology and enhance your inner healing intelligence, which results in extraordinary health and radiant beauty. If you violate these laws, you generate imbalances that obstruct the flow of your inner intelligence, and may progress to poor health and chronic diseases, as well as accelerated aging. Studies confirm that the healthiest lifestyle—one which also promotes longevity and radiant beauty—is based in the timeless truths of this ancient system of holistic medicine.

In my quest to find effective natural approaches to health and beauty,

I also discovered techniques in other traditional systems of medicine, such as Traditional Chinese Medicine. My investigations uncovered new technologies too, many of which are based in quantum physics—for example, subtle energy devices that can restore health by rebalancing and detoxifying the body.

As my knowledge of simple, effective, natural techniques to health, beauty, and longevity grew, so did my desire to let as many people as possible gain access to this information. For that reason, I approached the television stations in Cincinnati suggesting I be their on-air doctor, hosting a segment on natural health in the newscast. They said, "Yes!" So, from 1999 to 2002, I worked as the medical editor and host of a biweekly segment on the newscast that focused exclusively on complementary and alternative medicine (CAM), including natural approaches to staying healthy. The segment aired on (ABC) WCPO-TV and then on (NBC) WLW-TV, and in 2001, it was syndicated nationwide on the WISDOM Television Network.

The more segments I completed, the more I learned about natural approaches to health, and the greater my disappointment with Western medicine grew. Not surprisingly, I woke up one morning in 2002, realizing I could no longer practice medicine as I had. So I left my lucrative plastic surgery practice to dedicate myself full time to my soul's passion: teaching people how to achieve and maintain an extraordinary state of health—naturally.

This book is written out of my lifelong passion and commitment to health and beauty and out of my belief that anyone—regardless of age or current physical condition—can achieve radiant health. It is written from the culmination of more than twenty years of research and personal experiences. It blends the ancient wisdom from *Ayurveda* with the latest evidence-based, non-pharmaceutical and non-surgical approaches to help you dramatically improve your health, beauty, and longevity.

This book is my gift to you. My hope is that you feel inspired to incorporate all of its gems and pearls and that it blesses you with radiant health, ageless beauty, extraordinary longevity, and a profound connection to Spirit.

Many blessings!
Christine Horner, M.D.

*"Take care of your body with steadfast fidelity.
The soul must see through these eyes alone,
and if they are dim,
the whole world is clouded."*

~JOHANN WOLFGANG VON GOETHE

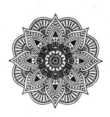

The Theories of
How and Why We Age

*B*efore you begin learning about all the factors that can help you achieve extraordinary health and longevity, I thought it would be helpful for you to be familiar with some of the basic theories of aging. These theories not only explain how and why we age, but also provide a framework for understanding how and why each item presented in this book is able to enhance your health and longevity.

The study of aging has been a fascination for the past several decades and generated more than 300 different theories explaining how and why we age. These theories are not exclusive from each other, but rather, aging is thought to be a result of many processes interacting simultaneously. In other words, all the theories are true. There isn't just one cause of aging, but rather many factors that simultaneously contribute to the process.

According to a review of the "Theories of Aging" published in the *Journal of Applied Physiology* in 2003 by researchers from the Department of Molecular and Cell Biology at the University of California, Berkeley, the most widely accepted theories of aging can be broadly viewed as either "programmed" or "error" theories. They also fall into one of four general categories: evolutionary, molecular, cellular, and system-based.

Programmed and Error Theories of Aging

The "programmed theories" of aging center on biological clocks regulating the timetable of your lifespan through the stages of growth, development, maturity, and old age. They depend on certain genes being switched on and off. Whereas, the "error theories" focus on the fact that your body is continuously being attacked by oxygen free radicals, as well as other factors that cause progressive damage to your tissues and cells. The structures inside your cells are also targets for this type of damage, especially your mitochondria (the power plants) and your DNA.

Evolutionary Theories of Aging

The evolutionary theories of aging involve the concept of "reproductive fitness." Based on Darwinian models of evolution, the evolutionary theories view longevity as a trait that is passed on *only* if it is beneficial to survival of the species. In other words, you are programmed for reproducing successfully, not for longevity. Living organisms only live longer if it helps them to produce more offspring.

Molecular Theories of Aging

The major molecular theory of aging is called the "Gene Regulation Theory." It explains that aging is due to changes in gene expression, and that lifespan is influenced by the turning on and off of genes that promote longevity. Said more simply, certain genes turn on and off as you age. Your lifespan can be lengthened by keeping your "youthful" genes turned on and your "aging" genes turned off.

In addition, there are specific genes that appear to be associated with exceptional longevity. For instance, studies have identified certain genes on chromosome 4 that may promote longevity. Scientists have also found three "super genes" that increase your likelihood of reaching 100 years of age by over twenty times. These genes reduce your chances of developing Alzheimer's disease by 80 percent, too. In one study, those who had these longevity genes had a one in 500 chance of reaching 100, compared with a one in 10,000 chance for those who did not.

Researchers in Bologna, Italy, found that centenarians also tend to have a more active tumor suppression gene p53, which may help to explain why they generally escape or postpone developing cancer.

Supporting the gene theories is the observation that exceptional longevity tends to run in families. Keep in mind, however, that members of the same families often eat the same foods, participate in the same lifestyle, and keep similar social support structures that are common in cultures with exceptional longevity. So, despite being genetically related, it's actually the environmental influences that are more responsible for their good health and longevity. In fact, a landmark Danish twin study documented that good health and longevity is 90 percent "environmental"—meaning diet and lifestyle—and only 10 percent genetic.

Cellular Theories of Aging

The cellular theories of aging include the "Cellular Senescence Theory," which highlights that normal human cells have a limited number of times they can divide. The limited number of cell replications has to do with special repeating DNA sequences at the end of chromosomes called "telomeres"—which shorten each time a cell divides. You may remember from high school biology that your cells regenerate themselves by replicating and dividing. First, the DNA lines up in the center of your cell, then it makes an exact copy of itself, and then the cell divides into two brand-new daughter cells. Each time your cells divide, the telomeres on the ends of your chromosomes become shorter.

There is a point where the telomere length becomes so short that the cell is unable to divide again. Consequently, the cell ages and eventually dies. An enzyme, called "telomerase," not only prevents your telomeres from shortening, but it can also cause them to grow longer. Longer telomeres prolong the life of the cell. When telomerase is activated in cells grown in the laboratory, the telomere length is preserved in the cells and they can be kept alive indefinitely—they never die!

You may be thinking right now, *Ah ha! The key to the fountain of youth is simply activating more telomerase,* but not so fast. Our biology is extremely complex. Attempting to manipulate it in a narrow way generally doesn't turn out well—as is the case with too much telomerase. One of the reasons that cancer cells grow out of control is that they produce abundant amounts of telomerase.

Telomere length is currently a major focus of anti-aging research. Countless studies have been performed on diet and lifestyle factors and the effect they have on telomere length. For instance, resveratrol, a substance from grape skins that is discussed in detail in chapter 4, has many health- and longevity-promoting benefits, including increasing the production of telomerase.

A study published in *The Lancet Oncology* in 2008 by cardiologist Dean Ornish, M.D., famous for showing that cardiovascular disease is reversible through diet and lifestyle changes, found that the same diet and lifestyle changes that reversed cardiovascular disease also increased telomerase activity in cells. Those changes included eating a plant-based diet, exercising regularly, practicing a daily stress-reducing technique, and participating in social support groups.

Telomere length has such a strong influence on longevity that it appears to be much greater than that of family environment and genetics. In a 2007 Swedish twin study, telomere length at advanced age predicted survival more than any other influence. Twins with the shorter telomeres had a three times greater risk of death during the follow-up period than their co-twins with the longer telomere length.

In a paper published in the *Journal of Gerontology: Biological and Medical Sciences* in April 2011, researchers at the University of Washington studied 1,136 participants in the Cardiovascular Health Study of adults aged sixty-five and older. Blood samples were taken upon enrollment to analyze telomere length. The participants were then followed for the next six years in which 468 deaths occurred. Those with the shortest telomeres had a 60 percent greater risk of dying during the follow-up time compared to those with the longest. The data strongly suggested that the major contributing factors to the erosion of the telomere length were oxidative stress and inflammation—the focus of two other cellular theories of aging: The "Free Radical Theory" and the "Inflammation Hypothesis."

The "Free Radical Theory" and the "Inflammation Hypothesis" theories state that aging is a result of the damage these processes cause to cells and DNA. The damage increases with age and leads to a progressive accumulation of biological "garbage" or waste material, including oxidized proteins, defective mitochondria (the power plants of the cell), lipofuscin (age pigment), and other debris. The waste material continues to build and the energy production in the cell gradually falls, until finally the cell dies. Not surprisingly, researchers have found that damage caused by both oxygen free radicals and inflammation also accelerates telomere shortening.

Systems-Based Theories of Aging

Finally, the "System-Based Theories" of aging state that declining function of essential systems in the body, such as the nervous, endocrine, and immune systems, is responsible for aging and death. During your lifespan, a multitude of physical, biological, and emotional stressors constantly tear down and weaken all of your biological systems until finally they can no longer sustain you. A study published in 2008 in the *Journal of Physiological Pharmacology* states that immunity decreases with aging, because of the decline of the numbers of T and B lymphocytes—a phenomenon that is also associated with shortening telomere length, as well as with oxidative damage and inflammation. Aging, according to these theories, is a result of "a decreasing ability to survive stress." Not surprisingly, the immune systems in those who live healthily past 100 years tend to stay strong.

Strategies for Extending Lifespan

In an effort to increase lifespan, scientists have developed a number of strategies to counteract each theory of aging. Researcher and scientist Aubrey de Grey, Ph.D., an expert on all forms of cellular and molecular damage involved in aging, believes that someday we will have biomedical technologies he calls SENS (Strategies for Engineered Senescence) that will be able to stop aging. But none of these are currently available, and it doesn't look like any of them will be in the near future. If you are interested in reading more about Dr. de Grey's work, you can do so in his book, *Ending Aging* (St. Martin Press, 2007).

Calorie Restriction

The most reproducible intervention that has been shown to extend lifespan is calorie restriction. A healthy calorie-restricted diet contains all the essential vitamins, minerals and other nutrients you need, but significantly restricts your calories by 30 to 70 percent. The anti-aging effects of calorie restriction have been studied for more than seventy years. Studies conducted on animals have found that it can increase their maximum lifespan by 30 to 40 percent. In humans, calorie restriction causes the same significant physiological improvements as it does in animals. For example, the most renowned study, called the "Biosphere 2" experiments, analyzed the effects of a calorie-restricted diet (30 percent fewer calories than the daily recommended) on eight individuals who lived in a closed system "biosphere" in the deserts of Arizona for two years. The physiological changes they experienced were similar to those that had been observed in mice and nonhuman primates. Their metabolic rates declined, as well as their body temperatures, systolic and diastolic blood pressures, blood glucose levels, and insulin and thyroid hormone levels.

Okinawans are famous for their exceptional good health and longevity, and researchers believe their low-calorie diet—based on vegetables, grains, soy, fruits, fish, and seaweed—may be one of the major reasons why. On average, their total daily calorie intake is 20 percent less than the average Japanese and 40 percent less than the average American. Interestingly, the type of diet Okinawans consume is very similar to the experimental calorie-restriction dietary models used for animals.

So how does calorie restriction work to improve health and extend lifespan? Researchers say there are a lot of different mechanisms at play. A study published in *JAMA* in 2007 notes that in adult men and women, calorie restriction causes a decrease in metabolic, hormonal, and inflammatory risk factors that increase the risk of diabetes, cardiovascular disease, and possibly cancer. Other physiological benefits associated with calorie restriction include:

- Increased tissue sensitivity to insulin

- The neuroendocrine and immune systems become more effective in defending against stress, infections, and cancer

- Reduced energy metabolism

- Increased production and turnover of proteins

- Reduced cholesterol, triglycerides, blood pressure, and arterial stiffness

- Increased HDL—the good type of cholesterol

- Improved balance of the sympathetic (fight-or-flight) and parasympathetic (relaxation) autonomic nervous systems

- Preserved telomere length

In addition, calorie restriction causes a reduction in white adipose (fat) tissue, which has also been shown to play a major role in extending lifespan. In fact, research shows there is a direct relationship between the percent of body fat you have and your health and longevity.

Aging Is a Complex Process

Keep in mind that aging is thought to be a result of many processes inter-acting simultaneously. In other words, there is truth to all the theories of aging. There isn't just one cause of aging, but rather many factors that simultaneously contribute to the overall aging process. Throughout this book, I will refer back to these basic theories to help explain how and why each item presented is able to improve your health and slow aging.

Most important, remember that no matter what the theories of aging say, you have tremendous influence on your health and longevity. This book will teach you everything you need to know to help counteract the various aging processes and achieve extraordinary health and exceptional longevity.

Collecting the Gems—
A Metaphor

*O*ne day while writing this book, I suddenly had the thought that the knowledge in this book could be thought of as "gems" and "pearls." Gems and pearls . . . hmmm. That thought led me to another: What if I used a metaphor for the book, which could help to make it more entertaining to read, just as I had done for my previous book, *Waking the Warrior Goddess?*

So, I sat down in meditation and asked to be shown what metaphor I should use. An image appeared in my mind of the breastplate of the high priest. I had never read anything about it previously, so I had no idea what it was. In my head I heard, *Go look it up!*

"Okay, I will!" I said and opened my eyes, ran to my computer, and googled "breastplate of the high priest." There I learned that in Exodus, God gave instruction to Moses to tell the Hebrew people to construct a breastplate for Aaron, the high priest. The purpose was to enhance this high holy man's ability to hear Divine guidance. Very specific instructions were given (Exodus 28:30), which included using twelve different gemstones arranged in three columns and four rows.

I realized that this book, serendipitously, is organized into twelve main chapters; the thirteenth puts all the important elements presented in the previous twelve chapters together into a 30-day program.

Well, doesn't that work out great? I thought. *One gemstone for each chapter.* As I contemplated this metaphor further, I saw how it also fit perfectly into the intentions of *Ayurveda.* The ultimate purpose of *Ayurveda* is "enlightenment," which simply put, means being as closely connected to God or Source as is humanly possible—the same purpose of the breastplate.

In addition, gemstones have been used for thousands of years for healing due to their energetic qualities, including their color. This might sound a little *woo-woo* to you, but quantum physics recognizes that all matter—including gems—produces energy, which can have a measurable influence on your physiology. Thousands of years ago, *Ayurveda* incorporated into its teachings that metals, gems, and stones held energetic qualities that could be used to counteract imbalances in the body. In his book *Ayurveda: The Science of Self-Healing*, Dr. Vasant Lad, one of the most renowned *Ayurvedic* physicians in the world, said, "Gems give off as well as draw in energy through their negative and positive vibrations," and can be used for physical, mental, and emotional healing. For example, lapis lazuli, which has a deep blue color, is said to be good for eye problems, as well as for sensitizing you to higher states of spiritual vibration.

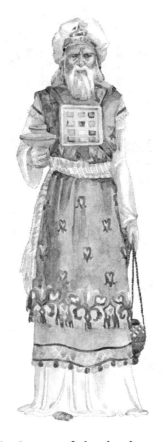

You can think of the information in each chapter of this book as a gemstone in a breastplate you are creating. As you read each chapter, you gather that gemstone and place it into your breastplate. After collecting all twelve of them, your breastplate is complete. Now you will have all the knowledge you need to achieve a state of *such* extraordinary health that you are able to connect easily to divine guidance—the ultimate purpose of this book.

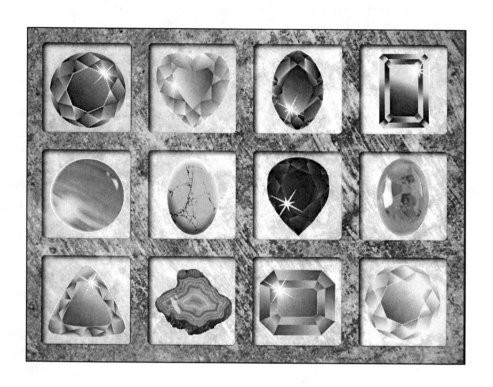

CHAPTER 1

Ayurveda

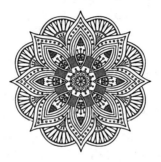

Rediscovering an Ancient System of Health and Longevity

*Vitality and beauty are gifts of nature
for those who live according to its laws.*

~LEONARDO DA VINCI

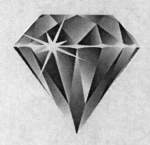

THE FIRST GEM: RUBY

Ayurveda represents the first gem in your breastplate of knowledge—a ruby. According to Eastern philosophies, the energy center called the "root chakra" or "base chakra" is the first and foundational energy center in the human body. Similarly, *Ayurveda* provides the foundation for your health and for understanding all of the information provided in this book.

The color of the root chakra is red, like that of a ruby. The color red is stimulating and represents fire and passion. When you bring your body into perfect balance by following the principals of *Ayurveda*, like the color red, you too will feel energized and inspired.

The energy of a ruby is said to assist you in the attainment of spiritual wisdom, health, knowledge, and your ultimate values—which is exactly what *Ayurveda* provides for you. Finally, a ruby is considered a shielding stone, and just like *Ayurveda*, it offers protection and encourages you to follow your bliss.

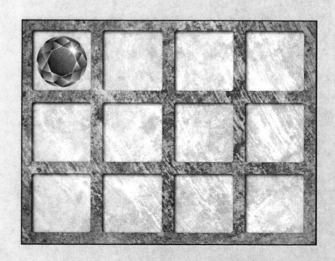

*A*fter eleven years of Western medical training, including medical school and residencies in general surgery and plastic surgery, I realized I had learned almost nothing about how to create good health and maintain it. Rather, my education had been focused on how to treat diseases and suppress their symptoms with medications and surgery. After a few years into my private plastic surgery practice, I discovered *Ayurveda,* a still vital 5,000-year-old prevention-oriented holistic system of health, and finally grasped the secrets to health and longevity.

When I was first introduced to *Ayurveda* and began to study it in 1996, I'm embarrassed to say that I had previously never heard of it, even though approximately one-sixth of the world's population uses it as their primary form of healthcare. I was so amazed by the incredible knowledge held by this system of medicine and the miraculous results it can achieve that I became certified in it and have continued to study and personally use *Ayurveda* ever since.

Ayur means life or lifespan and *veda* means knowledge, so *Ayurveda* literally means the *knowledge of life* or the *science of lifespan.* It's the science of how to live a long, radiantly healthy life—to its full potential—by achieving and maintaining a fine state of balance. This system of medicine details the eternal unchanging laws of Nature that when followed, support health, longevity, and beauty; and when disobeyed, destroy it. All the techniques and recommendations of *Ayurveda* are designed to bring you into balance and keep you there. *Ayurveda* underscores this core truth: *Perfect balance is the foundation and key to perfect health.*

A Holistic Approach

Ayurveda is a holistic system of health. This means, it embodies the paradigm that there is no separation between your mind, body, spirit, and consciousness or anything seemingly outside you in the universe. Quantum physics has shown that this is true. Everything inside you and everything outside you, at the most finite level, is intimately connected. So, everything affects everything. In other words, any technique—be it mental, physical, or spiritual—has profound effects on your entire physiology. Naturally, it follows that everything in your environment affects your health, as well.

17

Ayurveda also emphasizes the experience of higher states of consciousness, which are characterized by an expanded awareness. These higher states, which have been documented by changes in brain-wave activity, have been shown to create profound balance in the mind and body. Research shows that people who practice meditation techniques that enliven higher, more expanded states of consciousness regularly enjoy so much balance that they are dramatically healthier than the average American. For example, a Canadian study found that individuals who practice a form of meditation called "Transcendental Meditation" for just twenty minutes twice a day, use the healthcare system, overall, 50 percent less often and have 87 percent fewer hospital admissions for cardiovascular diseases!

But the ultimate intention of *Ayurveda* goes far beyond preventing disease. Not only is its goal to produce robust health for the mind and body, but also to support your ability to achieve higher states of consciousness—and, ultimately, "enlightenment." Enlightenment is considered the highest state of human awareness; it is the ability to see and know the reality of all things and to enjoy mastery over the physical state of being. Examples of well-known enlightened beings include Buddha, Mohammad, and Christ. But there have also been thousands of others who have lived in the past or who are currently alive who have achieved enlightenment. If you are interested in reading a classic book on this topic, I recommend *Autobiography of a Yogi,* written by the spiritual master Paramahansa Yogananda.

Clearly, the goals and objectives of *Ayurveda* are very different from the Western model of healthcare. I like to put it this way: Western medicine is about suppressing the symptoms of disease; *Ayurveda* is about creating profound health. Because we have grown up with a "disease-care" system of medicine (as opposed to "healthcare" system), most Americans have no idea how to create an extraordinary state of health—or even believe that it's possible—especially as we age. Fortunately, *Ayurveda* holds a reservoir of simple recommendations and techniques that can help each of us, including you, to experience radiant health at every age—including old age.

The History of *Ayurveda*

Ayurveda dates back at least 5,000 years and is thought to be the oldest comprehensive system of medicine still practiced today. The *Vedic* culture, a visionary society that lived in an area of the world that is now India, is credited with being the original source of this knowledge. Initially, all the wisdom held in *Ayurveda* was passed down through oral tradition. Then about 2,500 years ago, it was written down in two texts: the medical text the *Charaka Samhita* and the surgical text the *Sushruta Samhita*. Both of these astoundingly comprehensive repositories of ancient knowledge are still used by students of *Ayurveda* today.

Although *Ayurveda* is thousands of years old, it is an extremely sophisticated system of medicine with forty divisions—branches of medicine—that have lasted through time. In fact, many of them make up the fundamental structure of our medical system today, such as internal medicine, ENT (ear, nose, and throat), ophthalmology, obstetrics and gynecology, pediatrics, geriatrics, psychiatry, toxicology, and surgery. In addition, *Ayurveda* also has divisions in nutrition, meditation, massage, rejuvenation therapies, herbal mixtures, and a variety of mind/body/consciousness techniques.

As a plastic surgeon, I was fascinated to learn that the preferred surgical technique for reconstructing the nose after trauma or cancer that was taught to me during residency was first described in the *Sushruta Samhita* in the 6th century BC!

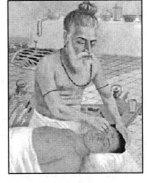

Written by a physician named *Sushruta*, the text includes descriptions of many surgical techniques performed today, ranging from hernia repairs, caesarian sections, and intestinal operations to cataract removal and the management of many types of bone fractures. Although the invention of the microscope would not occur for thousands of years, the importance of sterilization of medical and surgical instruments was described. In addition, *Sushruta* is thought to be the pioneer of anesthesia, because his text has the first written records of its use—recommending that wine with incense of cannabis be administered to patients before surgery.

The text also identifies hundreds of chronic diseases. For instance, *Sushruta* described diabetes and associated its development with obesity and a sedentary lifestyle. He also recommended dietary changes and exercise to help cure it.

After thousands of years of continuous practice, *Ayurveda* went through some extremely rocky times when the British invaded India, declared its practice illegal, and closed all the *Ayurvedic* medical schools. After India gained its independence in 1947, attempts were made to reestablish *Ayurveda*. Not surprisingly, much of the ancient knowledge had become fragmented, and some of it had been completely lost. The practice of *Ayurveda* had degenerated essentially into an herbalized form of Western medicine. Prevention and techniques of consciousness were no longer at its forefront.

Then, in the early 1980s, Maharishi Mahesh Yogi, the person who brought Transcendental Meditation (TM) to the West, recognized that the world was in desperate need of *Ayurveda*—in its original comprehensive form. He brought the top *Ayurvedic* doctors (called *vaidyas*) together to reconstruct the lost knowledge. They were given the task to carefully read the original *Ayurvedic* texts and then select the most effective techniques that would best suit our culture now. This form of *Ayurveda* is distinguished by being called Maharishi Ayurveda or Maharishi Vedic Approach to Health (MVAH).

Navigating Alternative Medicine

If you've ever looked into using complementary and alternative medicine (CAM), I'd be surprised if you didn't become confused and overwhelmed. On the surface, it appears to be a smorgasbord of hundreds of different health practices with no apparent link. Without expert guidance, the average person can't select the right combination of techniques or approaches to most effectively meet his or her individual needs.

Most of the techniques used in CAM today have their roots in *Ayurveda*, including such diverse treatments as yoga, massage, meditation, music therapy, sound therapy, aromatherapy, herbs, breathing techniques, special diets, and detoxification, to name just a few. So, an expert in *Ayurveda* is also masterful at creating a comprehensive program using these various techniques to best meet the unique needs of each individual patient.

Ayurveda also teaches a group of simple yet profound principles that provide a broad fundamental understanding of all the different techniques included in CAM. Its basic principles form a framework for understanding these techniques and how they fit together into a comprehensive model of healthcare. These timeless truths are actually laws of Nature that govern health. They reveal how and why certain techniques work to improve health.

Throughout this book, I will present *Ayurvedic* principles to help give you the "big picture"—a deeper and clearer understanding of each element of the program. If all the methods to achieve radiant health and ageless beauty were presented without teaching you about their underlying *Ayurvedic* principles, they would seem like a long list of unrelated items that you could easily forget. But when you understand them in relationship to the fundamental laws of Nature, you will understand them on a much deeper level. They will make sense to you and stay with you.

To give you an idea of what I'm talking about, let's look at an example. One *Ayurvedic* principle is: *Food is medicine.* Our culture doesn't usually think of food as medicine. Most Americans are unfamiliar with the medicinal qualities of foods, because Western doctors don't prescribe foods; they prescribe pharmaceutical medications. That's why we're all very familiar with how to approach common, uncomplicated health problems using medications, such as aspirin or antacids. But very few of us know the names of the spices, herbs, and foods that may be just as effective.

Ayurvedic physicians, on the other hand, prescribe food as one of the first lines of treatment. Instead of recommending aspirin for a painful swollen joint, a *vaidya* would instruct you to consume the cooking spices turmeric and ginger, and the vegetables asparagus and spinach. For acid indigestion, instead of recommending an antacid, rice, *mung dal* (lentil soup), pumpkin, squash, pomegranate, fennel, cumin, coriander, or turmeric would be prescribed.

Thousands of years ago, the intelligence contained in food was well recognized for its ability to induce balance and increase the healing intelligence of your body. Modern science is now confirming what ancient physicians knew: The right food *is powerful medicine.* In chapter 4, you'll learn about some of the best medicinal foods, as well as those foods you should avoid to dramatically improve your overall health, lower your risk of most chronic disorders associated with aging, and add years to your life.

Two Underlying Principles of *Ayurveda*

All the techniques and principles in *Ayurveda* boil down to two grand underlying principles. The first and foremost one is this:

Perfect balance brings perfect health.

Ayurveda emphasizes that everything you do or eat—every day—either brings you into balance or throws you out of balance. The trick is to know the difference. If you choose only those foods and activities that bring balance, you can create perfect health.

The second most important principle is this:

**Perfect health is achieved through
enlivening your inner healing intelligence.**

In other words, all the health-promoting foods, activities, and herbs that are recommended work by making your body *stronger* and *smarter* at repairing itself and resisting disease. At their most fundamental level, all the seemingly unrelated techniques presented in this book help you to achieve radiant health and ageless beauty by creating balance, which causes your body's inner healing intelligence to be enlivened.

It's equally important to recognize not only what brings you into balance, but also what throws you out of balance—what to avoid. These are the activities you do or the foods you eat that weaken you, because they violate the natural laws governing your mind and body. Knowing these laws of Nature in advance helps to keep you from making the mistakes or creating the habits that obstruct your inner healing intelligence.

The principles of *Ayurveda* are the keys to understanding all the rules that govern your health. When you know the rules and follow them, you thrive abundantly, avoid catastrophes, and pave the path to extraordinary health and longevity.

*"Sickness is the vengeance of nature
for violation of her laws."*

~CHARLES SIMMONS

The *Doshas*

Ayurveda describes three unique fundamental energies that govern all of life. There is no corresponding concept in Western medicine, so these energies, called the *doshas*, may seem foreign or possibly weird to you. Hang in there with me, because you will soon understand how they work and they will begin to make sense.

There are three major types of *doshas: vata, pitta,* and *kapha. Vata* manages movement, *pitta* controls metabolism and energy production, and *kapha* is responsible for cohesion and structure. Each *dosha* has various qualities and functions. *Vata* is light, quick, dry, cold, subtle, unstable, and rough. *Pitta* is hot, fluid, sharp, and sour. *Kapha* is slow, heavy, soft, sweet, cool, unctuous, and stable. A few examples of the functions of *vata* include movement, carrying impulses from the senses, separating waste from food, and expelling waste. *Pitta* is responsible for vision, digestion, heat production, appetite, thirst, and intelligence. *Kapha* provides oiliness, stability, strength, patience, and virility.

The three *doshas* occur in every person, but in varying amounts. If a person has a predominance of the *vata dosha,* he or she will have many of the following characteristics:

- Tall and thin
- Cold intolerant
- Dry rough skin
- Thin dry hair
- Longer, crooked teeth
- Good short-term memory and poor long-term memory
- Speaks quickly
- Light sleeper
- Very active
- Quick restless mind
- Tends to worry, frighten easily, and be anxious

FAMOUS VATA PEOPLE

Audrey Hepburn	Keira Knightley
Woody Allen	Courtney Cox
Fred Astaire	Don Knotts
Shelley Duvall	Christy Turlington
Calista Flockhart	Celine Dion

The characteristic of a person who is predominantly *pitta* include:

- Medium height and build
- Soft fair skin, light brown or reddish hair
- Small teeth
- Green to gray penetrating eyes
- Speaks clearly, but sharply
- Sound sleeper
- Intelligent
- Emotionally intense
- Tends to be aggressive, easily irritated, and quick to anger

FAMOUS PITTA PEOPLE

John F. Kennedy	Debra Messing
Jack Nicholson	Brad Pitt
Nicole Kidman	Tom Cruise
Sting	Bill Clinton
Julianne Moore	Cindy Crawford

A person who has a preponderance of the *kapha dosha* will have many of these traits:

- Larger framed or overweight
- Thick, pale, cool, oily skin
- Large mouth with full lips
- Big eyes
- Beautiful thick dark hair and lashes
- Speaks slowly
- Needs lots of sleep and time to think things through
- Loving and secure
- Slow learner, but great long-term memory

FAMOUS KAPHA PEOPLE

Oprah	George Clooney
Martin Luther King	Tom Hanks
Arnold Schwarzenegger	Kim Kardashian
Marlon Brando	Beyonce
Queen Latifah	Kate Winslet

Most people have a predominance of two *doshas*. Those who have only one or have a balance of all three, called *tri-doshic*, are relatively uncommon. Your dominant *dosha* type is called your "constitution" or, in Sanskrit, your *prikriti*. You are born with your constitution, and for most people, it never changes. There are ten different types of constitutions, or *prikritis*.

1. *Vata*
2. *Pitta*
3. *Kapha*
4. *Vata-pitta-kapha*
5. *Vata-pitta*
6. *Vata-kapha*
7. *Pitta-vata*
8. *Pitta-kapha*
9. *Kapha-pitta*
10. *Kapha-vata*

To discover your *dosha* constitution, you can take a simple quiz that asks you questions about your characteristics. Here is a link to a *dosha* quiz on Banyan Botanical's website, an excellent *Ayurvedic* herbal company. It only takes a minute or two to take: www.banyanbotanicals.com/info/prakriti-quiz/.

Understanding your body constitution is important, because it provides the specific guideline or "prescription" for you to create balance in your body. We are not all the same. One size does not fit all when it comes to recommendations for your ideal diet and lifestyle. What brings one person into balance may take another person out of balance. For instance, if you have a high amount of *pitta*, hot spicy foods may cause you to have indigestion and acid reflux, so you will want to avoid them. However, if you have a lot of *kapha*, hot spicy foods can be wonderfully stimulating and will not cause any unpleasant symptoms. Constitutional prescriptions not only include recommendations for the food you should favor or avoid, but also for what types of activities, exercise, weather, behavior, and routines that are best for you.

Your constitution also gives insight to the type of chronic diseases you may have a tendency toward developing. For instance, because *vata* governs movement and has a tendency to be dry, a *vata* dominant person is more prone to develop osteoarthritis or a nervous tremor. By contrast, a person with a large amount of *pitta*, which is characterized by heat, is more likely to develop inflammatory conditions, such as peptic ulcer disease or acne. Those who have a predominance of *kapha*, have more oiliness and a tendency for congestion and, therefore, are more prone to developing cysts or chronic bronchitis.

The Stages of Disease

According to *Ayurveda*, all diseases begin as imbalances of the *doshas*, which are caused by poor choices in diet and lifestyle. Imbalances are easily reversible in the early stages with some modest diet and lifestyle changes. The further advanced they become, the more difficult they are to reverse. If left unchecked, imbalances can progress to full-blown diseases, which are difficult and time consuming to correct.

Ayurveda recognizes six stages of disease:

1. Accumulation

2. Aggravation

3. Dissemination

4. Localization

5. Manifestation—symptoms first appear

6. Disruption—or full-blown disease

Stage one is the accumulation of an excess amount of a *dosha*. In stage two, the *dosha* becomes aggravated. It disseminates throughout the body in stage three. At stage four, the aggravated *dosha* becomes localized to one area of the body and causes prodromal nonspecific symptoms such as pain, indigestion, headaches, and general malaise. If the *dosha* imbalance progresses to stage five, structural changes occur in the body, which cause disease-specific symptoms. It is only in this last stage that a full-blown disease appears.

Western medicine does not have the sophistication to pick up imbalances in their early stages. It is only able to diagnose an imbalance once it has advanced to stage five. That's because Western medical tests can only find abnormalities caused by structural damage to your body. You might experience early mild or vague (prodromal) symptoms before any structural damage has occurred to your body (stage four) and seek help from your doctor. But the tests available by your doctor will not detect any problems. Therefore, your doctor will assure you that you are fine and may even tell you that all your symptoms are in your head—when, in fact, you are in an advanced stage of developing a disease. In contrast, *Ayurvedic* physicians, or *vaidyas*, are able to detect imbalances in their earliest stages and can provide simple, effective diet and lifestyle recommendations that can rapidly restore balance.

Pulse Diagnosis

You may be wondering how a *vaidya* is able to detect imbalances before you have any symptoms or structural changes to your body. The answer is—by feeling your pulse. Your pulse doesn't just reveal the rate of your heartbeat; it also contains a tremendous amount of more detailed information about your health, including your *dosha* constitution (*prikriti*), your *dosha* imbalances (*vikriti*), and the state of your various organs and tissues.

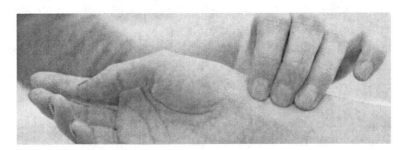

It may seem like magic, but the explanation for how a *vaidya* is able to do this is quite simple. Quantum physics tells us that the fundamental structure of the universe is nothing more than vibrations. Therefore, every structure and cell in your body produces a vibration. The vibration that each cell emits reflects its state of health. As your blood flows through your blood vessels, it comes in contact with every cell in your body and picks up its vibrational information. *Ayurvedic* physicians, as well as doctors in several other ancient holistic forms of medicine including Traditional Chinese Medicine, are trained to feel and interpret the vibrational information carried in your blood.

The 3 Pillars of Health

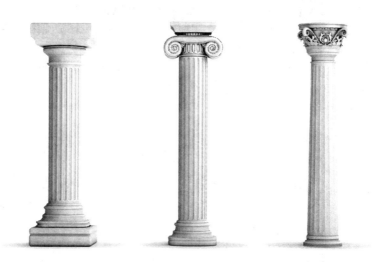

According to *Ayurveda*, there are three factors that are so crucial to health that they comprise what is called the "three pillars of health." The first pillar is diet and digestion, the second is sleep, and the third is control of the senses. Diet and digestion serve as the foundation to all prescriptions given by a *vaidya*. Regardless of what imbalances or disease you may have, the first recommendations the *vaidya* will give you will always include the foods you should avoid and the foods you should favor, as well as the behaviors, spices, and herbs that will enhance your digestion. Next, the *vaidya* will discuss with you ways to improve your quality of sleep. Lastly, you will be asked many details about your lifestyle to determine if your imbalances may also be caused by excesses—such as too much television watching or computer work, too much eating or drinking, or too much of any other activity that might be overstimulating your senses.

After addressing the three pillars, the *vaidya* will then go over other details that are also important to your health, such as your daily routines (discussed in the next section). If herbs are also recommended, they are always discussed at the end of your consultation. That's because herbs don't work well if you don't make the diet and lifestyle changes first. As one of my favorite sayings goes, "You can mop your floor, but you'll never get it dry if you don't turn off the faucet first."

Recommended Daily Routine

Following a healthy daily routine is also fundamental for good health. The ideal daily routine recommended by *Ayurveda* includes:

- Wake up before sunrise or 6 a.m.
- Do your cleanliness routine, including brushing your teeth, scraping your tongue, and going to the bathroom
- Give yourself an organic sesame oil massage (*abhyanga*)
- Perform yoga *asanas* (positions), including sun salutations in preparation for meditation
- Quiet your nervous system with nasal breathing exercises (*pranayama*) for at least ten minutes
- Meditate for a minimum of twenty minutes
- If desired, listen to pleasant/healing music or sounds immediately after meditating
- Exercise before 10 a.m., such as brisk walking
- Eat a light breakfast, such as cooked stewed fruits and oats
- Eat your main meal at noon
- In the early evening, repeat yoga, *pranayama,* and meditation
- Eat a light dinner, such as soup

- Go for a walk

- Participate in pleasant activities that are not overstimulating, such as conversations or reading

- Go to bed by 10 p.m.

In addition, at the change of seasons, *Ayurveda* recommends a week or two of purification. The purification program offered by *Ayurveda* is called *panchakarma* and is discussed in chapter 8.

Without a doubt, the medicine of the future will reincorporate these ancient truths. It's already happening. An integrated system of medicine— one that combines the best technologies of Western medicine with those of ancient holistic systems of medicine—will serve us best. Imagine a system of medicine that uses all of the best knowledge and techniques of health from every culture in the world, where rapidly advancing sophisticated technology is built on a base that includes everything we have learned about our bodies and health over thousands of years since the beginning of recorded time.

CHAPTER 2

All You Need Is Love

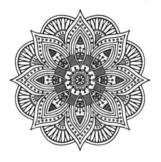

The Extraordinary Power of Love and Relationships

The heart that loves is forever young.

~GREEK PROVERB

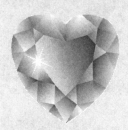

THE SECOND GEM—PINK TOURMALINE

Love is the second gem in your breastplate—a pink tourmaline. Pink is one of the colors of your heart chakra, or fourth chakra. The heart chakra is also the center of the human energy system. It represents unconditional love and compassion.

The color pink symbolizes unconditional love, compassion, femininity, calmness, intuition, and affection.

The energy of a pink tourmaline is said to stimulate both your heart and crown chakras and brings forth a synthesis of love and spirituality. It promotes joy and peace during periods of spiritual growth and change. Pink tourmaline also promotes the feeling of joy and enthusiasm for life by releasing destructive tendencies and helps you to trust in the power of love.

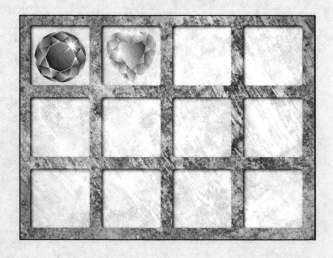

There's something that has more of an effect on your health and longevity than anything else—more than diet, smoking, or even your genetics. It's the feeling of being loved and emotionally supported. That's right—nothing has been shown to influence your health more powerfully than giving and receiving love.

What's Love Got to Do with It?

You might wonder why love has such a profound effect on your health and longevity. After all, love is just an emotion. However, research shows that emotions aren't something trivial or insignificant when it comes to your mind and body. All emotions interact with your mind and body through biochemical reactions, which can have a significant supportive or detrimental impact on your health.

Candice Pert, Ph.D., discovered that with each emotion you feel, there are specific chemicals released that can attach to receptors on many types of cells in your body, including your immune and nervous systems, and even to your DNA. In general, negative emotions such as fear and anger produce chemicals that are harmful for you. They can depress your immune system and interact with your genes in a way that increases your risk of chronic diseases, including cancer. Whereas, positive emotions have the opposite effect—they boost your immune system and influence genes that support and protect your health.

The Science of How Emotions Affect Your Immune System

When you feel an emotion, scientists have found that it's processed through your brain's limbic system and the hypothalamus. The hypothalamus releases neuropeptides, which then stimulate the pituitary gland to release hormones. All the endocrine glands, especially the adrenals, react to these hormones by producing other hormones that can weaken or strengthen the function of the immune system.

Anger, fear, and rage produce neurochemicals that strain your body and can damage your organs. On the other hand, positive emotions such as joy reduce the release of stress hormones—cortisol, norepinephrine, and epinephrine—from the adrenal glands. Laughter also stimulates the activity of the immune system. In a study published in *Alternative Therapies in Health and Medicine* in March 2002, researchers found that laughter increased a type of cell in the immune system called "natural killer (NK) cells," which kills foreign invaders, including bacteria, viruses, and cancer cells. Laughter also enhances many other types of immune-system cells. The immune-boosting effects of laughter were found to last for up to twelve hours.

Should You Avoid Negative Feelings?

You might think that with all the ill effects negative emotions can have, it would be best to try to never feel them. But suppressing your feelings is even more damaging to your health. The stress of repressed and suppressed emotions, especially unresolved anger, can take a huge toll. Ideally, you want to feel all of your emotions fully and then let them pass through you. Every emotion has a purpose, including the negative ones. Those that may be unpleasant can actually help you to become aware of some underlying emotional wound that needs to be healed or alert you to a situation that may hurt you. It is very helpful to learn a variety of techniques that can help you effectively process your emotions. Throughout this chapter, I will give examples of techniques, tools, and programs that I've had personal experience with and know are very effective.

The Purpose of Emotions

The human experience involves a wide range of feelings and emotions—from sadness, resentfulness, and hatred to compassion, forgiveness, and love. As human beings, it is part of our journey to continually feel and process emotions. Your emotions help to guide you to make the right decisions and to grow and evolve. Without them your life would have no meaning, depth, or purpose. Imagine if you felt nothing—no compassion, no desire, no joy, no sense of accomplishment, no pride, no pleasure, no pain. Nothing could move you to tears—not the most exquisite beauty of Nature, not the birth of your child, not the atrocities of war. Nothing! It's hard even to imagine.

Fields of Love

Emotions aren't just biochemical; they are also electrical and energetic. They affect your nervous system and actually generate a "field effect" outside of your body. In other words, when you feel love, a field of energy is produced that not only affects you, but also your environment and everyone in it. The same is true for all of your emotions, including the negative ones. For example, when you feel angry, you send negatively charged energy out into the environment. Whenever strong emotions have been produced in a room, especially with groups of people, the subtle energy in the room can be quite pronounced and easily felt. For example, think back to a time when you may have walked into a room after an intense disagreement occurred and felt "heaviness" in the air. Or when you visited a sacred place, such as a temple, where as soon as you walked through the door, you felt immediate peace and lightness.

Experiments using the field effect of love on non-human subjects, such as plants or bodies of water, have been amazing. These types of experiments are particularly valuable, because they do not involve any subjective human bias. For example, researchers conducted experiments on plants to see what, if any, influence love had on their growth. Half of the plants were the "control" plants grown in a neutral environment. The other half was grown in identical conditions, except every day, the researchers told those plants they were loved. The plants that received love grew significantly faster and were more robust than the control plants.

A world-renowned Japanese researcher, Dr. Masaru Emoto, was the first to document that the words we speak or think influences the molecular structure of water. In his experiments, words with either positive or negative meanings were taped to the outside of flasks of water. The water with

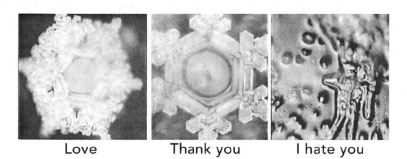

Love   Thank you   I hate you

the positive words, such as love or gratitude, formed unique beautiful crystalline structures. Whereas, water exposed to negative words, such as "I
hate you," formed ugly misshapen crystals.

Because the adult human body is made up of approximately 70 to 80
percent water, Dr. Emoto concluded that the words we say or think have an
enormous effect on our physiology and health. That's why Dr. Emoto says
he wakes up every morning, looks at himself in the mirror, and says, "I love
you, Dr. Emoto!" It's a simple practice that you, too, can do to profoundly
support your health.

In another experiment, Dr. Emoto showed that the molecular structure
of large bodies of water, such as lakes, can be changed by intentional
thoughts of groups of people. Samples of water were taken from the heavily
polluted Lake Biwa—a lake so revered it is called the "Womb of Japan."
Under the microscope, the water crystals appeared amorphous and visually
disturbing. He then had a group of people stand at the edge of the lake and
say prayers of love and thanks. Within a few short hours, the crystalline
structure of the lake significantly improved, becoming more defined and
visually pleasing.

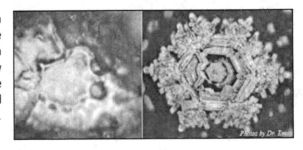

On the left is an ice crystal from
severly polluted water. On the
right is the same water refrozen
after having been blessed by
Dr. Emoto. One can see that we
have the ability to not only heal
ourselves but the Earth as well.

Photos by Dr. Emoto

All of this may sound like science fiction, but quantum physics has a
simple explanation. According to the quantum field theory, every particle
in the universe affects everything else in the universe. Even the flap of the
wing of a butterfly in South America is said to influence global weather.
Quantum physics has shown that a person's conscious thoughts also influence the behavior of subatomic particles. In other words, your thoughts not
only affect you on the inside, but everything outside of you too.

"Every act of kindness, every smile you give,
spreads a new consciousness around the world."

~J. J. GOLDWAG

Distant Healing

The influence of your emotions and thoughts isn't just limited to your immediate environment. In fact, your emotions and thoughts are not limited by time or space. For instance, research has shown that when people engage in prayer for a patient's well-being at a hospital thousands of miles away, measureable physiological improvements occur in that patient. In her book *The Intention Experiment*, Lynne McTaggart reports on a plethora of experiments on the effects of intentional thought. These experiments show beyond a doubt that your thoughts and emotions actually influence the world, and time and distance are irrelevant. If you are interested in learning more on this topic, I highly recommend this fascinating book.

When groups of people join together with the same focused intention and emotion, the effects are magnified exponentially. Several published studies show that when large groups of people simultaneously practice Transcendental Meditation (TM), a type of meditation, the calming effect in the surrounding environment is so powerful that it causes a significant measurable decrease in violent crime and accidents. For example, two studies published in the *Journal of Conflict Resolution* (1988, 1990) found that when large groups of TM meditators were brought to Lebanon during the war, there was a significant reduction in armed conflict and an improved quality of life.

The more people who join together, the more powerful the influence is. A study published in the *Journal of Mind and Behavior* in 1989 found a direct relationship between the number of people in the group practicing TM in Washington D.C. and the reduction in violent crime. Mathematical equations have been worked out, revealing that one percent of the population in joined intention, or consciousness, is required to cause a statistically significant influence on the surrounding population. When groups of individuals join together to practice a more advanced Transcendental Meditation technique, the TM-Sidhi program, only the square root of one percent of the population is necessary!

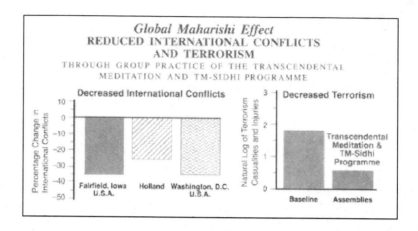

One of the missions of the organization involved with teaching TM is to reduce violence and enhance peace in the world by making use of this phenomenon. They have been gathering large groups of meditators in various locations, called "Peace Palaces," with the intent to powerfully infuse peace into the world. Currently, there are large Peace Palaces in India and Fairfield, Iowa, and many smaller ones in various locations throughout the world. To learn more, go to www.globalpeaceproject.net.

Lynne McTaggart is also working for world peace by using group intentions for peace. If you would like to participate in one of her experiments or are interested in more information about them, check out her website: www.theintentionexperiment.com.

Love Begins with Loving You

"You have been criticizing yourself for years and it hasn't worked. Try approving of yourself and see what happens."

~LOUISE HAY

I'm not sure why negative thoughts have the upper hand in most of us, but the fact is, they do. Ironically, some of the worst thoughts we have are directed against ourselves. If you pay attention to your self-talk, you more than likely will observe that you say mean and critical things to yourself that you would never say a close friend—every day and multiple times a day. I call those ugly voices my "inner mean committee." If your inner mean committee is anything like mine, they expect you to be perfect and hold you to standards that no human being could ever measure up to. They love to tell you that you are not loveable, because you are not enough of whatever: skinny, pretty, talented, smart, wealthy, or . . . (you fill in the blank).

The good news is, with some conscious diligence, you really can get the inner mean committee to pipe down. Pay attention to your self-talk, so that you can catch them as soon as they start criticizing you. Thank them for sharing and then tell them to shut up and go take a hike! Some people have found adding humor helps too. For instance, you could name your inner critic(s) something that makes you chuckle, such as *Bitchy Bertha*. Whenever you hear your inner critic, you don't need to compound the situation by criticizing yourself even more for having those thoughts; instead you could lightheartedly stop and laugh, "Oh, there's that *Bitchy Bertha* showing up again." We all do it. It's a part of being human. Your job is to find a gag that works for you.

Putting a gag on your inner critics is the first step; the next is creating rituals of self-love. If you haven't practiced self-love in the past, it may at first seem weird and narcissistic. However, self-love rituals are anything but. They help you to build a healthy self-esteem and allow you to authentically love others. You can't truly love another in a healthy way, unless you love yourself first.

An easy way to begin is to consider that each of us is unique, like a snowflake. There is no one exactly like you. Each of us has unique gifts to give to the world. That includes you. What are your special gifts? If you can't easily think of any, it's a sign your inner mean committee has gotten out of control. Ask a couple of your close friends what they appreciate about you. It's great to hear an outside perspective of what a difference you make in other people's lives. They may tell you about gifts you didn't even realize you had.

Don't compare your gifts to anyone else's. Don't devalue what is so special about you. That's *Bitchy Bertha* talking. No one's gifts are better or any more important than anyone else's. For instance, a doctor and a migrant farm worker who picks berries both contribute to helping people to keep well. Both are essential. One is not more important than the other.

Your unique gifts may have nothing to do with your job or occupation. Perhaps you are an extraordinary compassionate listener and friend. Perhaps you make people laugh or just your presence uplifts everyone when you walk in a room. For example, my brother has many extraordinary gifts. He is brilliant, great with numbers, and an amazing musician, to name a few. But what is most remarkable about him is that he is the most kind, supportive, and loving person I have ever met. Everyone I've introduced to him remarks about how much they instantly liked him. As one of my girlfriend's exclaimed, "Wow—he always makes me feel like I'm one of his long lost best friends!" He does that with everyone—cashiers at the grocery store, tellers at the bank, the mail carrier—everyone.

Compassion and Forgiveness

Another stumbling block to self-love is holding on to some judgment about yourself regarding something you did in the past of which you weren't proud. Practicing compassion and forgiveness for others is essential for harmony and inner peace. It is also essential that you do this with yourself. None of us is perfect, so quit expecting that you should be. When you ease up on the criticism of yourself, you will find you are less critical of others too. When you begin to love yourself more, you'll also find you are able to love others more.

One of my favorite self-help books is *Radical Forgiveness* by Colin Tipping (Sounds True, 2009). I took Colin's course almost twenty years ago and still use his techniques today. He presents an incredibly effective way of using powerful insights to transform judgments and complaints into gratitude, acceptance, and peace. Worksheets that take you step by step through the process can be downloaded from www.radicalforgiveness.com. It's easier to start with a complaint or upset you may have with someone else. Once you see how the magic of it works, try one for an issue you have with yourself.

> *"The practice of forgiveness is our most important*
> *contribution to the healing of the world."*
>
> ~Marianne Williamson

The Emotional Freedom Technique (EFT) is another very effective and popular way to help shift negative thoughts and diminish their charge. This technique, also referred to as "tapping," involves tapping your fingers on specific acupressure points while saying, "Even though I (state whatever is currently upsetting you), I deeply and completely love and respect myself." There are some great instructional videos for this technique on YouTube. Here is a link to one I recommend: www.youtube.com/watch?v= IWu3rSEddZI.

Showing the Love

Every day, it is important to practice self-love. Ask yourself each morning, "What can I do today to honor and love myself? What can I do to take care of myself?" One way I honor myself is by always having fresh flowers in my house. For you, it might be getting a massage, taking yourself out for dinner at a nice restaurant, or simply spending some quiet time thinking about a few things you appreciate about yourself. Think about what makes you feel good. Make a list. Make sure you do something on your list every day to express love to yourself.

I had a spiritual counselor recently who told me to set up a sacred space in my house to honor myself. The idea of it seemed pretty strange at first. It felt narcissistic. I initially even thought about putting it on the shelf in my closet because I would be embarrassed if anyone saw it. But then he said to use this display as a visual reminder to honor myself every day. It can also be used as a vision board. What are your hopes and dreams for your future? What do you want to create or do? Put pictures or symbols in your special area of what you want to call into your life.

Another option is to choose a symbol that reminds you to be more loving to you. Close your eyes and take a few deep slow breaths. Feel into your heart. Ask, "What symbol means self-love to me?" Allow a symbol to appear in your mind. Then put the symbol up in various locations in your house, car, or at work so that you will be constantly reminded to send love to yourself.

A couple of years ago, I watched a video featuring Stephen Sinatra, M.D., a holistic cardiologist, who said, "Did you ever notice that when you are in love you don't get sick?" That's because the emotions of being in love are the best immune boosters ever. Then I thought, *Why not try to generate those feelings about myself?* Every day I woke up and did a meditation where I focused on my heart and generated the feelings of being in love, and then repeated several times, "I am in love with myself!" I did this several times throughout the day and before I went to bed at night. Within a few days, I was amazed at how overcome I was with joy, peace, and happiness. When I shared this with some of my girlfriends, they tried it and said they couldn't believe how peaceful and happy they felt too. Give it a try! It can be magical.

There are many programs available that can help you with the self-love process. One of my favorites is by Christine Arylo called "Madly in Love with ME." She wrote a book with the same name and a guidebook, which you can download on www.madlyinlovewithme.com.

The field effect you learned about a few pages back means that the conversations you have in your head about yourself are also affecting those in your immediate environment and even at distances. Therefore, it is your responsibility to the world to "gag" your inner critics and transform your mind chatter to being mostly positive and uplifting. When you evolve yourself, you are contributing to global consciousness and the evolution of everyone!

The Impact of Your Relationships

Human beings are genetically designed to be social. In other words, you are wired to be in relationships with others. In fact, your physical and emotional health is directly linked to how social you are and the quality of your relationships. If you isolate yourself from others, feel unsupported and lonely, or suffer with toxic or abusive relationships, research shows your risk of chronic disease and depression are much higher, and your predicted lifespan considerably shorter. Conversely, if you have large network of loving supportive friends, you are much more likely to be healthier, happier, and live longer. If you develop a serious illness, such as cancer or heart disease, the greatest predictor of your survival is whether or not you feel loved and supported.

In cultures of extraordinary longevity where exceptional numbers of people live to be over 100 years of age, one of the commonalities is a strong social network. A great example of how powerful socialization can be on health is Murl, a teacher I had in high school, who is now ninety-six years old. When I lost both my mom and dad over twenty years ago, Murl became my surrogate dad. We still talk with each other at least once a week and sometimes more. His mind is as sharp as a whip. He is vibrant, brilliant, and always ready for an animated debate of current social and political events. Murl loves life, is upbeat, and laughs a lot. At the end of every conversation, he always tells me how much he cares about me.

But I'm not the only person who Murl talks with like this. He stays in touch with hundreds of friends and former students. After losing his wife to cancer, he remarried at the age of ninety-one to an equally feisty woman near his age. Murl still drives—and long distances. Not long ago, he chose to drive, rather than fly, thousands of miles from Ohio to Florida and back so that he could stop and visit with former students the whole way.

One day in the summer of 2013, Murl called me sounding like his normal upbeat, dynamic self. I asked him where he was—there was a lot of background noise, and I thought he might be at Starbucks. He said he was calling me on his cell phone from the cardiac intensive care unit. I almost dropped the phone. After having chest pain, he went to the hospital and the doctors found a problem with the aortic valve in his heart. He wanted them to operate and replace his valve. Because Murl's heart condition could have caused him to die suddenly at any moment, and because he was the most vibrant ninety-plus-year-old the doctors had ever met, the doctors decided to operate.

I booked the first flight to get there. When I walked in his hospital room, there was Murl holding court. Doctors and nurses were in his room, jaws dropped and mesmerized by this extraordinary man's energy and animated stories. The next day he went into surgery. I prepared his wife, son, and daughter for common complications that can occur after heart surgery. For example, more often than not, older people—decades younger than Murl—have temporary dementia as a side effect of being on the cardiac bypass machine. I also told them he would have lots of tubes and look swollen and pale immediately afterward.

Not only did Murl sail through his surgery, he looked better than anyone of any age I have ever seen after cardiac surgery. He wasn't pale or swollen. His mind stayed totally clear. Within a day or two, he was holding court again in his room. He hardly skipped a beat. This extraordinary man is the most social human beings I have even known, and I am convinced this is why he recovered so quickly and is still so remarkably vibrant and healthy at ninety-five.

Improving Your Relationships

Most of us don't learn good relationship skills at home or have any formal education concerning this topic. Therefore, the vast majority of us stumble along in our close relationships, unconsciously reacting from past wounds and programming. Then we wonder with frustration why we aren't able to create and maintain the type of smooth, close intimate relationships we desire. The high divorce rate in America is one of the dramatic illustrations of our general lack positive relationship and communication skills.

Fortunately, psychologists have been acutely aware of this problem for decades, and many have developed programs to teach simple, effective communication and relationship skills. For example, almost twenty years ago, I took a course in the PAIRS program. The six-month course taught dozens of techniques designed to help enhance intimacy and resolve conflicts. Through deeper self-awareness and the use of these techniques, I noticed an amazing shift in all of my relationships.

Another extraordinary relationship course I have experienced is called "An Adventure in Intimacy." Taught by psychologist Hedy Schleifer and her husband, Yumi Schleifer, this weekend workshop is filled with powerful transformative information and techniques that greatly enhance communication, intimacy, and satisfaction in relationships. As children who survived the concentration camps, Hedy and Yumi are deeply committed to a peaceful world. They continue to teach all over the world because they passionately believe peace begins with individuals. The more people they can reach, the more peaceful our world will become. Weekend workshops are currently being taught several times a year in Miami, Florida, and Monterey, California. For more information, visit www .hedyyumi.com.

I strongly encourage you to take a relationship course, so that you can gain insights and skills that will help you to enhance the love and joy in your relationships. Just one weekend course can be life-altering. Because your relationships play such a major role in your health and happiness, making yours the best they can be is one of the most important and powerful actions you can take.

The Spiritual Side of Love

Lastly, consider this: God, Spirit, the Divine, or whatever you prefer to call the creative source of the universe, is pure love. All of creation comes from love. You come from pure love. Your essence is love. The key to a happier, healthier life and a more peaceful world is for you to open your heart and let in as much love in as you possibly can.

"Teach only love for that is what you are."

~A COURSE IN MIRACLES

CHAPTER 3

Stress Busting
Subduing Stress with Grace

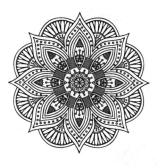

*Give your stress wings
and let it fly away.*

~TERRI GUILLEMETS

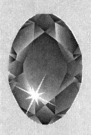

THE THIRD GEM—BLUE SAPPHIRE

The third gem in your breastplate is a blue sapphire and symbolizes the calming of stress. It is the color of your throat chakra and assists in communication. Relationship stress is the most damaging type of stress to your body. So, by cultivating great communication, you can help to keep your relationship stress to a minimum.

The color blue is cooling and anti-inflammatory. Situations and people who inflame you create stress in your life. The color blue can dowse the flames and cool you off. Blue is also relaxing and peaceful, so it can help to return you to a state of serenity.

Blue sapphire is said to reduce stress by quieting unwanted thoughts and supporting lightness, joy, and peace. It also assists in the healing of your entire body. *Ayurveda* says blue sapphire represents the planet Saturn. According to astrologists, Saturn can help reduce stress by bringing order and stability into your life.

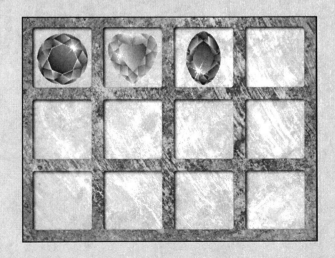

*D*oes this sound familiar? The moment you notice that your life seems to be going rather smoothly . . . *Wham!* All of a sudden a series of unexpected events come crashing down—all of which are completely out of your control. Perhaps you've experienced a time or two, or more . . . when there were so many extremely difficult circumstances converging on you at one time that you felt completely stressed out, overwhelmed, and wondered how you were going to make it through. At least one good-intentioned friend probably told you, "God never gives you more than you can handle," which only made you feel irritated and think, *Really? God definitely overestimated what I could handle this time!*

Even during the smoother times, minor stresses occur almost every day to everyone—from traffic jams, to unexpected bills, to work demands, to a cranky child, to an unintentional barb from a significant other. All of these minor tension-provoking incidents add up to chronic stress. Chronic stress is now a major issue for most Americans. In fact, the National Institutes of Health has said that stress is a major contributing factor in at least 90 percent of all chronic illness—mental and physical.

You may think there is very little you can do to minimize the damaging effects of stress. If so, the good news is, you are wrong. There are many simple and effective techniques that can powerfully diminish the destructive force of stress. But, before I tell you about them, I want to first give you some background information about stress, including what it is, its purpose, why it is important, and how certain types of stress can actually be good for you.

Stress: Necessary by Design

With all the bad press stress has gotten, you might think that all stress is bad. But the right kind of stress is essential to life. In reality, stress is the major motivational factor for growth: physical, mental, emotional, and spiritual. For example, weight lifters must stress their muscles with heavier weights to cause them to grow larger and stronger. Stressing your mind with new information and tasks, such as learning a new language or working on perplexing puzzles, is one of the best ways to keep your brain sharp and ward off dementia. Significant emotional stress can be the instigator for profound insights that lead to substantial growth in maturity and wisdom. Spiritual stress, especially which occurs during the "dark night of the soul" times—when life throws you its greatest challenges—can be the trigger for radical breakthroughs in your relationship with a higher power. For many, it takes being completely broken apart by life to learn how to surrender to a higher power and develop trust, faith, and grace.

Stress can also help save your life. The stress response, also known as the "fight-or-flight" response, gives you the extra energy, speed, and strength you may need to survive a life-threatening situation. For example, if a robber starts chasing you, the fight-or-flight response changes your physiology so that you have the extra strength and speed you need to potentially escape. Sometimes the amount of additional energy created by the neurochemical cascade during extreme acute stress is so great that you can develop "superhuman" powers. A good example is when a petite mother is able to lift a 2,000-pound car off her trapped child.

Chronic Stress

Stress only becomes a significant problem when it becomes chronic. In other words, instead of being present for only a short time to handle an emergency situation, it sticks around and keeps your body inappropriately in the fight-or-flight mode. When you allow stress to get the best of you, overflow its boundaries, and become pervasive and chronic, it becomes one of the most destructive forces known to your health and happiness. In fact, nothing has a more potent damaging influence on your physiology— not drugs, genetics, smoking, or a terrible diet—than a serious case of stress.

Chronic stress disrupts your endocrine, nervous, and immune systems, and stops your gastrointestinal tract from functioning properly. Over time, unremitting stress can have catastrophic consequences by leading to serious, even fatal diseases, such as hypertension, heart disease, diabetes, obesity, and cancer.

Defining Stress

Dr. Hans Selye is recognized as the pioneer in stress research. Born in Vienna in 1907, he received an M.D. and Ph.D. from the German University in Prague and published thousands of scientific articles and contributed to dozens of books. Dr. Selye defined stress as, "a psycho-physiological (mind/body) event that takes place when your system is overwhelmed by an experience: physical, mental or emotional." He said, "Stress is the non-specific response of the body to any demand, whether it is caused by, or results in, pleasant or unpleasant conditions."

Dr. Selye emphasized that stress is not something "out there." But rather it is purely subjective and internal. What might be considered stressful for one person may not be stressful for a different person. For instance, one person may become paralyzed with fear when asked to speak in front of a room, while another person may leap at the opportunity, because there's nothing they find more fun.

Top Stressors

Despite the subjectivity of stress, there are certain situations that most people find stressful. Some of the top common stressors include:

- Problems at work or job loss
- Financial difficulties
- Relationship tensions
- Death of a loved one
- Moving
- Being a caregiver for someone who is ill
- Personally having a significant health challenge

Symptoms of Chronic Stress

If you have more than one of the following symptoms, you may be showing the signs of too much chronic stress:

- Difficulty sleeping
- Daytime fatigue
- Failure to remember dreams
- Poor tolerance to heat or cold
- Muscle tension
- Indigestion
- High blood pressure
- Emotional disturbances, including anxiety, tension, depression, frustration, and anger

Pay attention to these warning signs. If you have several of them, you need to take significant action soon to lower your stress. If you don't, you will be at a high risk of developing a serious disease in the near future. At the end of this chapter, I'll tell you about several very effective stress-reducing techniques. Choose one to start with and add others over time. I also highly recommend that you see your physician for an evaluation. Many serious conditions that require medications do not have symptoms in their earlier stages.

The Stress Response

If you like to know all the technical details about how things work, this section is for you. If this type of information makes you glaze over, you can skip this part!

When you perceive a stressful situation, a chemical alarm signals your endocrine and nervous systems and causes your nervous system to go on high alert. A coordinated and interdependent response occurs in your endocrine system, ultimately leading to the release of stress hormones from your adrenal glands, which are located on top of your kidneys.

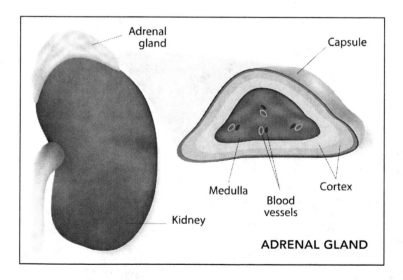

ADRENAL GLAND

The neurochemical stress-alarm signals first interact with your hypo-thalamus gland found deep in your brain and cause it to release a substance called "corticotropin-releasing factor" (CRF). CRF then activates your pituitary gland, which releases adrenocorticotropic hormone (ACTH). ACTH then travels to your adrenal glands and causes them to release cortisol and prostaglandin E_2 (PGE_2).

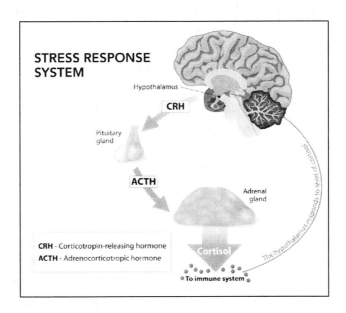

Adrenaline is released from the medulla, or central portion, of your adrenal glands within minutes. This hormone is the main force behind the fight-or-flight response. The burst of adrenaline activates your sympathetic nervous system, which increases your heart rate, blood pressure, and mental alertness, and shuts down your digestion. All of these actions are required for the most efficient and immediate fight-or-flight response.

Cortisol

Cortisol is considered the major stress hormone. It assists the fight-or-flight response by preventing blood glucose from being used for energy. A time-consuming process is required for your muscle cells to draw in blood glucose and use it for energy. First, insulin must attach to a receptor in your muscle cell's membrane so that it can facilitate moving the glucose from your blood, through your cell membranes, and into the interior of your cells. Once the glucose is inside, it must be converted into energy through a series of steps. Cortisol not only blocks your muscles from trying to use this slow energy source, but it also encourages your muscles to get their energy from the quickest source—itself. In other words, cortisol causes your muscle cells to break down so that they can get immediate energy from their own tissue.

Cortisol blocks the ability of glucose to get into your cells in two ways. First, cortisol causes your pancreas to produce less insulin. Next, it causes your cells to be less sensitive to this hormone. Because glucose can't get into your cells, it stays in your blood and its levels can begin to soar, especially when your cortisol levels stay consistently high due to chronic stress. Excess blood glucose is extremely damaging to your body. It lights the fires of inflammation and throws fuel on the development and progression of most chronic diseases, including arthritis, cardiovascular disease, diabetes, dementia, and certain cancers, especially cancers of the breast, prostate, and colon.

High glucose levels also increase the risk of a common metabolic condition known as "Syndrome X." Syndrome X is characterized by truncal obesity (apple shape), high blood pressure, and hyperlipidemia (high cholesterol and triglycerides). These physiological changes set the stage for type 2 diabetes, heart disease, and strokes.

The damaging effects of chronically high cortisol are not just limited to raising blood glucose. It also has numerous other detrimental effects that can result in devastating damage to your endocrine, gastrointestinal, immune, and neurological systems. They include:

- Bone mineral density loss and an increased risk of osteoporosis

- Muscle loss, especially of limbs

- Hypothyroidism characterized by fatigue, weight gain, dry skin, depression, mental apathy, and constipation

- Sympathetic nervous system overdrive, which triggers spasms in the smooth muscles in your digestive tract and blood vessels, resulting in high blood pressure, gastrointestinal spasticity, irritable bowel syndrome, and cardiac arrhythmias

- Excess abdominal fat

- Suppression of the immune system, especially natural killer (NK) cells

- Increased oxygen free radicals

- Increased risk of infections and autoimmune diseases

- Impaired wound healing

- Accelerated aging

- Shortened lifespan

Chronic Stress and Impaired Wound Healing

A study was conducted analyzing the effects of stress on wound healing by comparing people who had minimal stress to those who had high stress—specifically, caregivers of patients with Alzheimer's disease. Small wounds were created about the size of an eraser head on the arms of the subjects. The wound healing capacity of the caregivers was found to be so impaired that it took nine days longer for their wound to heal compared to those who had minimal stress!

Chronic Stress and Obesity

According to numerous studies, including a 2009 study published in the journal *Hormones* by researchers at the University of California, San Francisco, chronic stress contributes to obesity through a myriad of behavioral and biochemical pathways. For example, it can causes overeating, which drives cortisol and insulin levels up even higher and promotes the accumulation of abdominal fat. Abdominal fat is particularly dangerous, because it is metabolically active—meaning that it creates harmful hormones, inflammatory proteins, and oxygen free radicals.

"He who is of a calm and happy nature will hardly feel the pressure of age, but to him who is of an opposite disposition; youth and age are equally a burden."

~PLATO

Stress and Aging

The aging process is graphically accelerated during times of intense stress. For instance, those who serve as president of the United States typically dramatically age during their term.

Those who live in war-torn countries can age so rapidly that a forty-year-old-man may have deeply haggard lines on his face, usually only seen in men decades older. By comparison, a Buddhist monk who has participated in long daily sessions of meditation and has experienced low levels of stress for most of his life may age so slowly that his face may appear unlined and youthful into old age.

Stress and Lifespan

Scientists have found that chronic stress not only accelerates aging, but also shortens your lifespan. One way that stress shortens your lifespan is by negatively affecting telomeres, a section at the end of your chromosomes. As you may recall, the length of your telomeres is directly associated with the length of your life. The shorter they are, the shorter is your predicted lifespan. As you age, your telomeres naturally lose length. There are many factors that can cause your telomeres to prematurely shorten. Chronic stress is a major one.

The good news is, you can reverse some of the damage to your telomeres. The length of your telomeres can be preserved, or even increased, with certain healthy diet and lifestyle choices. Everything that causes your telomeres to lengthen does so by stimulating the production of the enzyme telomerase. In other words, telomerase is directly responsible for rebuilding your telomeres. On the contrary, when the production of telomerase is blocked by any of a number of factors, including stress, your telomeres will prematurely shorten.

Clinical Studies of Stress and Telomeres

In a study published in 2004 by researchers at the University of California, San Francisco, healthy premenopausal women with the highest levels of perceived stress had telomeres that were much shorter than women with low stress levels. In fact, their telomere lengths were equivalent to those normally found in women a decade older. In another study published in *Biological Research for Nursing* in 2011, telomere length was measured in sixty-one women who had a history of being victims of domestic violence and forty-one women who had never been abused. It should come as no surprise that the telomere length was significantly shorter in the women with a history of abuse.

Chronic Stress Reduces a Longevity Factor

Researchers discovered a longevity factor, called "klotho," which appears to help you live longer. Decreasing levels of klotho are associated with increasing symptoms of aging, including hardening of the arteries and loss of muscle mass and bone density. Researchers at the University of California, San Francisco, studied ninety high-stress female caregivers and eighty-eight low-stress controls, most of whom were in their thirties and forties and otherwise healthy. They found that the high-stress women had significant reductions in klotho compared to those with low stress. Even lower levels of klotho were found in those who also suffered with significant clinical depression.

Preventing Damage from Stress with Exercise

Regular exercise can be a great stress reliever and can add years to your life. There are many ways that regular exercise improves your health, slows aging, and lengthens lifespan, which are discussed in detail in Chapter 6. Preserving telomere length by diminishing stress is just one of the ways that exercise can help you live longer. In a study published in 2010, researchers at the University of California, San Francisco, examined sixty-three postmenopausal women and found that vigorous regular exercise protected against the telomere shortening that normally occurs with significant stress.

Minimizing the Stress Response

According to *Ayurveda,* stress occurs in your physiology when you don't respect the rhythms of nature. So, the first step to minimize stress is to *pay attention to the rhythms of the day, week, month, and year.* If you attune your-self to the rhythms of Nature and adjust your activities accordingly, your body will relax in the flow of Nature. When your body relaxes, all of your physiological functions run more efficiently. Your immune system strength-ens, your digestion is smooth, and your overall health is enhanced. Con-versely, if you go against the rhythms of Nature, your body develops tension and stress from fighting against the strong currents. As a result, your phys-iology is challenged, your immune system diminishes, your digestion becomes sluggish, and your overall health weakens.

Certain daily rhythms are obvious, such as the cycles of activity with the day and rest at night. For instance, if you stay up too late at night, your hormones will go out of balance, your physiology weakens, and your risk of numerous chronic diseases increases, including heart disease, diabetes, and cancer. On the other hand, if you follow the natural rhythms and for example, go to bed by 10 p.m. and get up by 6 a.m., you not only counter-act some of the damaging effects of stress, but also infuse your body with healing intelligence, which optimizes your hormonal balance, enhances your immune system, and balances your physiology.

According to *Ayurveda,* there are more subtle rhythms throughout the day, which cause physiological changes that either support or undermine various activities. Modern science has confirmed this ancient advice based on hormonal fluctuations and brainwave activity that occur throughout the day and night. If you would like to review *Ayurveda's* suggested ideal daily routine, turn back to page 29.

EFFECTIVE STRESS-REDUCING TECHNIQUES

Thousands of years ago, the ancient *Vedic* culture recognized that even if you follow the rhythms of Nature, live a healthy lifestyle, and eat nutritious balancing foods, it's not enough to protect yourself against all the normal daily stresses. The daily practice of a powerful effective stress-reducing technique is also required. If you want to stay healthy in our fast-paced, high-stress modern culture, in my opinion, practicing a daily effective stress-reducing technique is no longer an option—it is mandatory.

Meditation

Spending some quiet time each day connecting with your inner Self is one of the simplest and most effective things you can do to alleviate stress and to rebalance and recharge your health. At your center is your soul—the part of you that is connected to all other people and all other things. It is your *true* Self. But during your daily waking state, it is normal to be so caught up with surface activities and concerns that you forget your true Self, which lies deep within.

When you take the time to quiet your mind and reconnect with your true Self, you are also tapping into universal Source energy, because at your subtlest level, that's exactly who you are. Uniting with the Source is like touching Nature's tuning fork—you start to vibrate with its tremendous calming, rebalancing, and healing energy. The most effective way to connect with this energy is through the practice of meditation.

Research shows that the most effective stress-relieving, anxiety-reducing, and health-promoting form of meditation is Transcendental Meditation (TM). *Ayurveda* considers TM to be the single most important modality for inducing balance, integrating the mind and body, preventing disease, and restoring health.

THE FOURTH STATE OF CONSCIOUSNESS

To meditate means to think, contemplate, or concentrate on something. *To transcend* means to go beyond. During the practice of TM, a unique state of consciousness is reached by transcending thought. It is characterized by a state of restful alertness and deep silence. Typically, the only states of consciousness you routinely experience are waking, sleeping, and dreaming.

When you practice TM, your mind goes to a fourth distinct state of consciousness, appropriately named "transcendental consciousness," or pure consciousness. Brainwave recordings, called "electroencephalographs" (EEGs), reveal that this special state of consciousness produces patterns completely different from those seen when you are awake, dreaming, or sleeping. For instance, the left and right hemispheres of the brain are normally asynchronous, which means that they have very different rhythms in their brainwave patterns.

During transcendental consciousness, the two hemispheres begin to synchronize and alpha waves predominate. Alpha waves are associated with a state of restful alertness. Practitioners of this type of meditation report that when they "transcend," they experience feelings of rest, relaxation, calmness, peace, expansiveness, and unity with the world.

When I first learned this technique in 1996, I was absolutely amazed by what I experienced. From my very first experience meditating, I could feel myself plunging into a deep state of peaceful silence, my body and mind deeply relaxing in a way they never had before, and my energy levels being recharged.

I had been concerned about the toll the long hours and high stress of my job as a plastic surgeon was taking on me. But after I experienced the profound stress-reducing effects of this simple mental technique, I realized I had a powerful tool of protection in my pocket. For example, one morning I arrived at the hospital after a short night's sleep feeling completely exhausted. I looked in my rearview mirror and gasped when I saw how stressed, drained, and pale I looked. Checking my wrist watch, I saw that I was almost twenty minutes early—just enough time to get my meditation in before I had to start my day. So I sat in my driver's seat, closed my eyes, and began to meditate. Immediately, I felt my mind and body drinking up the deep state of relaxation. Twenty minutes later, I opened my eyes, checked the mirror again, and was shocked at how much better I looked. My previously pale face now had vibrant color, my skin texture looked suppler, the tension lines had relaxed, and there was brightness to my eyes. Seeing the dramatic physical changes that just twenty minutes of Transcendental Meditation can cause made such a deep impression on me that, twenty years later, I am still amazed.

Quantum Physics and Consciousness

Quantum physics has shown us that the world we perceive, the material world, is just an illusion. An atom—the smallest particle of an element—is made up of more space than matter. So what appears solid, such as a table, is actually mostly empty space. According to quantum physicists, underlying all the diversity of the material world is the real world: a homogeneous, unchanging, unified field composed of nothing but small vibrating strings.

If you're interested in reading more about this, I recommend a wonderful book that beautifully explains the "superstring theory" called *The Elegant Universe* by quantum physicist Brian Greene. Quantum physics is so strange and complex that physicists such as Niels Bohr said, "For those who are not shocked when they first come across quantum theory cannot possibly have understood it," and Richard Feynman said, "I think I can safely say that nobody understands quantum mechanics." Despite its being impossible to fully understand, *The Elegant Universe* does a great job explaining the basics of the theory and is sure to give you a whole new, life-altering perspective on the structure of the universe.

You might be wondering, "What lies beyond the vibrating strings? What controls the vibration of all these strings and how do they manifest the diversity of the material world?" According to scientists (and logic), there *must* be an underlying field of intelligence or consciousness that manages these strings. Scientists have called this field of intelligence the "Unified Field of Intelligence," or the "Unified Field of Consciousness." This field holds the power to orchestrate Nature; therefore, it contains all the laws of Nature.

When you experience transcendental consciousness, your mind merges with this unified field of consciousness. This merging powerfully establishes balance in your mind/body. In other words, when you tap into the Source that holds the knowledge of all the things you need to do to keep your body in perfect balance and perfect health (the laws of Nature), you are immersed in this knowledge and, at the same time, soothed and healed by its balancing effects.

Not surprisingly, when people first connect with this Source of knowledge, they discover that they spontaneously start making choices in alignment with good health. For example, their yearning to smoke cigarettes, drink alcohol, and partake in other disease-promoting activities decreases, and their desire to eat nourishing foods and engage in healthy activities increases. That's why research shows that regularly experiencing this unified field of consciousness produces powerful health benefits in mind, body, spirit, and emotions.

The History of Transcendental Meditation

Transcendental Meditation is not a new technique. In India, it was passed on from teacher (yogi) to student for thousands of years. It remained unavailable to the general public until the late 1950s when concern over the deteriorating health and collective consciousness of the world's people drove one yogi into action. Maharishi Mahesh Yogi adopted the task of teaching this technique to the public. He and his lineage of masters knew that the simple mental practice of TM was so powerful that if enough people were taught how to do it, it could substantially improve health, calm the collective consciousness, and promote world peace.

In the mid-twentieth century, the practice of meditation was radically foreign to most people in the West. In order to gain widespread acceptance and to encourage as many people as possible to learn it, a focus was also placed on research to prove and document TM's many astounding benefits. Studies were initiated all over the world. Today—thanks to the proliferation of studies that show that TM is a remarkably effective approach for boosting and fostering health and peace—millions of people throughout the world have learned this technique and practice it daily.

TM's Mind/Body Health Benefits

More than 600 studies have been conducted on TM at 200-plus independent institutions and universities in more than thirty different countries. These studies show that the health benefits of experiencing transcendental consciousness daily are nothing short of miraculous. It dramatically reduces stress and anxiety and promotes good health.

As you may recall, according to the National Institutes of Health (NIH), stress is the cause of, or a major contributing factor in, more than 90 percent of all illnesses. Because TM radically lowers stress, it also substantially lowers the risk of most diseases. For example, research shows that people who practice this form of meditation daily have 56 percent fewer hospital admissions for all diagnoses, including cancer and accidents, and 87 percent fewer admissions for cardiovascular diseases, including heart disease.

The research-proven health benefits of the regular daily practice of TM are numerous, diverse, and impressive. They include:

• Lower blood pressure

- Reversal of coronary artery disease
- Better mental capacity with improved academic performance
- Enhanced creativity
- Improved verbal and analytical thinking
- Fewer emotional disturbances including less worry, depression, and anxiety
- Better relationships
- Enhanced job performance
- Increased life satisfaction
- Reduction in all chronic illnesses, including cancer
- Slowed aging
- Longer lifespan

TM and Addictions

Addictions to drugs, alcohol, or other vices generally originate from a desire—albeit misguided—to reduce stress, anxiety, and depression. For many people, overcoming health-destroying addictions is one of the most difficult challenges they will face in their lifetime. Standard treatment programs are very successful for some, but for others, especially over the long term, they are not. Researchers have found that people have greater success in overcoming addictions if they replace a health-destroying habit with another habit—ideally one that is health-supporting, such as the practice of an effective stress-reducing meditation. A meta-analysis of 198 independent treatment outcomes for drug, alcohol, and cigarette addictions found that the daily practice of TM was more effective in helping people overcome these addictions than any of the standard treatment programs.

TM and Aging

One of the most astonishing findings about the regular practice of TM is that it can *reverse* the aging process. This mental technique is actually what *Ayurveda* calls a powerful behavioral *rasayana*, which means "that which negates old age and disease."

Research shows that individuals who have meditated for more than five years are physiologically about twelve years younger than those who haven't. These conclusions were based on measurements of near-point vision, hearing, and systolic blood pressure—all of which predictably worsen with age.

As you age, the levels of hormones in your body also change. For example, you produce much less of the hormone dehydroepiandrosterone sulfate (DHEA)—the most abundant hormone found in young adults. DHEA has many positive roles in the body, one of which is to help in the production of lean muscle mass. By the time you reach your mid-thirties, you start losing lean muscle mass and declining DHEA levels are thought to be largely responsible for this phenomenon. Research shows that you can slow down the rate at which DHEA levels drop and stay physiologically younger by exercising and practicing TM. In general, the level of DHEA in TM practitioners is the same as that normally found in people five to ten years younger.

Please note that I don't recommend taking supplemental DHEA because its long-term safety has not been adequately evaluated, and there is some cause for concern. Raising and maintaining your DHEA levels naturally seems to have a far different effect on your body than taking supplemental DHEA. DHEA is a steroid-type molecule that is converted to testosterone and estrogen in the body. Taking supplemental DHEA may abnormally raise the levels of these hormones and has been reported to cause unwanted hair growth, acne, and mood swings. Of even greater concern is that it may also increase the risk and accelerate the growth of breast and prostate cancer. In a study published in the *European Journal of Clinical Nutrition*, prolonged supplementation of DHEA, particularly by those who are obese, significantly increases the risk of postmenopausal breast cancer.

TM and Lifespan

In 2009, researchers at the University of California, San Francisco, found that TM slows the rate of cellular aging and lengthens telomeres. The next year, another study published in the journal *Psychoneuroendocrinology* found that subjects who participated in a meditation retreat or practiced for three months had significantly greater telomerase activity compared to the controls. In other words, regular daily meditation may help you live longer.

Learning TM

You can't learn TM from a book. As a long-time teacher of this technique said to me, "Think of it like flying a plane. You would never try to fly a plane if your only experience came from reading a flight-instruction manual. There are many variables and subtle nuances that can make the difference in a safe flight. Similarly, awareness of the refined subtleties of TM can make all the difference in successful practice. If you don't practice TM properly, you will not reap the full health benefits."

Like flight instructors, certified teachers of TM have gone through a long, rigorous training course to become proficient at teaching this technique. To locate a certified teacher in your area, call 1-800-LEARN-TM (1-800-532-7686) or go to www.TM.org. The Transcendental Meditation program is taught in seven steps over four days.

There are a couple of common concerns people have that interfere with learning and practicing this technique. The first is time. When will they find time in their already overloaded day to meditate? Rest assured, TM is practiced for only twenty minutes, twice a day. Anyone can squeeze two twenty-minute sessions into his or her day with relative ease. Here's how: Wake up twenty minutes earlier than you usually do, or meditate on your way to work if you take mass transit, or skip one half-hour television show in the evening and meditate instead.

Another common concern people have is that learning to meditate is difficult because you must force your mind to stop thinking. Many fear that they won't be able to meditate successfully because their mind is always racing. The TM technique is a simple, effortless, natural process that your mind easily follows. You don't have to *try* to do anything. There's no forcing, no concentrating, and no effort required. If you can think a thought, you can practice TM.

Taking the time to learn and practice TM is one of the best gifts you can give yourself. It's one of the most powerful daily habits you can do to improve your overall health and decrease your risk of disease.

(Pages 58–65 adapted from *Waking the Warrior Goddess* by Christine Horner, M.D., used with permission of Basic Health Publications.)

Other Forms of Meditation

Learning TM is expensive, and unfortunately, teachers are becoming more difficult to find. So, if you cannot arrange to learn TM, consider learning another form of meditation. Although other forms of meditation may not be as effective as TM, they certainly have their benefits. Be sure to research various techniques to find one that works for you. Certain types of concentration meditation may actually increase anxiety, so be careful in your choice of technique.

Pranayama—Using Your Breath

"Breathing deep with your arms spread wide fills you with prana, the energy of the air, and revitalizes your system. This simple technique is the foundation for ancient practices of maintaining health."

~ J. J. GOLDWAG

Breathing is synonymous with life. If you stop breathing, you stop living. But breathing has many finer aspects than the black and white of life and death. The way you breathe can affect your health for better or worse. *Ayurveda* uses a set of breathing techniques called *pranayama* to enhance health and lower stress.

Prana is a Sanskrit word that means "breath," but its full meaning goes way beyond that. In *Ayurveda*, *prana* is known as "life energy," paralleling the ancient notion of *chi* energy in China, "vital force" for the ancient Greeks, and *ki* in ancient Japanese medicine. *Prana* is the life force that governs all bodily functions and influences your mind, memory, thought, and emotions. By breathing with the techniques of *pranayama, Ayurveda* says you can strengthen your life force and induce balance, which enhances your health and lowers your risk of disease.

Pranayama literally means "regulating the breath." The techniques of *pranayama* are numerous, but usually involve breathing through alternating nostrils. The technique of breathing through alternating nostrils is said to create balance in the physiology, improve the function of the nervous system, and benefit many specific organs.

A *PRANAYAMA* TECHNIQUE

Pranayama is usually practiced just before meditation to settle the body and mind and facilitate transcending. You can also use *pranayama* to help calm yourself whenever you are upset. Here's a simple way to practice:

1. Sit upright, and close your eyes.

2. Use your right thumb to gently close your right nostril.

3. Breathe out through your left nostril slowly and naturally until you breathe your breath completely out. Don't force it.

4. Breathe slowly back in the same (left) nostril.

5. Close your left nostril with the long finger or ring finger on your right hand.

6. Release your thumb on your right nostril, and breathe out slowly and easily.

7. Breathe back in through the same (right) nostril.

Repeat this process for about five to ten minutes. You should notice an almost immediate calming effect.

Research has documented that the regular practice of *pranayama* increases the depth and the length of time you're able to hold your breath and enlarges the vital capacity of your lungs. It improves stress-hormone balance and decreases pulse rate, blood pressure, and blood fats such as cholesterol. *Pranayama* can also be extremely beneficial for improving asthma.

New Realities

Other good stress-reducing and health-promoting practices include yoga, tai chi, qigong, and even laughter. There are also various devices you can use that contain music or guided meditations that can provide tremendous protection against stress. A few years ago I discovered one wonderful relaxation device that I absolutely love. Made by New Realities, guided meditations are recorded on a digital iPod-type device. It is important to use headphones or earphones, instead of speakers, to get the right effect.

What makes this device so special is that subliminal binaural beats accompany each meditation. The unperceivable alternating beats in your ears cause your brainwaves to synchronize—just as they do when practicing TM. The device also comes with goggles with light-emitting diode (LED) lights designed to stimulate your retina through closed eyelids. The LED lights help to facilitate the meditative state. The first time I tried it, I became a big fan. Anyone can use it, and no training or classes are needed. It's a very simple, affordable, and effective way to receive the benefits of meditation. You can read more about the New Realities device on my website: www.drchristinehorner.com.

> *"Tension is who you think you should be.*
> *Relaxation is who you are."*
>
> ~CHINESE PROVERB

Functional Education

Another important approach to reduce the stress in your life is to become more self-aware and improve your relationship skills with something I call "functional education." There is a literal cornucopia of classes available that teach techniques that help you to function with yourself and others in a more evolved, balanced, and less stressful manner. Some of the training and development courses I have done and highly recommend include courses taught through Landmark Education Corporation (www.landmarkworldwide.com), *Radical Forgiveness* by Colin Tipping (www.radicalforgiveness.com), relationships-focused courses called "PAIRS" (www.pairs.com), and "An Adventure in Intimacy," taught by Hedy and Yumi Schleifer (www.hedyyumi.com). If you would like, go to page 44 in the previous chapter to review the more detailed description of these courses.

There are also many other types of one-on-one and relationship therapies that can be very helpful. All of these courses can help you to develop a greater self-awareness and acceptance, improve your communication skills, and help you to cultivate compassion, patience, and grace.

Releasing the Stress of Traumatic Events

The emotional charge from traumatic events can continue to stay with you and add to your underlying level of stress. Post-traumatic stress disorder involves abnormal neural pathways that occur at the time of the event when creating the memory. When anything occurs in your life that reminds something in your nervous system of the original event, such as a loud noise, it can cause you to have a supercharged response that is inappropriate for the current situation.

What may seem like relatively minor traumas can also cause lasting negative effects in your body. Emotional memories are not only recorded in your brain, but also by your body. There are a variety of very effective techniques that can quickly release the stress of the past events. Four techniques that I have experienced and was amazed by their effects include Eye Movement Dissociate Reprogramming (www.emdr.com); Emotional Freedom Technique (www.eftuniverse.com); Body Memory Recall (www.body memory.com); and EVOX (www.zyto.com/Products/EVOX).

Eye Movement Dissociate Reprogramming (EMDR)

There are many techniques that rapidly "reprogram" neural pathways in the brain and extinguish abnormal heightened emotional and stress responses. Those responses can range from isolated minor emotional upsets to full-blown post-traumatic stress disorder. Francine Shapiro, Ph.D., one of the first researchers to discover that an emotionally charged memory can be transformed to carry little to no reaction instantaneously and permanently by engaging both sides of the brain while discussing the memory, developed the technique Eye Movement Dissociate Reprogramming (EMDR). In the classic form of the technique, a therapist guides a client to move their eyes from left to right while discussing the emotionally upsetting memory. The abnormal emotionally charged neural pathway immediately becomes "reprogrammed" or rewired in the brain. The new pathway for the memory carries no emotional charge.

Emotional Freedom Technique (EFT)

One of the simplest and best techniques that can help you to instantly shift or release your negative emotions—whether they have been long-standing or have just arisen—is the Emotional Freedom Technique (EFT) or "tapping." Nothing fancy is required—it only takes a few minutes to learn, is free, and can be done anywhere. This technique takes advantage of the brain's ability to reprogram itself when both hemispheres are engaged. Tapping can be done by anyone, at any time, and does not require a therapist. Using acupressure points on the face and upper body, this quick and simple technique rapidly relieves the "emotional" charge of a situation. Talking about your emotional upset while tapping on a set series of points has been found to "rewire" the nervous system pathways similar to EMDR and discharge aggravated emotions, restoring emotional peace. There are some great instructional videos on YouTube.

Body Memory Recall (BMR)

Trapped stressful emotions and traumatic memories can be responsible for a spectrum of chronic health problems—for example, chronic pain, fibromyalgia, and recurring emotional upsets. There are several types of treatments that help to release these trapped emotions. The most effective one I have personally experienced is Body Memory Recall (BMR). Developed by Jonathan Tripodi, stored memories and their emotions are released from the body using a unique method of energy work and physical touch similar to myofascial release. I recommend reading Tripodi's book *Freedom from Body Memory* to learn more about this technique. He has trained practitioners in BMR all over the country. To find someone who is certified in your area, go to www.freedomfrombodymemory.com.

EVOX

EVOX is a computer-based device designed to alleviate emotional stress by "rewiring" your brain. It uses a multisensory approach that includes light, sound, and electromagnetic frequencies, which quickly, gently, and effectively repatterns the mind and body. A therapist guides you through issues that may have emotional charges, while a computer simultaneously maps out subtle qualities in your voice. The EVOX program then provides the frequencies of light and sound needed for subconsciously repatterning your brain. The changes it produces allows you to quickly release negative patterns, such as depression, anger, sadness, grief, fears, and phobias.

Energy Medicine

Various techniques that fall under the umbrella of "energy" medicine—discussed in detail in chapter 10—can be highly effective in quelling anxiety and other emotions associated with stress. Examples include Therapeutic Touch (TT), Reiki therapy, acupuncture, and flower essences such as Bach Flower Remedies, and essential oils. Research shows that all of these techniques can be effective in lowering anxiety and stress:

- **Therapeutic Touch**: A double-blind, randomized study published in 2008 found that TT on infants improved measurements of the parasympathetic nervous system responsible for the relaxation response.

- **Acupuncture**: With a history of use that dates back thousands of years, acupuncture is one of the most researched CAM techniques. Hundreds of studies have shown that it can be effective for anxiety and stress, including a 2014 meta-analysis published in the journal *Evidence-Based Complementary and Alternative Medicine.*

- **Bach Flower Remedies**: A study conducted by researchers at the University of Miami in the January 2007 issue of the journal *Complementary Health Practice Review* found that Rescue Remedy, a blend of five Bach Flowers, caused a statistically significant reduction in stress in test subjects.

- **Essential Oils**: A 2002 Japanese study found that certain essential oils, such as rose and patchouli oil, can significantly calm your nervous system. Other studies show that lavender and jasmine oils can sooth your mood and decrease anxiety. The research-proven essential oils for reducing stress include lavender, lemon, bergamot, peppermint, vetiver, pine, and ylang ylang.

Nutritional Supplements

Stress depletes you of certain vitamins and minerals and increases oxygen free radicals. Supplying your body with the supplemental nutrients it needs during times of stress help you to recover more quickly and decrease your risk of becoming ill. Key vitamins and nutrients include:

- Vitamin C: normalizes cortisol

- Vitamin B1: protects adrenals
- Vitamin B6: improves glucocorticoid secretion
- Vitamin B5: enhances adrenal cortex function
- Alpha-lipoic acid: prevents catecholamine accumulation
- L-tyrosine: replenishes catecholamines

Supplemental antioxidants are also very important. A stress reaction creates excess oxygen free radicals, which have been linked to most chronic degenerative disorders, including Alzheimer's disease, cancer, and accelerated aging. Important antioxidants include vitamin C, vitamin E, selenium, and CoQ10.

The *Ayurvedic* herbal mixture *Amrit Kalash*, according to research, may be the best antioxidant of all. Dr. Yukie Niwa, a Japanese researcher, studied more than 500 different antioxidants over a period of thirty years. He found that the most powerful and effective antioxidant of all those tested was *Amrit Kalash*.

Antioxidant Supplements

- Vitamin C
- Vitamin E
- Selenium

- CoQ10
- *Amrit Kalash*

Herbal Adaptogens

Certain herbs have been shown to effectively reduce the stress response through a variety of mechanisms. They are termed "adaptogens" because they help you to adapt to stress. For example, research shows that holy basil, an *Ayurvedic* herb, which has a 5,000-year-plus history of use, protects against and reduces stress. It decreases the release of the stress hormone cortisol. It also enhances stamina and endurance, increases the body's effective use of oxygen, and boosts the immune system when you're under stress. In addition, it slows aging and provides a rich supply of antioxidants, as well as a multitude of other benefits. Two other standout herbal adaptogens include ginseng and ashwagandha.

The Stress-Reducing Actions of Holy Basil

Decreases:

- cortisol
- biochemical changes in the brain
- recovery time
- blood sugar in type 2 diabetics
- cholesterol
- blood pressure

Improves:

- physical endurance
- performance
- mood
- neutrophil function and numbers

None of us are immune from the damaging effects of chronic stress. Life throws us curve balls on a regular basis. Even when life seems to be going relatively smoothly, in our fast-paced culture, a series of minor stresses happen almost every day—to everyone. Because chronic stress contributes to every chronic disease and accelerates aging, it is important that you do everything you can to minimize its damaging effects. Choose an effective stress-reducing technique and commit to practicing it every day. During those times when your stress is particularly high, take time to nurture yourself even more by getting regular massages or other relaxing treatments. Make sure to arm yourself with protective nutritional supplement and adaptogenic herbs, such as holy basil. Remember that even though you may not have much control over many of the stressful events that occur in your life, you do have an arsenal of tools to help you minimize the damage that chronic stress can cause.

Summary of Techniques to Reduce Stress

- Respecting rhythms of Nature
- Regular schedule
- Good quality sleep
- Regular exercise
- Fresh, organic, whole-foods plant-based diet
- Meditation
- Breathing exercises
- Relaxing music/massage
- Nature walks
- Laughter
- Loving relationships

- Functional education
- Emotional release techniques and devices:
  - EMDR
  - Emotional Freedom Technique (EFT); tapping
  - BMR
  - EVOX
- Subtle energy approaches:
  - Energy work such as Reiki
  - Bach Flower Remedies
  - Acupuncture
- Nutritional supplements and herbs

CHAPTER 4

Foods for Health

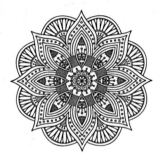

Nourishing Your Body for Extraordinary Beauty and Longevity

*Let food be your medicine
and medicine be your food.*

~AYURVEDIC PROVERB

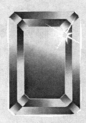

THE FOURTH GEM—EMERALD

The foods for health and beauty are embodied by an emerald—the fourth gem of your breastplate. Green is another color associated with the heart chakra. An emerald is said to be "the stone of successful love." There is no greater expression of self-love or love for others than nourishing yourself and your loved ones with highly nutritious organically grown plants. According to *Ayurveda* and modern science, the foods you eat have one of the most profound influences on your health and longevity.

The color green has a soothing influence on your mind and body. Green brings peace, rest, hope, comfort, nurturing, calmness and harmony. This color also contains the inherent strength and symbolism of fertility, growth, rejuvenation, resilience, healing, harvest, abundance and prosperity. Fresh organic plants are imbued with all of these qualities. Green can aid in any condition in need of healing—just as the plants with this hue are known to do.

An emerald is said to help guide you to the "right" choice. Therefore, it helps you to make all the right choices in food that will support your health and spiritual growth.

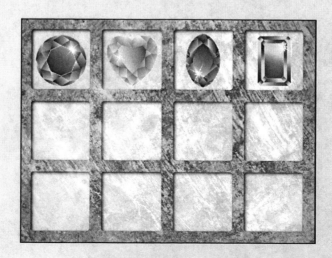

*O*f all the factors that impact your health, the foods you chose to eat, or not eat, have one of the most powerful influences. When I went to medical school in the early eighties, I didn't have a single course in basic nutrition. Twenty years later, when I returned to my medical school to give a lecture on *Ayurveda*, I asked the medical students if they had a nutrition course—their answer was alarmingly, "No!"

Despite the fact that the medical literature is filled with thousands of studies documenting that the foods you consume are critically important to your health and longevity, very little of this information is taught in Western medical training. Most Western-trained physicians—including most likely your doctor, too—only know the most rudimentary basics of nutrition. The extent of their knowledge is generally limited to knowing that it's a good idea to eat more fruits and vegetables and avoid junk foods. What I find disturbing is that our medical system has such a blind eye to the health effects of diet that not uncommonly hospitals house fast-food restaurants and still serve green Jell-O and glazed donuts to patients for breakfast!

Unlike Western-trained physicians, physicians trained in *Ayurveda* possess an extremely sophisticated knowledge of the medicinal and energetic qualities of plants. Because of this, they prescribe fruits, vegetables, grains, seeds, spices, and herbs as the initial approach for the prevention or treatment of any health condition. Not only do they know the medicines and energetic qualities contained within each plant, but they also know the ideal harvesting, processing, and mixing procedures to maximize the plant's healing potential.

In fact, *Ayurveda* places so much importance on not only diet, but also digestion, that together they form the first of the three pillars of health. The second pillar is sleep, and the third is "managing the senses" (lifestyle). When you meet with an *Ayurvedic* physician or *vaidya*, at the end of your consultation, he or she will discuss a holistic health plan for you, which always begins with recommendations for the specific foods that should be favored and the foods that should be avoided. The food prescription is very individualized based your unique constitution (*prikriti*) and imbalances (*vikriti*).

Although a plant-based diet is generally recommended, a *vaidya's* recommendations are much more specific based on their sophisticated knowledge of the properties of each plant. These properties are not limited to only the nutritional content that you typically find on American food labels, but go way beyond that. The plants are prescribed primarily based on the medicines they contain, the energetic qualities they express, their category of taste, and their influence on the *doshas*. For instance, if you have an excess of *vata,* sweet, sour, and salty foods will be prescribed to help to bring it back into balance. A *vaidya* will also recommend that you favor foods that are warm, heavy, and oily, and avoid foods that are cold, dry, and light. Cooked asparagus, sweet potatoes, bananas, avocados, mangoes, and nuts are *vata* pacifying, while cold salads with sprouts or cabbage will make your imbalance worse.

Ayurveda recognizes six different tastes, which are listed in the chart below, along with examples of foods in each category. The next chart lists the influence that each taste has on each *dosha,* followed by the general dietary recommendations that help to balance them.

Ayurveda Six Tastes

1. **Sweet:** sugar, milk, butter, rice, breads, pasta

2. **Sour:** yogurt, lemon, cheese

3. **Salty:** salt

4. **Pungent:** spicy foods, ginger, hot peppers, cumin

5. **Bitter:** green leafy vegetables, turmeric

6. **Astringent:** beans, lentils, pomegranate

How to use the six tastes to balance the *doshas:*

TO DECREASE:

Vata: sweet, sour, salty

Pitta: sweet, bitter, astringent

Kapha: pungent, bitter, astringent

TO INCREASE:

Vata: pungent, bitter, astringent

Pitta: pungent, sour, salty

Kapha: sweet, sour, salty

Vata **Pacifying Diet**

- Favor foods that are warm, heavy, and oily. Minimize foods that are cold, dry, and light.

- Favor sweet, sour, or heavy fruits such as oranges, bananas, avocados, cherries, peaches, plums, mangoes, and papayas. Reduce apples, pears, pomegranates, cranberries, and dried fruits.

- Reduce beans except mung dahl.

Pitta **Pacifying Diet**

- Favor foods that are cool and liquid; minimize hot foods.

- Favor olive oil and coconut oil; reduce sesame and almond oils.

- Fruits: Favor grapes, cherries, melons, coconuts, pomegranates, and sweet plums; reduce grapefruits, olives, papayas, and sour plums.

- Vegetables: Favor asparagus and cucumbers.

- Avoid ginger, cinnamon, cumin, black pepper, clove, mustard seed, chili peppers, and cayenne.

Kapha **Pacifying Diet**

- Favor light, dry, and warm; minimize heavy, oily, and cold.

- Favor the spices bitter and astringent; minimize sweet, salty, and sour.

- Minimize dairy.

- Favor lighter fruits, such as apples and pears; reduce heavy fruits, such as bananas, pineapples, figs, dates, avocados, coconuts, melons, and nuts.

The Energetics of Food

Ayurveda also takes into consideration the energy held by a food. This "energy" does not refer to the calories in the food, but rather the amount of "life force," or *prana,* it holds. For example, recently harvested fresh organic produce has the strongest *prana,* while foods that are frozen, canned, chemically preserved, or packaged are said to have little to no *prana,* and therefore, should be avoided. Remember that *Ayurveda's* ultimate goal is "enlightenment"; therefore, the fundamental intent of nourishing your body is to raise its energetic vibration so high that you can easily experience higher states of consciousness or, in other words, feel as close to Creative Source, or God, as humanly possible.

Why a Plant-Based Diet Is Best for Health and Longevity

Thousands of studies show that a diet rich in plants—especially fresh organically grown fruits, vegetables, and whole grains—is the most supportive for warding off disease and creating and maintaining extraordinary health, beauty, and longevity. *Ayurveda* explains that the reason these plants are so protective is that they contain a high amount of "intelligence." They transfer this intelligence into your body, increasing its natural healing intelligence and its ability to keep you healthy.

Western scientists have studied many of these plants to determine what causes them to be so protective for your health. Research shows they are low in calories, high in fiber, and nutrient dense. Fruits, vegetables, grains, seeds, spices, and herbs are also packed full of vitamins, minerals, nutrients, and antioxidants that are crucial to good health. In addition, they contain hundreds of plant chemicals, or phytochemicals, that have no nutritional value or caloric value, but act as "natural medicines" with a remarkable array of healing benefits.

One commonality among all cultures with extraordinary longevity is that their diet is primarily plant-based. Their food is usually fresh and locally gown. Many have their own gardens. A multitude of studies, including one published in the journal *Nutrition* in February 2003, supports that the recipe for a long healthy life is:

- Consuming fewer calories
- Being physically active
- Eating more plant foods

And avoiding:

- Red meat
- Sugar
- Saturated animal fats
- Alcohol
- Junk foods
- Smoking

A prospective study by John Hopkins Bloomberg School of Public Health published in the *American Journal of Epidemiology* in 2004 followed participants from 1974 to 2002 and examined the association of fruit, vegetable, and antioxidant intake with all-cause, cancer, and cardiovascular disease death. The researchers found that overall, a greater intake of fruits and vegetables was associated with a lower risk of death from any cause. In 2010, a study published in the *Annals of Internal Medicine,* which collected data from more than 85,000 women enrolled in the Nurse's Health Study (ages thirty-four to fifty-nine) who provided dietary data for twenty-six years; and 44,500 men enrolled in the Health Professional's Follow-Up Study (ages forty to seventy) who provided dietary information for twenty years found similar findings. Those who adhered to a diet low in carbohydrates, but rich in animal-based fats and proteins increased their risk of death, especially by cancer. On the other hand, those who followed a low-carbohydrate diet, but rich in plant-based fats and proteins were associated with a lower risk of all-cause and cancer mortality.

Plant Protection Against Age-Related Diseases

"The doctor of the future will no longer treat
the human frame with drugs, but rather will
cure and prevent disease with nutrition."

~THOMAS EDISON

In a study entitled "Dietary Approaches That Delay Age-Related Diseases," published in the journal *Clinical Interventions in Aging* in 2006, Australian researchers concluded that the best diet to delay age-related diseases, such as cardiovascular disease, diabetes, dementia, and certain cancers is one that is low in calories and saturated animal fats, and high in whole grains, legumes, fruits, and vegetables. In 2008, Italian researchers analyzed the relationship of plasma carotenoids and skeletal muscle strength in subjects ages sixty-five and over. They found that higher intake of fruits and vegetables appears to protect against inflammation, poor physical performance, and disability. They also found that older adults with lower plasma carotenoids levels, a marker of poor fruit and vegetable intake, are at a higher risk of decline in skeletal muscle strength over time, which can lead to disability and a reduced quality of life.

These same Italian researchers published another study in 2008, which focused on the total plasma carotenoids level in older adults and the development of walking disabilities over time. They found that those with higher total plasma carotenoids had a significantly lower risk of developing a severe walking disability over the six-year follow-up period.

FAMOUS VEGETARIANS

Jane Goodall, world's foremost expert on chimpanzees

Susan B. Anthony, leader of the women's suffrage movement

Aung San Suu Kyi, Nobel Peace Prize winner

Rosa Parks, African-American Civil Rights activist

Cesar Chavez, Latino-American Civil Rights activist

Thich Nhat Hanh, Vietnamese Buddhist monk, teacher, author, poet, and peace activist

Dennis Kucinich, former U.S. Representative from Ohio

Coretta Scott King, wife of Martin Luther King, African American activist and peace activist

Princess Diana, former Princess of Wales and the first wife of Prince Charles

Albert Einstein, theoretical physicist and winner of the Nobel Prize in Physics

Leonardo da Vinci, Italian genius, inventor, painter, mathematician

Nikola Tesla, inventor of 700 devices

Srinivasa Ramanujan, one of India's greatest mathematicians

Mahatma Gandhi, leader of the Indian independence movement in British-ruled India

Vincent van Gogh, Dutch Post-Impressionist painter

Thomas Edison, American inventor

Pythagoras, Greek philosopher and mathematician

Mark Twain, American author and humorist

Franz Kafka, German novelist

Plant Protection Against Cancer

According to a review study published in 1991 in the *American Journal of Clinical Nutrition*, eating vegetables and fruit lowers the risk of cancers of the mouth, pharynx, larynx, esophagus, stomach, colon, rectum, bladder, cervix, and lung. A Norwegian study in 1998 concurred with this study and went on to say that high fruit and vegetable intake lowers the risk of several other cancers, including those of the pancreas and breast.

Supplier of Antioxidants

Oxygen free radicals are unstable molecules of oxygen created as a natural byproduct of cellular metabolism. They are necessary to drive every chemical reaction in your body. What makes them unstable is that they are missing one electron. So, they try to find an electron from another source. When they steal an electron from certain biologically active molecules in your body, they perform a vital beneficial function by helping to drive essential chemical reactions in your body. However, if there are too many oxygen free radicals in your body, they can cause a lot of damage by stealing electrons from your cell membranes and DNA. In fact, excess oxygen free radicals cause so much damage that they are one of the primary forces responsible for initiating and fueling the development of most chronic diseases, including heart disease, arthritis, dementia, and certain cancers. They also accelerate aging by damaging your organs and tissues, including your skin.

The antidote to excess oxygen free radicals are antioxidants. Antioxidants donate electrons to oxygen free radicals and prevent them from taking them from, and consequently damaging, your cells and DNA. The best source of antioxidants is fresh, organically grown plants: vegetables, fruits, spices, whole grains, nuts, seeds, and essential oils. Below is a table listing the top antioxidant foods according to the U.S. Department of Agriculture. The level of antioxidants found in a food is reported as its "Oxygen Radical Absorbance Capacity" or ORAC value.

TOP 20 FOODS WITH THE HIGHEST ORAC VALUES

	FOOD	ORAC VALUE (PER 100 GMS)
1	Cloves, ground	314,446
2	Sumac bran	312,400
3	Cinnamon, ground	267,536
4	Sorghum, bran, raw	240,000
5	Oregano, dried	200,129
6	Turmeric, ground	159,277
7	Acai berry, freeze-dried	102,700
8	Sorghum, bran, black	100,800
9	Sumac, grain, raw	86,800
10	Cocoa powder, unsweetened	80,933
11	Cumin seed	76,800
12	Maqui berry, powder	75,000
13	Parsley, dried	74,349
14	Sorghum, bran, red	71,000
15	Basil, dried	67,553
16	Baking chocolate, unsweetened	49,926
17	Curry powder	48,504
18	Sorghum, grain, high-tannin	45,400
19	Chocolate, Dutched powder	40,200
20	Maqui berry, juice	40,000

Data sourced from the U.S. Department of Agriculture during 2010. The USDA recommends an ORAC unit ingestion of about 3000 to 5000 units daily.

Chronic Inflammation

Like oxygen free radicals, inflammation plays a critical role in the normal physiological processes of your body. But when it occurs in excess, it becomes a powerful promoter of chronic disease and aging. For example, inflammation is required for the initial stages of wound healing. It helps to clear the debris of dead tissue, signals for the immune system cells to come to the area, helps to fend off foreign invaders such as bacteria and infections, and initiates tissue repair. But when inflammation becomes persistent, it turns into a formidable and destructive force. In fact, excess oxygen free radicals and chronic inflammation are thought to be the two most dominant processes that drive all chronic diseases and speed up aging. In addition, each increases the production of the other: oxygen free radicals escalate inflammation, and inflammation gives rise to more oxygen free radicals.

A few examples of chronic diseases strongly associated with chronic inflammation include:

Alzheimer's disease	Depression and anxiety	Multiple sclerosis
Aging (unhealthy)	Dry eye syndrome	Osteoporosis
Acne	Eczema	Pain
Allergies	Dysmenorrhea	Parkinson's disease
Arthritis	Hypertension	Psoriasis
Asthma	Kidney stones	Renal insufficiency
Cancer	Macular degeneration	Skin cancer
Cardiovascular disease	Malaise/fatigue	Stroke
Cognitive decline	Migraine headaches	Ulcerative colitis
Crohn's disease		

Source: Cleveland Clinic

You might have noticed that all of these inflammatory-associated diseases are common in the American culture. It is not a fluke or a mystery as to why. Researchers have concluded that the American diet is largely responsible. Most of the foods that make up a typical American diet cause inflammation. In fact, an estimated 72 percent of daily calories come from the pro-inflammatory food listed in the following table:

PERCENT OF DAILY CALORIES	FOOD GROUP
1–2%	alcohol
10–11%	dairy products (milk, cheese, butter)
20.4%	refined grains (various flour products [bread, pasta, etc.]; cereals)
18.6%	refined sugars (sucrose, high fructose corn syrup, glucose, etc.)
17.6%	refined omega-6 oils (salad/cooking oils, shortening, margarine)

By contrast, organically grown plants not only supply large amounts of antioxidants, vitamins, minerals, and other nutrients essential for health, but they also contain powerful anti-inflammatories. Below is a table listing the foods with the highest amounts of anti-inflammatory power listed from the highest to the lowest. The inflammatory or anti-inflammatory potential of foods is reported as its "Inflammation Factor" (IF) Ratings. Foods with positive IF Ratings are considered anti-inflammatory, and those with negative IF Ratings are considered inflammatory—the higher the number, the stronger the effect.

IF RATING	FOOD
60,860	pepper, serrano, raw
43,611	tabasco sauce
18,790	garlic powder
15,889	ginger powder
14,079	ginger root, raw
12,745	turmeric, ground
2,521	chives
2,252	spinach

IF RATING	FOOD
2,000	turnip greens
1,901	onions, spring or scallions (includes tops and bulb), raw
1,882	lettuce, romaine
1,534	collards
1,490	basil, fresh
1,453	coriander (cilantro) leaves, raw
1,210	salmon, wild caught alaskan
965	carrots
690	asparagus
600	vegetables, mixed (corn, lima beans, peas, green beans, carrots)
453	broccoli
420	sweet potato
340	parsley, dried
316	Brussels sprouts
290	thyme, dried
265	cabbage
254	melons, cantaloupe
217	pickles, cucumber, sour
199	oregano, dried
163	celery
156	pineapple
143	cauliflower

Best Anti-Inflammatory Spices

- Hot chile peppers
- Garlic powder
- Cayenne pepper
- Ginger root
- Turmeric powder
- Onion powder
- Curry
- Fresh garlic
- Basil
- Coriander (cilantro)
- Parsley
- Thyme
- Oregano

Best Anti-Inflammatory Vegetables

- Parsley
- Carrots
- Chives
- Pumpkin
- Collard
- Spinach
- Turnip leaves
- Onions
- Romaine lettuce
- Asparagus
- Broccoli
- Beets
- Tomatoes
- Sweet potato
- Brussels sprouts
- Cabbage

Best Anti-Inflammatory Fruits

- Berries: blueberries, raspberries
- Tart cherries
- Melons
- Pineapple
- Papayas
- Strawberries
- Grapefruit

Best Anti-Inflammatory Nuts and Seeds

- Flaxseeds
- Macadamia nuts
- Hazelnuts or filberts
- Mixed nuts
- Chia seeds
- Pecans
- Almonds
- Walnuts
- Brazil nuts

Food pH and Your Health

Food pH refers to whether a food is alkaline or acidic forming. In general, acid-forming foods create inflammation and promote chronic disease. Whereas, alkaline foods have the opposite effect—they create an environment that quells inflammation and discourages chronic diseases. As you might have guessed, the foods that are pro-inflammatory are generally acidic, and the foods that are high in antioxidants and anti-inflammatories tend to be alkaline.

What Makes a Stellar Vegetable and Fruit So Special

All fruits and vegetables contain a wide array of incredible health-promoting qualities. But there are some that stand out due to their unusually high concentration of nutrients. For example, let's take a closer look at one vegetable and one fruit that top the nutritional charts. Most dark leafy green vegetables are nutrient dense, contain high amounts of antioxidants, are anti-inflammatory, and have an alkaline pH. Of all the leafy greens, kale contains the highest concentration of many nutrients, which is why it has become so popular. For instance, kale contains large amounts of vitamin C and A, and calcium. In fact, one cup of kale has more calcium than one cup of milk.

Kale is also rich in carotenoids, which are powerful antioxidants. Lutein and zeaxanthins are two of the major carotenoids found in kale. Both of these substances help to prevent macular degeneration—the most common pathology leading to adult-onset blindness. A 2008 study published in the journal *Nutritional Review* states that these two carotenoids also reduce the risk of cataracts in healthy postmenopausal women.

Research shows that the substances in kale help to lower your risk of heart disease, too. For example, a study published in *Biomedical and Environmental Science* in 2008 evaluated the effects of consuming kale juice, every day, for three months on coronary artery disease risk factors in men with high cholesterol. The researchers found that those who consumed a half cup of kale juice per day had a 27 percent increase of the "good" cholesterol (HDL) and a 10 percent decrease in the "bad" type of cholesterol (LDL).

Kale belongs to the cruciferous family. There are approximately twenty other members of this family, including broccoli, cauliflower, Brussels sprouts, cabbage, bok choy, radishes, and watercress. Cruciferous vegetables have been the subject of thousands of studies, because they contain many exceptional health benefits. All the members of the cruciferous family contain significant amounts of several powerful cancer-fighting nutrients, including beta-carotene, sulforaphane, indole-3-carbinol, calcium D-glucarate, and folate (a B vitamin needed for the repair mechanisms of your DNA). Not only does folate help to reduce the risk of cancer, but research shows that it can drastically improve short-term memory. Indole-3-carbinol has many different actions that help to reduce the risk of a variety of cancers, including breast, prostate, colon, and lung.

According to nutritionist Linda Posh, kale has seven times the beta-carotene of broccoli and ten times more lutein. Kale is also high in vitamin K1 and K2, fat-soluble vitamins that serve in a variety of essential functions, including helping your blood to clot normally; strengthening your bones; and lowering your risk of heart disease, Alzheimer's disease, and certain cancers. The K vitamins also help to regulate your insulin and blood sugar levels and reduce your risk of type 2 diabetes.

THE NUTRITIONAL CONTENT OF KALE

One cup of cooked kale contains only 36 calories and supplies the following percentage of daily required nutrients:

Nutrient	%	Nutrient	%
Vitamin K	1,180%	Vitamin E	7%
Vitamin A	98%	Vitamin B2	7%
Vitamin C	71%	Magnesium	6%
Manganese	27%	Vitamin B1	6%
Copper	22%	Protein	5%
Vitamin B6	11%	Phosphorus	5%
Fiber	10%	Omega-3 fatty acids	5%
Calcium	9%	Vitamin B3	4%
Potassium	8%	Folate	4%
Iron	7%		

A Power-Packed Berry

When it comes to fruit, blueberries are one of the healthiest choices you can make. Like kale, blueberries contain an unusually high concentration of nutrients. Some of the most health-promoting substances found in blueberries are proanthocyanidins. These are powerful antioxidants that are both water soluble and fat soluble, which means they can provide protection from the damage caused by oxygen free radicals to all the tissues in your body. For example, because they are able to dissolve in your blood, as well as easily pass through the fatty membranes of your cells, proanthocyanidins are able to protect you against virtually all age-related chronic disorders, including arthritis, heart disease, diabetes, dementia, and certain cancers. They also help to slow down aging and diminish wrinkles.

Researchers from the University of Maine, Northwestern University, and the University of Louisville published a study in 2010 in the *Journal of Agricultural and Food Chemistry,* which found that wild blueberries may reduce blood pressure by increasing nitric oxide. Nitric oxide is a naturally occurring gas in your body that causes the walls of your blood vessels to relax and dilate, which if you have high blood pressure will cause your blood pressure to go down.

Blueberries contain another nutrient, ellagic acid, which has strong anticancer properties. It protects your DNA from damage that can lead to cancer and encourages apoptosis, or the death of damaged cells and cancer cells. If you are undergoing radiation treatments, you'll be interested in knowing that according to a study published in 2010 in the journal *Cancer Investigation,* ellagic acid improves its cancer-cell killing effects. Ellagic acid has also been found to inhibit the growth of a variety of cancer cells, including those that occur in the breast, pancreas, prostate, and brain (neuroblastoma).

Quercetin is yet another powerful flavonoid antioxidant found in blueberries with many research-proven health benefits. An Argentinean study published in 2010 found that quercetin enhances nitric oxide and causes your blood pressure to drop if you have high blood pressure. According to several studies, including a 2009 study by the University of South Carolina, quercetin also increases endurance capacity and performance in athletes. This study also reported that quercetin has anti-inflammatory, antioxidant, and psychostimulant activity, and stimulates the growth of new mitochondria (the energy producers in cells), which greatly improves overall health and disease resistance. Another study published in 2008 from the Netherlands notes that quercetin protects against osteoporosis, certain forms of cancer, pulmonary and cardiovascular diseases, and aging.

Blueberries contain dense amounts of several vitamins and minerals, including vitamin C, vitamin E, riboflavin, niacin, folate, iron, magnesium, manganese, and potassium. If that weren't impressive enough, they also have potent antioxidants called "catechins." Catechins not only protect against the damage of oxygen free radicals, but they have also been found to assist weight loss—especially belly fat—by activating fat-burning genes in abdominal fat cells. In a 2008 study published in the *Journal of Nutrition*, researchers at Tufts University state that regularly ingesting catechins can increase abdominal fat loss by 77 percent and double total weight loss.

According to a study published in the *Journal of Nutrition* in September 2010, blueberries decrease cardiovascular risk factors in obese men and women with metabolic syndrome. Forty-eight participants with metabolic syndrome (four males and forty-four females) consumed a freeze-dried blueberry beverage (50 grams freeze-dried blueberries, approximately 350 grams fresh blueberries) daily for eight weeks. By the end of the study, the majority of the participants experienced a drop in systolic and diastolic blood pressure, as well as the amount of oxidized LDL—the "bad" type of cholesterol.

Eating blueberries may also help learning and memory. In a study published in the journal *Age* in 2008, age-related deficits in a cellular substrate for learning and memory called "NMDAR-dependent LTP" were prevented in rats fed a blueberry-enriched diet.

Finally, blueberries can reduce pain and improve your mood. They contain salicylic acid, the active substance in aspirin and also increase the production of dopamine, which elevates mood.

If your favorite way to consume blueberries is with milk on your morning cereal, you may want to consider eating them in another way. A 2009 study published in *Free Radical Biology & Medicine* found that when subjects consumed blueberries with milk, their antioxidant levels did not go up. The researchers theorized that the antioxidants in blueberries must have an affinity for proteins found in milk, which prevents them from being available to your body.

THE NUTRITIONAL CONTENT OF BLUEBERRIES

One cup of blueberries contains 1.1 grams of protein, 84 calories and 3.6 grams of dietary fiber and the following amounts of minerals and vitamins:

Potassium	114 mg	Vitamin B1 (thiamine)	0.055 mg
Phosphorus	18 mg	Vitamin B2 (riboflavin)	0.061 mg
Magnesium	9 mg	Niacin	0.08 mg
Calcium	9 mg	Folate	9 mcg
Sodium	1 mg	Pantothenic Acid	0.184 mg
Iron	0.41 mg	Vitamin B6	0.077 mg
Selenium	0.1 mcg	Vitamin C	14.4 mg
Manganese	0.497 mg	Vitamin E	2.29 mg
Zinc	0.24 mg	Vitamin K	28.6 mcg
Vitamin A	217 IU		

Whole Grains

Whole grains have been a primary food staple in the diet of many cultures for thousands of years. But some very prominent physicians are now saying that you should avoid all grains. They claim that grains increase your glucose levels, make your cells more insulin resistant, and promote inflammation. With all due respect, this generalization is simply not true. It is true for refined grains, which have had most of their nutrients and fiber stripped out during processing. But unprocessed whole grains contain a multitude of nutrients, which research shows have tremendous health benefits.

Whole Grains Decrease Risk of Chronic Disease

Studies consistently show that those who consume diets high in whole grains have a much lower risk—up to 50 percent lower—of many common chronic diseases including obesity; type 2 diabetes; and cardiovascular diseases such as high blood pressure, strokes, heart attacks, and metabolic syndrome. In addition, the incidence of several different types of cancer is much lower in those who consume several servings of whole grains per day—particularly cancers of the stomach, colon, prostate, and breast.

Why Are Whole Grains So Protective?

Scientists have found a multitude of nutrients in whole grains that have beneficial health effects. According to a 2003 study published in the *Proceedings of the Nutrition Society,* whole grains contain fiber, including oligosaccharide carbohydrates, which are starches that are resistant to digestion. The bacteria in your intestines will ferment them, producing short-chain fatty acids (SCFA) known to lower the pH in the colon, which is good for colon health. SCFA also decrease blood lipids, provide an energy source for cells in the colon, and promote the growth of beneficial gut bacteria, which strengthen your immune system.

A study published in 2010 in the journal *Nutrition Research Reviews* includes a long list of all the other nutritional components in whole grains:

- Antioxidants: alpha-lipoic acid and polyphenols

- Vitamins: B complex and E

- Trace minerals: selenium, zinc, copper, magnesium

- Carotenoids

- Melatonin, the sleep hormone: a powerful antioxidant and immune booster

- DNA-protecting sulfur compounds

- Lignans: compounds that contain over a dozen anticancer properties

- Plant stanols and sterols: lower cholesterol

- Oligosaccharides: a type of indigestible carbohydrate that improves constipation, mineral absorption, lipid and glucose metabolism, and immune function

- Methyl-donating molecules: methionine, betaine, choline, inositol, and folate—which prevent cancer-promoting DNA changes and also protects the liver and cardiovascular system

Each of the major nutrients in whole grains has been isolated and extensively studied for its individual health benefits. However, when the nutrients are combined together—as they occur naturally—they have synergistic effects with each other, causing their beneficial health effects to be much greater than any of the isolated ingredients alone. There are also many nutrients found in whole grains that occur in much higher concentrations than that found in fruits and vegetables.

Grains and Belly Fat

In a recent study, scientists reviewed the diets of approximately 3,000 men and women and found a strong correlation between belly fat and grain choice. The whole-grain lovers tended to have less belly fat and smaller waist measurements compared to those who consumed refined grains. Of note, however, is the fat-curbing effect of whole grains was canceled out if refined grains were also consumed. In other words, the whole-grain cereal you eat at breakfast won't help keep your belly fat low if your breakfast also includes white toast or a bagel.

The Skinny About Fat

Fat is a macronutrient that is absolutely essential for your body to function properly. For decades, fat was vilified and blamed for causing obesity and cardiovascular diseases. In response, the food industry began making "low-fat" foods. To make them palatable, they made the disastrous decision to replace the fat with sugar. Instead of seeing a drop in the incidence of obesity and chronic disease in the 1990s when the low-fat craze peaked, the numbers soared. Thousands of studies have confirmed that sugar, not fat, is in fact the major culprit in the obesity and chronic disease epidemic.

Yes, there are certain types of fat that are very bad for you, especially saturated animal fats and man-manipulated *trans* fats. In fact, *trans* fats cause such a profound surge in inflammation and oxygen free radical production that consuming only a very small amount of them can cause the incidence of heart disease and other chronic disorders to skyrocket. This is why in the summer of 2015, the U.S. government stepped in and legislated that all *trans* fats must be phased out of foods produced in the U.S. by 2018.

Trans fats are fats that have been chemically altered by having hydrogen ions added to them. The purpose of creating these fats was twofold: First, to increase the shelf-life of processed foods, such as potato chips, cookies, and crackers; and second, to make their texture crispier. On a food label, *trans* fats may appear as hydrogenated or partially hydrogenated fats. Until the phase-out date of 2018, be sure to avoid foods containing these fats.

On the other hand, there are other types of fat that are so essential for the structure and function of your body that you cannot survive without a regular supply of them. Fat is the major substance that composes the membranes of every cell in your body. In addition, your entire nervous system, including your brain, is coated in a layer of fat. Without this fatty sheath, electrical impulses cannot travel down your nerves. For instance, if a problem develops with this fatty sheath—as it does with multiple sclerosis— the ability of the electrical impulses to move along nerves becomes impaired, and therefore, so does your ability to move.

Fat also assists in wound healing, helps with the absorption of vitamins and other nutrients, creates hormones, provides insulation (which helps to maintain your body temperature and protect you from trauma), and stores and provides energy.

Essential Fat Acids (EFAs)

Fats are made up of smaller units of molecules called "fatty acids." There are several types of fatty acids that your body cannot make, but are crucial for your health. So, you must supply your body with them through your diet. These fatty acids are long-chain polyunsaturated fatty acids made from carbon atoms. They are categorized based on the position of a double bond that occurs between carbon atoms. For instance, fatty acids that have a double bond located at the sixth position from the end of the molecule are classified as omega-6 fatty acids. The other essential fatty acids are classified as omega-3, 7, and 9, and have a double bond in the third, seventh, and ninth position, respectively.

Omega-6 Fatty Acids

There are a variety of different types of omega-6 fatty acids. Some are pro-inflammatory, or cause inflammation to increase. They also increase the risk of chronic diseases, especially if consumed in excess. Other types of omega-6 fatty acids have the opposite effect—they powerfully reduce inflammation and the risk of chronic diseases. Borage oil and evening primrose oil are two good examples.

The following is a partial list of the foods and oils that are high in omega-6 fatty acids, which increase inflammation and should be consumed in only small quantities:

- grape seed oil
- commercial salad dressings
- margarine
- safflower oil
- corn oil

- mayonnaise
- sesame oil
- cottonseed oil
- peanut oil
- soybean oil

Omega-3 Fatty Acids

Omega-3 fatty acids are the most health-promoting types of fat you can eat. Omega-3s are vital for brain function, as well as for normal growth and development. Symptoms of omega-3 fatty acid deficiency include fatigue, poor memory, dry skin, heart problems, mood swings, depression, and poor circulation.

Research shows that omega-3s have strong anti-inflammatory properties and may help lower the risk of chronic diseases such as heart disease, cancer, periodontitis, and arthritis. In a study published in the journal *Cell* in September 2010, researchers at the University of California, San Diego, discovered that the anti-inflammatory effects of omega-3s are more potent than any other anti-inflammatory substance ever tested!

Omega-3s also have strong antioxidant capabilities. In a study published in August 2010 in the journal *Free Radical Research,* scientists from the University of Western Australia and the University of Montpellier in France reported that the subjects in the study—all of whom were either overweight or had type 2 diabetes—had a significant reduction in free radicals after six weeks supplementation of the omega-3 fatty acids, eicosapentaenoic acid (EPA) or docosahexaenoic acid (DHA).

Researchers at the University of California, San Francisco, discovered that omega-3s are linked to a younger biological age. They looked at the length of telomeres in test subjects, which occur at the end of chromosomes and shorten as cells replicate and age. They discovered an inverse relationship between baseline blood levels of omega-3 fatty acids and the rate of telomere shortening over five years. Those with the lowest levels of DHA and EPA experienced the most rapid rate of telomere shortening, while those with the highest average blood levels experienced the slowest rate of telomere shortening. The researchers found a linear relationship between the levels of omega-3s and telomere length. For each one standard deviation in DHA and EPA levels, there was a 32 percent reduction in the odds of telomere shortening.

Omega-3s are highly concentrated in the brain and appear to be important for cognitive function, such as memory, performance, and behavioral function. A report from National Institutes of Health's website (ods.od.nih.gov/factsheets/Omega3FattyAcidsandHealth) concluded that omega-3 fatty acids:

- Reduce all-cause mortality and various cardiovascular outcomes, such as heart attacks and sudden death

- Normalize heart rate (reduces variability and arrhythmias) and improve coronary blood flow

- Lower triglycerides

- Lower blood pressure in people with hypertension

- Improve exercise capacity in patients with coronary artery disease

- Reduce joint tenderness and need for corticosteroid drugs with rheumatoid arthritis

According to a report from the University of Maryland Medical Center, the clinical evidence for omega-3s is strongest for cardiovascular disease, but they may also be beneficial for:

- High cholesterol: People who eat diets high in omega-3s, including walnuts, which are rich in alpha-linolenic acid (a type of omega-3) have higher HDL, or "good" cholesterol, decreased triglycerides, and lower total cholesterol.

- High blood pressure: A team of researchers at Japan's Shiga University studied 4,680 men and women ages forty to fifty-nine in Japan, China, the U.K., and the U.S. Those with the highest intake of omega-3 fatty acids tended to have the lowest blood pressure.

- Heart disease: Lowers risk of death, heart attack, stroke, and abnormal heart rhythms in those who have already had a heart attack. Omega-3s

also helps to prevent and treat atherosclerosis by slowing plaque formation and blood clots. A Harvard study published in March 2010 found
that people who replaced saturated fats with omega-3s cut coronary
heart disease by 19 percent. In another study published in the *Journal of
Nutrition* in April 2010, researchers in the Netherlands found that people
with low fish intakes but who took omega-3 fatty acid supplements cut
their risk of heart disease by 50 percent.

- Strokes: Eating two servings of fish per week can lower the risk of
  strokes by up to 50 percent.

- Diabetes: Improves lipid profile. A study published in the November
  2010 issue of the *Journal of Nutritional Biochemistry* suggests that supplementation with fish oils activates a gene that regulates fat cells and
  blood glucose.

- Rheumatoid arthritis: Improves joint pain and morning stiffness.

- Systemic lupus erythematosus: Reduces autoimmune symptoms of
  fatigue and joint pain.

- Osteoporosis: May help increase levels of calcium and improve bone
  strength.

- Depression: Omega-3s may improve mood.

- Macular degeneration: Those who consume higher omega-3s have a
  lower incidence.

- Cancer: Higher dietary omega-3s are associated with a lower risk of cancers of the breast, prostate, and colon.

The Fred Hutchinson Cancer Research Center in Seattle conducted a
study published in the *European Journal of Clinical Nutrition* in 2011 of
330 Eskimos living in Alaska, whose average consumption of omega-3s
from fish is twenty times higher than people in the lower forty-eight states.
Seventy percent of the study subjects were overweight or obese. In those
with lower blood levels of DHA and EPA, obesity increased triglycerides
and C-reactive protein (CRP)—a measurement of inflammation in the
body. However, obesity did not increase those factors in those who had
high levels of DHA and EPA. Therefore, the researchers concluded that

taking high amounts of omega-3s reduces the risk of obesity-related diseases.

Consuming high amounts of omega-3s has also been shown to potentially reduce the risk of Alzheimer's disease. In a study published in *Neurobiology of Aging* in 2005, researchers found that omega-3s limited amyloid plaques, oxidative damage, and cognitive deficits in mice.

According to a study conducted by Harvard Medical School and published in the *Journal of the American Dietetic Association* in November 2010, higher intakes of DHA, and to a lesser degree EPA, are associated with lower prevalence of periodontitis, or gum disease.

Foods High in Omega-3 Fatty Acids

Some of the best sources of omega-3s include certain fatty fish, such as wild caught salmon, mackerel, anchovies and sardines. Good plant sources include flaxseeds, chia seeds, hemp seeds, and walnuts.

Omega-9 Fatty Acids

Omega-9 fatty acids are another type of healthy fats found in high amounts in olive oil. Virgin olive oil is produced through a cold-pressing method that uses no chemicals and only small amounts of heat. Researchers have found that it is the biologically active phenols, including hydroxytyrosol, tyrosol, and oleuropein, that are responsible for many of health benefits and the reduced mortality and morbidity associated with olive oil.

Here is a summary of olive oil's health benefits:

- Lowers the risk of cardiovascular disease

- Decreases total cholesterol, LDL, and triglycerides, and increases HDL ("good" cholesterol)

- Decreases LDL oxidation and platelet activity and aggregation, which are major risk factor for atherosclerosis and cardiovascular disease

- Improves inflammatory markers: decreases thromboxane B2 (TXB2), Leukotriene B4 (LTB4), arachidonic acid release, and COX-1 and COX-2 activity

- Improves cellular function

- Lowers the risk of cancer: kills cancer cells and inhibits cell proliferation of leukemia, and cancers of the colon, prostate, and breast

- Increases bone formation and density

- Antimicrobial activity: kills bacterial pathogens, such as *H. pylori* associated with stomach ulcers

- Protects against Alzheimer's disease: inhibits aggregation of microtubules, protects neurons from amyloid beta, and promotes clearance of amyloid beta by antibodies

- Lowers the risk of diabetes by improving insulin sensitivity

- Protects the liver from toxins: A study published in 2010 in the journal *Nutrition and Metabolism* found that rats fed a diet of olive oil were partially protected from liver damage after being exposed to a moderately toxic herbicide.

- Promotes healthier aging, a higher quality of life, and increased longevity

When you purchase olive oil, *always* remember to buy certified organic. If your local grocery store doesn't carry it, ask the manager to order it.

Omega-7 Fatty Acids

Omega-7 fatty acids are best known for helping to repair mucosal membranes and skin, and reduce wrinkles. Palmitoleic fatty acid is a type of omega-7 found in high quantities in the plant sea buckthorn. Omega-7s also have a variety of other beneficial effects, including:

- Promotes skin heath: Studies from China show that sea buckthorn retards skin aging, smooths skin wrinkling, and cures or alleviates acne, impetigo, atopic dermatitis, and dry skin.

- Improves wound healing: Studies show that sea buckthorn causes wounds to heal faster, including burn wounds and ulcers. A 1990 study found that sea buckthorn significantly decreased damage to DNA caused by highly toxic agents, indicating that it may also protect the DNA in our skin from environmental toxins.

- Improves vaginal dryness and inflammation: A study conducted at the University of Turku Central Hospital found that oral sea buckthorn given to women with chronic vaginal inflammation significantly improved their condition (itching, burning, pain, discharge, and dryness) after twelve weeks.

- Protects against cardiovascular disease: Research shows omega-7s lower total serum cholesterol and LDL (the "bad" type), and raises HDL (the "good" type). Animal studies indicate it may also decrease the incidence of strokes.

- May improve diabetes: In a study published in 2001, researchers found that omega-7 fatty acids had several beneficial effects on the insulin-secreting beta cells of the pancreas. According to a Swedish study published in 1994 in the journal *Diabetes*, omega-7s may also help lower the risk of non-insulin-dependent diabetes by altering the fatty acid composition of the serum cholesterol.

- May help to prevent cancer: Researchers at Okayama University in Japan found that palmitoleic acid helps to prevent the formation of cancer. In animal studies it was also found to prolong the life of mice with advanced cancer.

Nuts

Nuts are an excellent source of many different types of healthy fats and have been associated with extraordinary longevity. In a study published in the *New England Journal of Medicine* in 2013, people who ate a handful of nuts a day (approximately one ounce) were found to live longer than people who rarely consumed nuts.

Numerous studies show that regular consumption of small amounts of nuts can decrease the risk of heart disease, certain cancers, gallstones, type 2 diabetes, and a variety of other health problems. In a study published in the *Archives of Internal Medicine* in May 2010, researchers from Loma Linda University in California examined twenty-five different studies that evaluated nut consumption and cholesterol levels. They found eating an average of 2.4 ounces of nuts a day reduced total cholesterol by an average of 5 percent, lowered LDL cholesterol by 7 percent, and improved the ratio of HDL to LDL. The effect was stronger on thinner people and people with baseline higher LDL.

A comparative study of nine different types of nuts presented at the 241st National Meeting & Exposition of the American Chemical Society on March 27, 2011, found that walnuts came out on top as containing the highest amounts of antioxidants.

Nuts are high in calories, so it is recommended to eat no more than 3 ounces a day—enough to get their health benefits, but not enough to put on weight. The good news is limiting the amounts of nuts you eat may be easier than you think. In a study published in the *European Journal of Clinical Nutrition* in 2015, people who added 1.5 ounces of almonds to their diet each day reported reduced hunger. After one month of eating almonds each day, the participants did not gain weight.

SUPERFOODS

Open a magazine, turn on your television, or log on to the Internet and you'll find people talking about "superfoods." You might be wondering, *What exactly are they? What's all the hoopla about? Are they really something you should be consuming? Is what's being said about them mostly hype?*

Superfoods are real. A "superfood" is a term given to a plant that contains exceptional amounts of nutrients and health-promoting properties. As an example, let's take a close look at one of the most remarkable superfoods, spirulina (*Arthrospira platensis*), a blue-green microalga (cyanobacterium) that grows in water. In fact, researchers state that spirulina is "nature's richest and most complete source of nutrition," because it contains a "unique blend of nutrients that no other single source has to offer."

What's in Spirulina That Makes It So Super?

Spirulina contains a rich amount of a wide spectrum of health-promoting and therapeutic nutrients including B-complex vitamins, minerals, proteins, amino acids, trace elements, and gamma-linolenic acid (a healthy type of omega-6 fatty acid also found in evening primrose oil). It also possesses potent antioxidants such as beta-carotene and vitamin E.

All of these nutrients add up to give spirulina substantial preventative and healing benefits. Best known for its ability to help the body detoxify, spirulina also has antibacterial, antiviral, anticancer, anti-inflammatory, antiallergenic, and antidiabetic properties. In addition, research shows that spirulina protects the liver and kidneys from damage by toxins and promotes the growth of healthy intestinal bacteria.

Spirulina Lowers Lipids

One of the most clinically researched benefits of spirulina is its outstanding ability to lower blood lipids, including triglycerides and cholesterol. For example, in a prospective study published in 2013 in the *Journal of Science of Food and Agriculture,* fifty-two adults recently diagnosed with hyperlipidemia (elevated blood lipids) were given one gram of spirulina daily for twelve weeks. At the end of this three-month period, a significant decrease was found in the average levels of triglycerides, LDL cholesterol (the "bad" kind), and total cholesterol.

In another study, thirty-six Mexican adults were given 4.5 grams of spirulina daily for six weeks. These subjects experienced a statistically significant drop in blood lipids, as well as systolic and diastolic blood pressure. A third randomized double-blind and placebo-controlled study looked at the effects of spirulina in elderly Koreans. The seniors were given either 8 grams of spirulina per day or a placebo. After four months, those taking spirulina were found to have a significant reduction in plasma cholesterol and a noteworthy increase in total antioxidants and immune function.

Spirulina Is Great for Diabetics

Type 2 diabetes mellitus is now near epidemic proportions in our population. This disease is fraught with numerous life-threatening complications, including cardiovascular disease caused primarily from elevated blood lipids and inflammation. Korean researchers conducted a randomized study in 2008 to establish the effects of spirulina on type 2 diabetics. Patients were given either 8 grams of spirulina per day or a placebo for twelve weeks. Those taking spirulina were found to have significantly lower triglycerides, total cholesterol, and LDL cholesterol. The greatest benefits were seen in those who initially had the highest blood lipid levels. Researchers also noted that spirulina caused an improvement in inflammatory markers and antioxidant levels.

How to Take Spirulina

Spirulina can be taken in capsules or in a green drink, including All Day Energy Drinks from the Institute for Vibrant Living (IVL). The taste of pure spirulina can be challenging for some, which is why consuming it in the delicious tasting All Day Energy Greens is a great choice. Spanish researchers have another yummy suggestion—combine spirulina with cocoa powder! They point out that the Kuna Indians of Panama, who regularly consume large amounts of flavonoid-rich cocoa, are virtually free of hypertension and strokes—even though they salt their food. Therefore, they submit that cocoa powder would not only add to the health benefits of spirulina, but would also mask the "somewhat disagreeable" flavor of the algae. The therapeutic dose of spirulina ranges from 1–8 grams per day.

Chlorella

Chlorella is a single-celled, fresh-water green algae native to Taiwan and Japan. This superfood, like the blue green algae spirulina, is rich with nutrients, including amino acids, chlorophyll, beta-carotene, potassium, phosphorus, biotin, magnesium, all the B vitamins, vitamin C, vitamin E, and vitamin K. Chlorella is particularly good for vegetarians since it is extremely high in protein and is considered a "complete protein," because it contains all the essential amino acids your body needs. In fact, it has more protein by weight than meat—being about 60 percent protein. A beef steak is 28 percent protein and a burger contains only 14 percent protein. Just one ounce of chlorella contains 16 grams of protein.

Because chlorella has a thick cell wall that is nearly impossible for you to digest, it must be processed by having its cell wall broken open. You can only get the nutrients from chlorella that is termed "cracked walled" or "broken cell walled."

Chlorella has been extensively researched and found to have a long list of health benefits, including:

• Reduces oxidative stress

• Decreases inflammation

• Boosts the immune system

- Normalizes blood sugar
- Supports healthy hormonal balance
- Improves cardiovascular health by lowering blood pressure and cholesterol
- Helps the body detoxify, particularly by helping to remove heavy metals
- Improves digestion
- Helps with constipation
- Promotes higher levels of energy
- Reduces pain in fibromyalgia
- Detoxifies harmful radiation
- Reduces body odor
- May reduce cancer risk
- Helps to protect against the dangerous side effects of chemotherapy and radiation
- Helps tissue growth and repair
- May help weight loss: In a study published in the *Journal of Medicinal Food*, the researchers stated, "Chlorella intake resulted in noticeable reductions in body fat percentage, serum total cholesterol, and fasting blood glucose levels."

Green Tea

More than 4,000 years ago, the Chinese began brewing the leaves of a plant and drinking it as a hot beverage. They called the infusion "tea." More tea is now consumed every day by people all over the world than any other liquid—except water. Research shows drinking tea, especially green tea, is a wise choice because green tea has been found to have many potent health benefits.

The Number-One Anticancer Beverage

Research shows that green tea is very effective in hampering the growth of at least eleven different types of cancer, including cancers of the esophagus, stomach, colon, bladder, prostate, skin, ovaries, and breast. It also reduces the risk of leukemia, non-Hodgkin's lymphoma, and lung cancer in smokers. That's why green tea is considered the number-one anticancer beverage. You may think the impact of drinking a few cups of tea each day on lowering the risk of these cancers is small. It's not. Cancers of the digestive tract are as much as 68 percent lower in tea drinkers.

Part of the reason why green tea reduces the risk of so many cancers is because it contains an exceptional blend of powerful anti-inflammatories and antioxidants. It also holds within it the remarkable ability to amplify the power of enzymes in your liver that detoxify toxins and carcinogens. Researchers believe most of the health benefits of tea come from substances in it called "polyphenols." There are three polyphenols that are considered most important: gallocatechin (GC), epigallocatechin (EGC), and epigallocatechin gallate (EGCG). Of these, EGCG is the most potent.

Major Health Benefits of Green Tea

Hundreds of studies show this verdant beverage has many other impressive health benefits, including:

- Decreases your risk of heart attacks and strokes by decreasing cholesterol, blood pressure, and atherosclerosis, or hardening of the arteries.

- Kills certain bacteria, especially in the bladder. Tea drinkers have a 40 percent lower incidence of urinary tract infections.

- Is a recognized thermogenic—it speeds up your metabolism and helps you lose weight.

- Preserves bone density and protects against osteoporosis—a study published in the *American Journal of Clinical Nutrition* in April 2000 found that women ages sixty-five to seventy-five who drank at least one cup of tea a day had significantly higher bone densities than women who didn't drink tea.

- Increases beneficial bacteria in your intestines and decreases the harmful ones.

The therapeutic dose of green tea for protecting against cancer is eight to ten cups of green tea a day. If you can't drink this much tea each day, you can take a green tea supplement. At least 500 mg per day are recommended.

Caffeinated Coffee

You might not think of caffeinated coffee as a superfood, but research shows it actually has an impressive array of health benefits. It has been associated with a lower incidence of Alzheimer's disease, Parkinson's disease, type 2 diabetes, heart disease, and strokes, as well as cancers of the colon, kidney, brain, mouth, throat, uterus, prostate, breast, and skin. Coffee can also improve cognitive and athletic performance, and may be beneficial for weight loss.

Coffee and Alzheimer's Disease

Many epidemiological studies show that coffee is therapeutic against Alzheimer's disease. For example, researchers at the Florida Alzheimer's Disease Research Center in Tampa, Florida, published a study in the *Journal of Alzheimer's Disease* in 2010 concluding that coffee protects against memory impairment and reduces the level of abnormal proteins found in the disease, including amyloid beta (Abeta). After only one to two months of coffee consumption, some of the cognitive impairments associated with Alzheimer's disease, such as memory, have been shown to *reverse*. The researchers believe that caffeine is also responsible for these benefits because they were not seen with decaffeinated coffee.

Coffee and Other Forms of Dementia

In a systemic review and meta-analysis study published in 2010 in the *Journal of Alzheimer's Disease,* caffeine intake was found to be related to lower incidences of Alzheimer's disease, as well other forms of cognitive impairment and cognitive decline.

Coffee and Parkinson's Disease

A study published in journal *Movement Disorder* in 2007 examined the association between tea and coffee consumption and the risk of Parkinson's disease among 29,335 Finnish men and women ages twenty-five to seventy-four. The men and women who drank three or more cups of coffee a day were found to have a substantially lower incidence of Parkinson's disease.

Coffee and Type 2 Diabetes

A Harvard review study published in 2006 reviewed twelve cohort studies conducted in Europe, the United States, and Japan, and found that the risk of type 2 diabetes is substantially lower in those who drink high amounts of coffee. The findings were similar for both caffeinated and non-caffeinated coffees, which lead the researchers to conclude that the non-caffeine components of coffee may be responsible.

Coffee contains hundreds of substances, including chlorogenic acid, quinides, lignans, and trigonelline, which in animal studies have all been shown to improve glucose metabolism. In a study published in *Diabetologia* in 2010 from Canada, caffeinated coffee improved insulin sensitivity and decaffeinated coffee improved the function of the beta cells in the pancreas—the cells that make insulin.

Coffee and Cognitive Function

A 2010 study conducted by the Center for Cognitive Ageing and Cognitive Epidemiology at the University of Edinburgh, Scotland, found that there was a significant positive association between total caffeine intake and general cognitive ability and memory. Drinking caffeinated coffee was also associated with a significantly better performance on the National Adult Reading Test and the Wechsler Test of Adult Reading. Another study published in the *European Journal of Clinical Nutrition* in 2007 found that coffee consumption is inversely associated with cognitive decline in elderly European men. Other studies show that coffee increases alertness and improves accuracy on attention-switching tasks

Coffee and Athletic Performance

Many studies show that caffeine and coffee consumption improves athletic performance, endurance, concentration, fatigue, alertness, and response time. It may also be beneficial for short-term, high-intensity athletic performance.

Coffee and Cancer

More than 1,500 published studies to date have investigated coffee drinking and the risk of cancer. The studies have shown that coffee can lower the risk of many types of cancer, including:

- Brain, mouth, and throat cancer: A 2010 study found that consuming five or more cups of coffee a day was associated with a 40 percent decrease in three different cancers: oral, throat, and glioma (a type of brain tumor).

- Colon cancer: Research from Gifu University in Japan in 2003 found that at least one cup of coffee a day may reduce a woman's risk of colon cancer by 50 percent.

- Uterine cancer: The Nurses' Health Study found women who drank more than four cups of coffee a day had a 25 percent lower risk of endometrial cancer.

- Prostate cancer: Harvard University researchers found that men who drank the most coffee were 60 percent less likely to get an aggressive form of prostate cancer.

- Breast cancer: A 2006 Canadian study published in the *International Journal of Cancer* found that the more coffee women who are at high risk for breast cancer (because they carry the BRCA1 mutation) drank per day, the lower was their risk of breast cancer. In this study, 1,690 women with the BRCA1 or BRCA2 mutations from forty centers in four countries were analyzed. Women (with the BRCA1 mutation, *not* the BRCA2 mutation) who habitually drank one to three cups of caffeinated coffee a day, four to five cups, or six or more cups had a 10, 25, and 69 percent reduction in their risk of breast cancer respectively, compared to women who didn't drink coffee. Women without this genetic mutation have up to a 40 percent lower risk of breast cancer.

Other studies confirm coffee's protective effect and shed light on specifically how this beverage lowers the risk of breast cancer. In the study above, researchers explain that coffee is an important source of phytoestrogens— weak plant estrogens that have a beneficial effect by blocking the ability of strong estrogens to bind to the estrogen receptors in the breast. Researchers at the Roswell Park Cancer Institute in Buffalo, New York, point out that coffee also contains polyphenols, which have anticarcinogenic effects.

In another study published in 2006, yet another breast cancer–defensive effect of coffee was found. Women who drank three or more cups of coffee a day were found to have a significantly higher ratio of 2-hydroxyestrogen (a "good" protective type of estrogen) compared to 16-alpha-hydroxyestrone (a "bad" cancer-promoting type of estrogen). Finally, a 1998 Japanese study discovered that high intakes of caffeinated beverages, including coffee, caused the amount of sex-hormone-binding globulin to increase. This serum protein binds estradiol—the most abundant and strongest form of natural estrogen in the body and the one most associated with an increased risk of breast cancer—and prevents it from attaching to and turning on the estrogen receptor in breast cells.

(Pages 106–111 adapted from *Waking the Warrior Goddess* by Christine Horner, M.D., used with permission of Basic Health Publications.)

Coffee and Cardiovascular Disease

A fifteen-year study published in the *American Journal of Clinical Nutrition* in May 2006, which collected data on 27,312 postmenopausal women who took part of the Iowa Women's Health Study, discovered that post-menopausal women who reported drinking at least one to three cups of coffee daily were 24 percent less likely to die of heart disease compared to those who didn't drink coffee. They were also 28 percent less likely to die of other non-cancerous inflammatory diseases.

Although some studies show that heavy coffee drinking may be associated with an elevated blood pressure, many other studies show a protective effect. A study published in 2008 in *Vascular Health Risk Management* reviewed the current epidemiological evidence of coffee consumption and blood pressure. They concluded that regular caffeinated coffee does not increase the risk of hypertension.

An article published in the journal *Stroke* reports the findings of a Swedish study of 34,670 women enrolled in the Swedish Mammography Cohort who were followed for ten years. The researchers found a 22 to 25 percent lower risk of stroke, cerebral infarction, and subarachnoid hemorrhage among women who drank at least one cup of coffee a day.

Coffee and Liver Disease

According to a study published by Oregon State University in the journal *Critical Reviews in Food Science and Nutrition* in 2006, numerous studies show that a caffeinated coffee reduces the risk of several different kinds of liver disease, including cirrhosis and hepatocellular carcinoma. Other studies have found that coffee slows the progression in chronic hepatitis C and decreases liver fibrosis.

Coffee may also prevent gallstones. In a study by Harvard University School of Health in Boston, men who drank two to three cups of caffeinated coffee a day had a 40 to 45 percent lower gallstone risk than men who drank none.

Coffee and Weight Loss

Coffee and caffeine has long been used to improve weight loss. In fact, the "active" ingredient in many diet pills is caffeine. But does it really work? In a meta-analysis published in *Gastroenterology Research and Practice* in 2011, several studies were reviewed which showed that coffee has a moderate influence on weight loss.

The Potential Drawbacks of Coffee

Yes, it's true that coffee can have some drawbacks. Caffeine can trigger anxiety attacks, jitteriness, impatience, mood swings, and cardiac arrhythmias; increase stress hormones; and cause insomnia. It also increases the amount of calcium your body excretes in your urine and decreases the amount you absorb from your intestines, which puts you at higher risk for osteoporosis. If you are pregnant, you will want to avoid consuming large amount of caffeine because it increases your chances of having a miscarriage.

Everyone is different, and it is important to use your own judgment when it comes to consuming coffee or other caffeinated beverages. If you don't feel good when you drink it—don't! But if you love coffee and have worried about it damaging your health, research shows you can relax a bit. It may not really be as bad a vice as you might have thought.

Cacao

In the early 1900s, a physician and researcher at Brigham & Women's Hospital and Harvard Medical School, Dr. Norman K. Hollenberg, observed that the Kuna Indians, the indigenous residents of the San Blas Islands of Panama, rarely developed high blood pressure—even as they aged. Neither

salt intake nor obesity appeared to have any influence. Genetics also proved
to be irrelevant, because when the islanders moved to the mainland, their
incidence of hypertension soared up to the levels of the rest of the population. Dr. Hollenberg noticed that the major difference between the Kuna
who lived in San Blas Island and those who lived on the mainland was that
the islanders drank about five cups a day of cocoa made from locally grown
cacao beans, which were high flavonol antioxidants.

There are more than 1,000 studies in the medical literature to date that
show chocolate made from cacao beans—in small doses (chocolate is high
in calories, so eating large amounts can cause you to gain weight)—can
be actually quite good for you. Chocolate has actually been revered for
thousands of years. There are records of the Maya drinking it more than
2,000 years ago. Aztec folklore said that the god Quetzalcoatl provided
chocolate to humanity as a divine beverage. When eighteenth-century
Swedish scientist Carl von Linné decided on the botanical name for chocolate, he no doubt agreed with the Aztecs. *Theobroma cacao* literally means,
"Food of the Gods."

In 2007, it was estimated that Americans ate 3.5 billion pounds of
chocolate a year. This may sound as if this might be a bad statistic—well,
yes and no. As it turns out, chocolate in its purest form (that is, dark chocolate without added sugar, butter, and other unhealthy ingredients) has a
remarkable number of nutrients that help to promote and protect your
health. For instance, chocolate is high in the minerals calcium, potassium,
iron, phosphorus, copper, and magnesium.

Chocolate also contains polyphenols, which are powerful antioxidants.
Polyphenols are known to reduce the risk of heart disease, aging, and cancer. One type of polyphenol found in chocolate, epicatechins, is also found
abundantly in tea. A Holland study published in the *Lancet* found that the
amount of epicatechins in chocolate is actually four times more concentrated than that in tea. Researchers at University of California, Davis, conducted an experiment in which they had healthy volunteers eat M&M
semisweet chocolate mini baking bits. (This is not the type of chocolate I
recommend! High-quality organic dark chocolate is your best choice.) The
researchers found that the epicatechin levels in the blood of the volunteers
increased exponentially in the first two hours after eating the chocolate and
faded by six hours.

There is another type of polyphenols called "flavonoids," specifically oligomeric procyanidins, which is also found in chocolate. It is the same substance found in red wine and tea. You might be surprised that Cornell University researchers found that a cup of hot cocoa has nearly twice the antioxidants of a glass of red wine and up to three times more than those found in a cup of green tea. Studies show flavonoids inhibit the oxidation of LDL cholesterol, which is one of the main risk factors contributing to atherosclerosis and heart disease.

The best type of chocolate to eat is dark, because it contains 50 to 70 percent cacao. Milk chocolate may contain only 5 percent and white chocolate contains none! The type of fat in dark chocolate, cocoa butter, is also considered to be healthy. Cocoa butter is a stearic acid and doesn't increase cholesterol or other cardiac risk factors. It also has been shown to promote healthy, smooth skin.

Here is a summary of all the health benefits of chocolate discovered so far:

- Decreases heart disease: It does this by decreasing cholesterol, LDL oxidation, platelet aggregation, blood pressure, and angiotensin-converting enzyme; and increasing HDL, nitric oxide, and endothelial function. Research shows a 39 percent lower risk of heart attacks and strokes for those who consume higher quantities of chocolate.

- Decreases heart failure: A 2010 study by Harvard Medical School published in the journal *Circulation and Health Failure* studied 31,823 women ages forty-eight to eighty-three and found a moderate chocolate intake was associated with a lower rate of heart failure and death.

- Decreases preeclampsia and gestational hypertension

- Reduces myocardial inflammation

- Protects the heart from ischemia-reperfusion injury

- Enhances mood: It is a mild aphrodisiac and antidepressant, and enhances bliss.

- Improves symptoms of chronic fatigue

- Decreases inflammation

- Increases antioxidant enzymes

- Decreases oxidases

- Protects against myocardial inflammation caused by air pollution

- Antimalarial

- Improves immune system function

- Antibacterial

- Anticarcinogenic: Studies show a 70 percent decreased growth of colon cancer cells.

- Antiproliferative

- Decreases the stress hormones cortisol and catecholamines

- Improves gut bacteria and eases diarrhea

- Decreases fasting blood sugar

- Enhances longevity: Men who eat chocolate live longer, according to a survey of healthy sixty-five-year-old men conducted by the Harvard School of Public Health. During the study, mortality was lowest among those who consumed chocolate one to three times a month and higher among those who indulged in the habit three or more times a week. Surprisingly, those who never ate chocolate had the highest mortality of all.

Super Spices

Spices just don't make your food taste great, most of them also contain powerful medicinal qualities. For example, turmeric has dozens of remarkable anticancer benefits, garlic is a strong antibiotic and lowers the risk of heart disease, and cinnamon protects against diabetes and lowers blood sugar in diabetics. Let's take a closer look at turmeric as an example.

Of all the spices, turmeric has been the most studied. There are currently over 9,000 studies in the medical research, which have found more than 150 ways that turmeric improves your health. Its benefits are diverse and nothing short of miraculous with dozens of diseases it significantly protects against.

Scientists attribute many of turmeric's profound health effects to its extraordinary antioxidant and anti-inflammatory properties. In fact, turmeric has 300 times the antioxidant power of vitamin E. Turmeric blocks dozens of mediators in the inflammatory process including NF-kappa B; the cytokines TNF, IL-1, -2, -6, -8, and -12; chemokines; and the enzymes COX-2 (cyclooxygenase-2) and LOX (lipoxygenase). Because most chronic degenerative diseases, including cardiovascular disease, diabetes, arthritis, and cancer, are fueled by excessive oxygen free radicals and inflammation, turmeric has been shown to be very effective at helping to prevent, treat, and even reverse many of these diseases.

Turmeric lowers your risk of heart disease by decreasing cholesterol and the formation of plaque in your arteries. It also reduces your risk of diabetes by improving insulin sensitivity and glucose transport, and protects against damage caused by oxygen free radicals and inflammation, which can lead to diabetic retinopathy, kidney disease, and brain injuries.

If you have gallstones, this amazing spice encourages your gallbladder to expel them. Turmeric aids digestion by increasing stomach secretions and decreasing the amount of gas produced in the intestines. It also protects against stomach ulcers.

Turmeric promotes wound healing by decreasing inflammation and stimulating the growth of new blood vessels. One of the more fascinating features of turmeric is that it clearly expresses its own intelligence. Turmeric *blocks* new blood-vessel growth to tumors, which slows the growth, while it *stimulates* new blood-vessel growth in wounds, which helps to speed healing. The key is that turmeric "knows" when to do each one. It can tell the difference between cancerous tissue and normal tissue and respond appropriately

In addition, turmeric shields your organs from chemical attack. It minimizes the damage to your brain caused by alcohol, as well as chemical damage to your liver. Elevated liver enzymes are an indication of liver injury. The higher the enzyme level, the more extensive the injury is. When turmeric is ingested, liver enzymes drop, indicating that it effectively helps the liver repair itself. Turmeric also strengthens your connective tissue and prevents the formation of adhesions or scar tissue. And it stimulates muscles to regenerate after trauma.

You can apply turmeric topically to your skin for another whole set of benefits. Turmeric can kill bacteria. If it's exposed to sunlight, its talent for exterminating bacteria improves. It is also effective for treating fungal infections, such as athlete's foot, and skin conditions, such as psoriasis. It is effective against viruses too.

Here is a short list of conditions that turmeric is known to help:

- Atherosclerosis/cardiovascular diseases
- Diabetes
- Cancer
- Respiratory illnesses, including acute and chronic lung injury, radiation injury, fibrosis, chronic obstructive pulmonary disease (COPD), asthma, and respiratory distress syndrome
- Arthritis
- Liver diseases, including cirrhosis
- Gallstones
- Obesity
- Pancreatic diseases, such as diabetes and cancer
- Intestinal issues, including poor digestion, bloating, and inflammatory conditions, such as Crohn's disease, and gastric ulcers
- Chronic renal diseases
- Neurological problems, such as Alzheimer 's disease
- Metabolic conditions
- Eye disorders: delays cataracts and helps to prevent retinopathy in diabetics
- Boosts the immune system: activates T and B cells, macrophages, lymphoid cells, dendritic cells, natural killer cells, both antigen and humoral cell-mediated immunity, enhances antibody response
- Antibacterial
- Antiviral
- Antifungal
- Skin diseases and aging: inhibits UVB damage, promotes wound healing, treats psoriasis and scleroderma

Turmeric is prepared by soaking and then drying the root. The dried root is then ground into a fine powder. Turmeric powder can be found in the spice section of most grocery stores. Remember, organic is always best. *Ayurvedic* physicians recommend adding about one-quarter teaspoon to your food near the end of cooking. Turmeric works more in harmony with your body when it is cooked—but not overcooked.

You can also take turmeric as a supplement. The recommended dose is at least 1,000 mg per day.

Super Fruits and Veggies from Around the World

Fruits and vegetables that are exceptionally nutrient-dense grow in nearly every type of climate—from inhospitable high altitudes battered by extreme winds and low temperatures, to the lush Amazon rainforest. Some of the most well-researched "super" fruits and vegetables include the following.

Maqui

The maqui berry plant only grows in the harsh environment of Patagonia, a southern region of Chile, and in a small area of Argentina. Research shows this small purple berry contains one of the highest amounts of antioxidants of any plant. According to a study published in the journal *Phytochemical Analysis,* fresh maqui berries contain on average 138 mgs of anthocyanins per 100 grams, and dried maqui berries contain up to 212 mgs per 100 grams. Maqui berries also contain strong anti-inflammatories and inhibits the COX-2 enzyme. For that reason, research shows that it reduces the risk of many chronic diseases, including cancer, and can help to decrease pain and increase flexibility and mobility in people with even severe arthritis and fibromyalgia. Maqui berries have also been be prized for their anti-aging and longevity-enhancing properties.

Other research-proven health benefits include:

- Promotes detoxification
- Aids weight loss
- Protects against heart disease by lowering cholesterol and blood pressure
- Lowers the risk of diabetes

Goji Berries

Goji berries, also known as wolfberries, are the fruits of the *Lycium bar-barum* and *Lycium chinense* plants. Used in Traditional Chinese Medicine for 2,000 years, these dried berries are high in antioxidants, vitamin C, and beta-carotene. In fact, goji berries have an "Oxygen Radical Absorbance Capacity" (ORAC) score of 3,290, which is higher than most fruits and vegetables. They contain approximately 500 times more vitamin C per weight than oranges, and have considerably more beta-carotene than carrots. As with all foods that have earned the designation of a superfood, these nutrient dense berries have numerous health benefits, including:

- Improve overall well-being. According to a study published in May 2008 in the *Journal of Alternative and Complementary Medicine,* drinking juice derived from goji berries has a positive effect on overall well-being. Study participants drank goji berry juice daily for a period of fifteen days, reporting improved levels of energy, quality of sleep, and feelings of happiness.

- Reduce damage by ultraviolet radiation

- Promote healthy skin

- Protect against macular degeneration

- Decrease the risk of certain cancers

- Improve male fertility

Acai Berries

This exotic relative of blueberries and cranberries contain some of the highest amounts of antioxidants found in any plant. In fact, one acai berry has ten to twenty times the amount of antioxidants as grapes, and two times the amount found in blueberries. Indigenous to the Amazon rainforests, acai berries have been heralded for centuries as a healing, immune-stimulating, and energy-boosting fruit. Some of the major health benefits of acai include:

- Supports heart health: In addition to the antioxidants and cholesterol-lowering effects, acai berries are also rich in plant sterols, which protect your heart by preventing blood clots, improving overall blood circulation, and relaxing blood vessels.

- Helps weight loss
- Promotes healthy skin: Brazilians have used acai berries topically or internally for centuries to treat skin conditions and improve complexion.
- Improves digestion
- Reduces inflammation
- Improves cellular health by protecting against oxygen free radical damage
- May reduce the risk of certain cancers: Acai is very high in vitamin C, ellagic acid, and anthocyanins—all of which have been shown to suppress the growth of cancer. A study published in the *Journal of Agricultural and Food Chemistry* found that acai reduced cancer cell proliferation by 56 to 86 percent.
- Slows aging: Because of acai's strong antioxidant and anti-inflammatory properties, it may help to slow or reverse the process of aging.
- Increases energy and stamina
- Improves sexual drive and function in men
- Improves menopausal brain fog

Camu Camu

This lemon-sized, light orange to purplish fruit grows on a shrub found in the rain forests of Peru and Brazil. It is known for having the highest amount of vitamin C found in any plant every recorded. In addition, it is rich in antioxidants such as beta-carotene and anti-inflammatories. Camu camu contains an abundance of minerals, including potassium, iron, niacin, phosphorus, as well as the amino acids threonine, leucine, and valine. The other health benefits of camu camu include:

- Increases energy
- Improves mood
- Strengthens the immune system
- Balances mood and helps improve depression
- Supports a health nervous system, including the eyes and brain

- Protects against arthritis by reducing inflammation
- Kills viruses

Pomegranate

With a history of use that goes back thousands of years, pomegranates have gained recent attention for their high antioxidant content and ability to ward off disease. The juice from pomegranates has been shown to be particularly beneficial for protecting against heart disease. Studies show it may improve blood flow to the heart and reduce plaque buildup in blood vessels. In animal studies, oral consumption of pomegranate extract inhibited growth of lung, skin, colon, and prostate tumors. According to research from UCLA, pomegranate juice may also slow the growth of prostate cancer. It has also been to shown to have the following benefits:

- Antiviral effects, including against herpes, Epstein-Barr, mononucleosis, and cold sores
- Protective actions against liver disease, including hepatitis and liver cancer
- Anti-inflammatory effects that reduce inflammation and joint pain in those with arthritis

The modern cosmetic industry has discovered that topical application of products containing this fruit may help to reduce wrinkles. Pomegranate contains a rare omega-5 fatty acid called "punicic acid," which has been shown to improve skin tone. Traditional Chinese Medicine used pomegranate juice for a longevity treatment.

According to a 2008 study, with pomegranate juice's high amount of antioxidant polyphenols, including tannin, anthocyanins, and ellagic acid, it scored the highest among ten different antioxidant-rich beverages, beating out the juices of grapes, acai, and blueberries.

Mangosteen

This fruit, which is indigenous to Southeast Asia, is another superfood known for its extraordinary anti-inflammatory and antioxidant properties, as well as a plethora of health problems that it helps to ward off. Polyphenol compounds, called "xanthones," are thought to be responsible for many of mangosteen's medicinal effects. There are two types of xanthones in this fruit: alpha-mangostin and gamma-mangostin. Mangosteen is best known for:

- Reducing free radical damage

- Protecting against cardiovascular diseases

- Slowing down aging

- Helping to maintain healthy skin: Due to its anti-inflammatory, anti-bacterial, antifungal, anti-allergy and antioxidant properties, research shows mangosteen helps to reduce the risk of various conditions, such as skin inflammation, skin aging, eczema, allergies, bacterial infections, and skin cancers.

- Boosting the immune system

Lychee

Lychee (*Litchi chinensis*) is a small tropical exotic fruit that is considered a prized delicacy in Asia. It has been used in Chinese medicine for hundreds of years for many conditions, such as sore throats and digestion. Lychee is known for its strong antioxidant, anti-inflammatory, antiviral, and antimicrobial qualities. Recent research reveals it has a broad spectrum of health benefits. For example, it lowers the risk of diabetes and certain cancers, and also has anti-aging properties. A study in the *Journal of Nutrition* found that of all fruits tested, lychee has one of the highest levels of heart-healthy polyphenols. Lychee also contains a unique polyphenol, "oligonol," which has been the focus of over thirty human clinical trials. Research shows oligonol:

- Improves circulation

- Has strong antioxidant and anti-inflammatory properties

- Reduces belly fat

- Improves metabolic syndrome

- Lessens fatigue and enhances endurance

- Supports cardiovascular health

- Protects skin against UV damage

- Reduces oxidative damage to collagen and elastin
- Improves skin wrinkling, elasticity, and pigmentation

Maca

Maca is a cruciferous vegetable and relative of a radish that grows high in the Andes in Peru. It has gained considerable attention for its ability to balance hormones and improve libido, fertility, energy, and endurance. It is also provides relief of menopausal symptoms, including hot flashes, mood swings, anxiety, and depression. In addition, maca is beneficial for skin issues, helping to clear acne and blemishes and decreasing sensitivity. The powdered root is rich in vitamins B, C, and E, as well as calcium, zinc, iron, magnesium, phosphorus, and amino acids.

Fermented Foods

Although fermented foods have been used for thousands of years, they have just recently gained popularity because of their important health benefits. These foods are all made with bacterial cultures—the "good" type your body needs to function well—so in essence, they are natural "probiotics." Good examples include tempeh, miso soup, sauerkraut, kefir, kombucha, and yogurt. Some of their health benefits include:

- Helping to balance the production of stomach acid: Fermented foods have the unique ability to ease digestive discomfort related to having either too much or too little stomach acid. When the production of hydrochloric acid by the stomach is low, fermented foods help increase the acidity of gastric juices. On the other hand, when the stomach produces too much acid, fermented foods help protect the stomach and intestinal lining from its caustic effects.

- Aiding digestion by increasing the production acetylcholine: Acetylcholine is a neurotransmitter and, therefore, helps with the transmission of nerve impulses. By increasing peristalsis, or movement, of the bowel wall, it helps to prevent constipation. Acetylcholine also increases the release of digestive juices and enzymes from your stomach, pancreas, and gallbladder.

- Populating your colon with beneficial bacteria and killing pathogenic bacteria: Scientists have discovered that the type of bacteria you have in your colon plays a huge role on your health. Beneficial bacteria are required to keep the lining of your bowel healthy and prevent infections and disease. They also play a critical role in your immune system and the production of neurotransmitters. In fact, because they are involved in neurotransmitter production, they can affect your mood. For instance, studies have found that taking probiotics can improve symptoms of depression.

WHY CHOOSE ORGANIC

Choosing to eat only organically produced foods is important for a number of reasons. Here are a few of them:

- Conventional agriculture uses chemicals harmful to you and the environment.

- Pesticides kill our soil and beneficial bugs, and are carcinogenic.

- More than 90 percent of the pesticides that Americans consume in food are found in the fat and tissue of meat and dairy products. According to the Union of Concerned Scientists, 70 percent of all antibiotics are fed to conventionally grown animals.

- To avoid potential health problems from genetically modified organisms (GMOs).

- Pesticides used in conventional agriculture are known to kill bees.

- Organic foods taste better, which is why many chefs prefer it.

- Organic foods contain higher amounts of antioxidants: A study conducted at the University of California, Davis, found that organic corn had a 58 percent higher antioxidant level compared to conventionally grown corn.

- Animals fed organic foods tend to have higher reproductive capacity and better recovery from illness and survival.

Every fruit and vegetable has its own unique pharmacy of natural medicines. You'll want to take advantage of all the extraordinary gifts that nature gives to us through our foods. So, instead of overloading with one type of fruit or vegetable, which many companies try to push—such as certain "miracle" fruit juices—consider every plant a miracle and consume a wide diversity of them.

The Maya included 1,200 plants in their diet. On the other hand, many Americans tend to have just one: French fries. You laugh, but it's true. It's no wonder that our health suffers so much. As your mother said and I will repeat, "Eat your vegetables and fruits!" Remember to get them fresh, organically grown, and locally grown whenever possible.

AVOID PESTICIDES WHEN BUYING PRODUCE

The Environmental Working Group tested forty-three different fruits and vegetables to determine the level of pesticide residue present on each plant. Their *Shoppers' Guide to Pesticides in Produce* reports that the following twelve fruits and vegetables ("the dirty dozen") had the highest pesticide load, making them the most important to buy or grow organic:

1. Peaches
2. Apples
3. Sweet bell peppers
4. Celery
5. Nectarines
6. Strawberries
7. Cherries
8. Lettuce
9. Grapes (imported)
10. Pears
11. Spinach
12. Potatoes

In contrast, the following twelve foods were found to have the lowest residual pesticide load, making them the safest bet among conventionally grown fruits and vegetables:

1. Broccoli
2. Eggplant
3. Cabbage
4. Banana
5. Kiwi
6. Asparagus
7. Sweet peas (frozen)
8. Mango
9. Pineapple
10. Sweet corn (frozen)
11. Avocado
12. Onion

ENHANCING DIGESTION

Even if you consume the best foods in the world, it won't make you healthier if your digestion in poor. That's why *Ayurveda* says the first pillar of health is both diet AND digestion.

The number of American adults with digestive problems is alarming. According to a recent survey, almost 75 percent of the population complains of digestive problems. These problems include gas, bloating, cramping, constipation, diarrhea, abdominal pain, and heartburn. The Western medical approach to these problems is pharmaceutical drugs. In fact, pharmaceutical companies run television commercials that say if you are at war with your food and suffering with heartburn and indigestion—the solution to all your digestive problems is to simply take their medication and keep on eating whatever you'd like.

Ayurveda takes a different and much healthier approach. It addresses the source of your indigestion by adjusting your diet and giving you tips to enhance your digestion. By eliminating foods that take you out of balance, and instead consuming only highly nutritious foods that bring you into balance, most of your digestive complaints will easily resolve. You can enjoy even smoother digestion by also incorporating *Ayurveda's* guidelines for enhancing digestion.

Ayurveda's Top-12 Aids to Digestion

1. Eat your main meal at noon.
2. Don't eat again until your previous meal has been digested (about three hours).
3. Keep regular mealtimes.
4. Don't overeat. Eat to fill three-quarters of your stomach's capacity.
5. Eat in a settled atmosphere.
6. Don't eat when you are upset.
7. Always sit down to eat.
8. Don't talk while chewing.

9. Favor lightly cooked foods over raw foods.

10. Avoid cold drinks.

11. Favor fresh wholesome foods, such as organic fruits, vegetables, and whole grains.

12. Put your full attention on your food.

Most of these recommendations are self-explanatory, but a few of them need further clarification. *Ayurveda* recommends that you *eat your main meal at noon* because your "digestive fires" are at their peak from 10:00 a.m. to 2:00 p.m. In other words, your body's metabolism is revved up during these hours, and you can digest your food better than you can early in the morning or later at night.

If you eat a big meal late at night, it won't digest well, and your sleep will be disturbed. I'm sure you've had this unpleasant experience at least once or twice. However, the times you've *eaten light in the evening and gone to bed early,* you more than likely woke up feeling great. Most of the principles and recommendations of *Ayurveda* are as simple as this one, but don't let their simplicity fool you. Their effects can be *very* profound.

Cold drinks should be avoided, especially during a meal, because according to *Ayurveda,* a cool drink cools down and dilutes the digestive fires. In Western scientific terms, cool drinks slow down the action of your stomach's digestive enzymes, which work best at body temperature or a little above. At the temperature of an iced drink, the effectiveness of your digestive enzymes is cut almost in half. If you want to drink something with your meals, *Ayurveda* recommends that you have sips of hot water only. Don't drink too much water with your meal, either, because water will dilute the enzymes in the stomach, making them less effective.

The *Ayurvedic* recommendation to favor fresh wholesome foods is a key principle of diet, and it plays a big role in lowering the risk of breast cancer. The 2,500-year-old text of *Ayurveda,* called the *Charaka Samhita,* proclaims the importance of a wholesome diet: "The distinction between health and disease arises as the result of the difference between wholesome and unwholesome diet." Wholesome foods are considered to be primarily fresh organic fruits, vegetables, and whole grains.

According to *Ayurveda,* when foods are lightly cooked they are easier to digest, and, therefore, more nutrients are absorbed. Overcooking foods or cooking foods at high temperatures should be avoided because it destroys nutrients and creates harmful substances.

Finally, when you eat a meal, it is ideal to put your full attention on your food. Don't watch TV or read the newspaper. When your full attention is on your meal, you're more likely to chew your food well, eat smaller portions, and digest your food better.

Ayurveda also recommends that you add spices to your food that assist digestion. Some of the top digestive spices include ginger, fennel, cumin, coriander, and cardamom.

If you eat highly nutritious foods and follow these simple recommendations, you can provide your body with the best building materials to construct and maintain the foundation of your health. If you choose poor materials, your foundation will be weak and no matter what else you do to support your health, it will crumble. With a strong foundation, you can build a structure so solid it will resist disease, and stay vibrantly healthy and beautiful—no matter what your age.

(Pages 126–128 adapted from *Waking the Warrior Goddess* by Christine Horner, M.D., used with permission of Basic Health Publications.)

CHAPTER 5

Filling in the Gaps

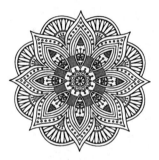

Key Nutritional Supplements
for Healthy Aging

Never be afraid to try something new.
Remember, amateurs built the ark;
professionals built the Titanic.

~AUTHOR UNKNOWN

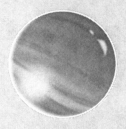

THE FIFTH GEM—JASPER

The fifth stone of your breastplate is orange jasper and signifies the dietary supplements that help to fill in your nutritional gaps and boost your health and longevity. Your sacral chakra, located on your lower abdomen just below your belly button, is associated with the color orange. It governs creativity, sexuality, power, relationships, and nurturing. Certain supplemental nutrients can supply you with the creative and nurturing power you need to become vibrantly healthy and add years to your life.

The color orange is warm and cheering. It has a freeing action upon your body and mind. Orange helps to show you new possibilities and options for your life, such as finding the nutritional supplements that can help to transform your health.

Jasper is known as the "supreme nurturer," and offers protection—just as the right supplements can supremely nurture and protect you too.

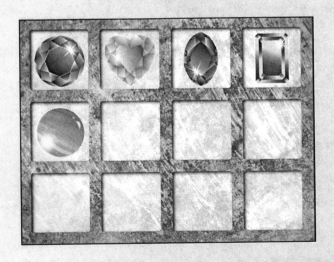

The fact is: You can't fulfill all of your nutritional needs from your food. Even if you eat a diet high in organically grown fruits and vegetables, you still need a few key supplements to get all the vital nutrients needed for extraordinary health and longevity. Nutritional supplements are not a replacement for nutritious foods. As their name implies, they are meant to *supplement* your healthy diet. The results of studies comparing the effects of nutrients given as a supplement verses consumed as food almost always show that nutrients from food sources are far superior. There are some exceptions, however, which is the focus of this chapter.

Multivitamins: To Be or Not to Be

Should you take them; should you not? This question has been debated for decades, because the results of controlled trials on individual nutrients and their effects on health are all over the map. Some studies show they are helpful, some show no effect at all, and others even suggest that they may be harmful. No doubt you must be thinking, *What the heck is the problem that researchers and doctors can't seem to figure this one out?*

One reason for these seemingly nonsensical results is that it is impossible to completely isolate certain vitamins and minerals in your diet, because they are present in all the food you eat—especially plants. Equally impossible is eliminating all the factors that affect your health, such as lifestyle. So what does this mean? It means that it's extremely difficult, if not impossible, to conduct good human studies on individual nutrient intake and accurately assess their influence on healthy aging.

But what we do know from observational studies is that eating lots of fruits and vegetables, which are packed with vitamins, minerals, and other nutrients, is associated with a lower risk of chronic disease and a higher probability of good health and longevity. When individuals with extraordinary longevity have been studied, they have generally been found to have blood levels of certain nutrients—such as antioxidants, selenium, manganese, iron, copper and zinc—that are much higher than in those who die younger. Again, consuming nutrients through a healthy plant-based diet is always best. However, for individuals with certain disease conditions or who are at high risk for a vitamin deficiency, a multivitamin/mineral supplement appears to be helpful.

Adequate amounts of vitamins (A, B complex, C, D, E, and K) and minerals (including selenium, potassium, magnesium, manganese, zinc, and chromium picolinate), as well as amino acids such as l-carnitine, are essential for your body to stay healthy and resistant to disease. Research shows that these substances reduce the incidence of diabetes, cardiovascular disease, hypertension, and congestive heart failure, as well as other age-related health problems, including deterioration of vision, brain, and immune function.

There are numerous studies showing that taking a multivitamin and mineral supplement may reduce the risk of many of these age-related chronic diseases and disorders. For instance, several studies show that daily multivitamin use may reduce the risk of heart attacks. A Swedish study in October 2010 prospectively investigated the use of multivitamins by 30,000 Swedish women between ages forty-nine and eighty-three. In women with no history of coronary artery disease, the incidence of heart attacks was 27 percent lower in those who took a multivitamin. A Dutch study published in the *American Journal of Clinical Nutrition* found almost twice that reduction. Those who took multivitamins had a 51 percent lower incidence of heart attacks than those who didn't. An American study also noted a lower incidence of coronary heart disease mortality in vitamin takers—a reduction of 25 percent.

Animal studies on specific nutrients are far easier to conduct, but there can be problems applying those results to humans. However, they are worth reviewing because the information we gleam from them generally correlates with human physiology. A Canadian study published in the *FASEB Journal* in 2010 tested the effects of vitamin C supplementation on mice with a genetic premature-aging disorder. The researchers found that vitamin C reduced inflammation and beneficially worked on certain genes, which caused the reversal of several age-related abnormalities and increased the lifespan of the mice.

According to a 2010 Canadian study published in *Experimental Biology and Medicine,* nutritional supplements may also slow aging and extend lifespan in normal mice. Mice fed a supplemental cocktail of thirty different vitamins, minerals, and herbs experienced a delay in the aging process and a 10 percent longer lifespan. The researchers used physical movements as a marker for aging and mortality risk. Mice fed a normal diet experienced a

50 percent loss of daily movement compared to those who were given supplements. These mice also had a loss of brain-signaling chemicals. There was no decline in movement or brain chemicals noted in the animals that were given supplements.

If you decide you would like to take a multivitamin and mineral supplement, be sure to choose one that is sourced from whole organic foods and avoid one that is synthetic because your body will not absorb it well. For instance, New Chapter makes multivitamins from whole organic foods called "Every Woman" and "Every Man."

Make Vitamin D Your Friend for Life

Vitamin D has been the subject of thousands of studies in the last several years, because it has been found to play a critical role in maintaining good health and preventing dozens of diseases. This vitamin acts more like a steroid hormone and is used by virtually every cell in your body. Vitamin D has more than 2,000 gene interactions, contributes to good muscle and bone formation, supports the immune system, has anticancer effects, and reduces inflammation.

Low levels of vitamin D are associated with a myriad of diseases, including:

- Heart disease
- Strokes
- Diabetes
- Multiple sclerosis
- Osteoarthritis
- Parkinson's disease
- Alzheimer's disease
- Cancer (seventeen different types), including breast, prostate, and colon cancers.

Mice with a genetic deficiency in vitamin D show a broad spectrum of abnormalities revealing that this vitamin is essential for countless structures and functions in the body. The abnormalities include:

- Growth retardation
- Osteoporosis
- Skin thickening and wrinkling
- Kyphosis (abnormal curvature of the upper spine)
- Alopecia (hair loss)
- Calcium deposits
- Hearing loss
- Balance loss
- Shortened lifespan

Supplemental vitamin D has been found to help all of these conditions. Vitamin D supplementation can have such a profound effect on your health—for example, studies have found that it lowers your risk of breast, prostate, and colon cancer by as much as 50 percent.

How Much Vitamin D Is Right for You?

Vitamin D is unique, because your body can make its own supply from a chemical reaction in your skin that is activated by ultraviolet rays from sunlight. Additional chemical reactions in other areas of your body convert the form of vitamin D made in your skin to its active form called "cholecalciferol," or vitamin D3. When choosing a vitamin D supplement, be sure to only take the D3 active form.

How much vitamin D3 you should take can vary greatly depending on many factors including your age, weight, percent of body fat, skin color, the season of the year, your sunblock usage, the latitude at which you live, and your state of health. If you are older, weigh more, and have a higher percent of fat than is ideal; live in northern latitudes; have darker skin color; and use sunblock or are ill, you'll generally require higher doses of vitamin D, which are also needed during the winter months. The Food and Nutrition Board at the U.S. Institute of Medicine recommends 200–600 IU of vitamin D3 per day. Many physicians and experts in the field of vitamin D, including myself, believe that these recommendations are far too low. Most specialists say that the amount of supplemental vitamin D that is more likely needed for optimum health each day is 2,000 IU or greater.

There is no perfect way to determine the right amount of vitamin D3 you should take. Currently the best method available is a blood test, which measures the level of a metabolite of vitamin D3 called "25-OH vitamin D." There are many metabolites of vitamin D, so it is probable that measuring only this one alone may not accurately reflect the total amount of vitamin D in your body. Also, vitamin D stores in your fat cells and the blood test only measure the amount of 25-OH vitamin D in your blood—not the vitamin D in your fat. However, as I mentioned, this is the best measurement currently available, and it does seem to show a strong relationship with the total amount of vitamin D you have in your body.

The range of normal for 25-OH vitamin D in your blood is 20–55 ng/ml. Some experts say that these levels are far too low, because they are based only on optimal bone health—not on any of the many other diseases known to be associated with low vitamin D. For instance, this amount may prevent rickets and osteomalacia, but it may not be enough to help prevent other diseases such as cancer, heart disease, and multiple sclerosis. Dr. Frank Lipman, an internationally recognized expert in Integrative and Functional Medicine, says that the ideal range should be 50–80 ng/ml. Based on these levels, an estimated 30 to 80 percent of Americans are deficient in vitamin D. A study conducted of young healthy women in California—a sunny and outdoor-activity-centered environment—found that 59 percent were low in vitamin D. Twenty-five percent were found to have seriously low levels of 20 ng/ml or less. Because so many Americans are deficient in this essential vitamin, experts say that everyone should consider taking supplemental vitamin D.

ANTIOXIDANTS: NEUTRALIZING A FORCE OF DESTRUCTION

As you may recall from earlier, oxygen free radicals are tiny molecules of oxygen that are unstable because they are missing an electron. In an effort to become stable, they steal electrons from other molecules. This process helps to drive all the chemical reactions in your body. But if there are too many oxygen free radicals in your body—usually as a result too much stress, bad food, and toxins—they damage your cells and DNA by stealing electrons from them. The destruction they cause is a major source for the development of chronic diseases and accelerated aging. That's why most experts recommend that you take supplemental antioxidants.

Antioxidants neutralize oxygen free radicals by donating an electron and, therefore, protect against the damage and diseases. There are a number of vitamins that have good antioxidant capabilities such as vitamins A, C, and E. However, research shows there are many other substances with far superior antioxidant power. For instance, *Amrit Kalash,* an ancient *Ayurvedic* herbal preparation, has an antioxidant power greater than any substance ever tested—more than 25,000 times more powerful than vitamin E.

Thousands of years ago, *Ayurvedic* physicians created *Amrit Kalash* to be the most powerful *rasayana*—meaning "that which negates old age and disease." A *rasayana* is defined as any herb, food, or activity that confers youthfulness and cures diseases. The purpose of a *rasayana* is to prevent disease and to impart strength, immunity, vitality, willpower, and determination. If taken properly, *Ayurveda* says a *rasayana* prevents early aging and keeps you young and active, both physically and mentally. Studies have found that *Amrit Kalash* appears to do just that—it slows aging and protects against numerous diseases including cancer. For example, a double-blind study was conducted to test the effect of *Maharishi Amrit Kalash* (MAK) on an age-related alertness task. Forty-eight men over thirty-five years of age were randomly assigned to receive MAK tablets, or a closely matched placebo, twice daily for six weeks. Those who took MAK scored significantly better in their performance on the alertness task after three and six weeks of treatment relative to the placebo group. The researchers concluded that MAK may enhance the capacity for attention or alertness, thus reversing some of the detrimental cognitive effects of aging.

Numerous animal studies have documented that MAK causes reversal of several age-related changes in the brain associated with oxygen free radical damage, including a study on the brains of Guinea pigs published in 2001 by the journal *Drug Metabolism and Drug Interactions*. This formula has also been shown to prevent many other deteriorative age-related changes. For example, it improves immune function and ameliorates several cardiovascular risk factors.

Other Powerful Antioxidants Defenders

There are a number of other strong antioxidants available as dietary supplements. Three of the most commonly recommended are CoQ10, alpha-lipoic acid, and resveratrol.

Coenzyme Q10 (CoQ10)

Also known as ubiquinone, this fat-soluble vitamin-like substance is found in nearly every cell in your body. It is used by the mitochondria in your cells to drive the chemical reactions that produce energy. Although CoQ10 is found in all of your cells, it is most concentrated in organs that use a lot of energy, such as your heart, kidneys, liver, and lungs. Your body makes its own supply of CoQ10, but after age thirty-five, the production of it begins to decline. If levels drop too low, your overall energy will feel depleted and your risk of numerous diseases will significantly increase. Low CoQ10 levels have been associated with congestive heart failure, high blood pressure, periodontal (gum) disease, type 2 diabetes, male infertility, chronic fatigue syndrome, sickle-cell anemia, certain cancers, immune system diseases (such as AIDS), and neurological disorders (such as Parkinson's disease).

CoQ10 has been the subject of thousands of studies, which show taking it as a supplement will:

- Improve congestive heart failure

- Help to produce more energy for your cells

- Support your immune system

- Decrease blood pressure in those with hypertension

- Reduce oxygen free radical damage to your skin

- Help to protect against organ damage caused by chemotherapy

- Reduce the risk of certain cancers

- Improve asthma and chronic lung disease

- Decrease migraine headaches—Studies of CoQ10 supplementation in children, adolescents, and adults show substantial decreases in the frequency of migraine episodes, number of days with migraine symptoms, headache disability, and frequency of nausea.

- Improve depression—A study of depression in older adults with bipolar disorder found a significant reduction in the severity of symptoms.

- Improve Parkinson's disease and slow its progression

- Directly influence the expression of multiple genes involved in aging, especially those regulating inflammation

- Decrease skin aging by protecting against UV light damage, oxygen free radical damage to the mitochondria, and by activating protective genes

- May extend lifespan—Research demonstrates that mice supplemented with CoQ10 live longer. In one case, supplemented animals experienced an 11.7 percent increase in mean lifespan, and a 24 percent increase in maximum lifespan.

CoQ10 at doses of 300–1,200 mg per day have been used in clinical research. In healthy human blood, more than 90 percent of CoQ10 exists in its reduced form called "ubiquinol." Research shows that ubiquinol is a more biologically active form of CoQ10—meaning that it absorbs into your cells better and its actions are stronger. Most CoQ10 supplements, however, contain the ubiquinone form, because it remains stable longer in capsules. Ubiquinone is converted to ubiquinol in the body, and research confirms that both forms work. Many experts are now recommending ubiquinol, because it doesn't require conversion and ubiquinone does. The recommended dose of ubiquinol is the same as ubiquinone, about 100–300 mg per day.

My opinion is that both forms work and it doesn't make that much difference which you choose. If you choose to take ubiquinone, a fermented product is definitely superior to a synthetic one. CoQ10 can also be applied topically to protect against skin aging, which is why it is an ingredient in many moisturizing formulas.

Alpha-Lipoic Acid (ALA)

This antioxidant is called the "universal antioxidant," because it is both fat soluble and water soluble. That means, it not only dissolves and transport well in your blood, but also passes easily through the fatty layers of your cell membranes and into the interior of your cells. Unlike the majority of other antioxidants, ALA can also pass through your blood brain barrier and reach your brain. Of all the antioxidants, ALA has the most consistent beneficial findings. In other words, the vast majority of studies on supplemental ALA find it is advantageous to your health.

Based on evidence from animal and human studies, alpha-lipoic acid offers the following health benefits:

- Reduces oxidative stress in the body via powerful antioxidant activity
- Improves several components of metabolic syndrome, which reduces the risk for diabetes
- Reduces blood pressure
- Improves the lipid profile
- Reduces weight
- Increases insulin sensitivity

- Improves diabetic neuropathy
- Protects against cataract formation
- Improves visual function in glaucoma
- Helps prevents retinal cell death when combined with vitamin E in retinitis pigmentosa
- Reduces brain damage after a stroke
- Prevents bone loss, possibly through an anti-inflammatory effect
- Removes toxic metals from the body, such as arsenic, cadmium, lead, and mercury
- Reduces frequency and intensity of migraines
- Improves skin texture
- Amplifies the effects of other antioxidants, including glutathione, coenzyme Q10, and vitamins C and E
- Helps energy production by protecting mitochondria from oxygen free radical damage and by working with the B-vitamin family to store energy from food

The dose of ALA used in medical studies ranges from 300–1,800 mg per day.

Resveratrol

This polyphenol is found in grape skins, cocoa, and certain berries and vegetables. It has been a subject of more than 7,000 published studies to date, not only for its antioxidant qualities, but also because of its anti-aging properties. Resveratrol has a unique ability to mimic the gene expression effects of caloric restriction, the only intervention that has been shown in peer-reviewed studies to prolong maximum lifespan and/or produce anti-aging effects. Not only does resveratrol have these effects in mice, but also in dogs and monkeys, which share more of our DNA. Therefore, researchers believe that resveratrol may have similar health and longevity benefits in humans. Studies show that resveratrol:

- Lowers blood pressure
- Improves insulin sensitivity

- Reduces the risk of certain cancers, such as cancers of the breast, prostate, colon, liver, thyroid, stomach, ovary, and skin (melanoma)

- Decreases the risk of metastasis of colon, prostate, and breast cancer

- Enhances the killing effects of radiation and chemotherapy

- Protects against the organ damage from chemotherapy

- Decreases inflammation by blocking the COX-2 enzyme

- Improves heart health and elasticity of blood vessels

- Stimulates the production of SIRT1, a protein that blocks many different diseases by speeding up the mitochondria, the cell's energy production centers

- Improves endurance levels during exercise

- Protects against Alzheimer's disease

- Reduces the risk of Parkinson's disease

- May be beneficial for weight control

The dosages of resveratrol used in studies vary considerable. So, the recommended daily amount has a very broad range. The brand I take, Integrative Therapeutics, contains 125 mg and is only available through a physician's office. To put this in perspective, one glass of red wine contains only 0.2–2.2 mg of resveratrol. Recently, a study received a lot of media attention by declaring that resveratrol didn't have any health benefits. However, the study did not evaluate therapeutic doses of resveratrol given as a supplement. Instead, it based its findings on comparing individuals who drank wine versus those who did not. The therapeutic dose of resveratrol is the equivalent of sixty glasses or more of wine! To get the amount of resveratrol you need to gain all of its benefits, you obviously can't get it from drinking wine and must take it as a supplement.

Anti-inflammatories: Dowsing Nature's Flames

Inflammation, like oxygen free radicals, plays an important role in your body. It is involved in normal wound healing and helps to fight infections. The inflammatory response is triggered anytime your body's tissues are damaged from physical trauma, excessive heat, irritating chemicals, or infections caused by bacteria and viruses. The chemicals released by the inflammatory process signal for cells from the immune system to come to the area. These chemicals also help to prevent the spread of damaging substances to nearby tissues, dispose of cell debris and bacteria, and initiate wound healing.

Inflammation only becomes a problem when there is too much of it, and it doesn't go away. In fact, chronic inflammation creates such a powerful force of destruction that it fuels the initiation and progression of every chronic disease and accelerates aging. Inflammation and oxygen free radicals are nearly identical twins: They both are necessary for the body in small doses, but in large doses, they are extremely destructive. They never go anywhere without each other. Where there is inflammation, there are oxygen free radicals and vice versa. That's because inflammation produces oxygen free radicals, and oxygen free radicals produce inflammation. Chronic excess inflammation and oxygen free radicals are such good friends that together they are the primary forces behind all chronic diseases and accelerated aging.

In a 2009 study published in the journal *Cancer Immunology and Immunotherapy,* centenarians were found to have high levels of anti-inflammatory cytokines in their blood. These proteins produced by the immune system indicate a lower than normal state of inflammation, which may help to explain the genetic reasons for their reduced incidence of chronic diseases, such as cancer, as well as their extraordinary longevity.

Virtually all of the diet and lifestyle factors that increase oxygen free radicals also increase inflammation and vice versa. For example, high stress, staying up too late at night, smoking, excessive alcohol, and ingesting toxins and junk food increase both inflammation and oxygen free radicals. Whereas, a diet rich in antioxidants found in fresh organically grown fruits and vegetables, olive oil, and omega-3 fatty acids, as well as practicing a stress-reducing technique, such as meditation, reduces both.

The best way to keep inflammation contained and prevent it from getting out of control is to follow all the diet and lifestyle advice presented in this book. All of the antioxidant supplements discussed in the previous section also have strong anti-inflammatory properties. There are certain foods, spices, and supplements with such outstanding anti-inflammatory

BASIC ANTI-INFLAMMATORY DIET

Avoid:

- Red meat
- Pork
- Poultry
- Processed Meats
- Butter

- Dairy
- Sugar
- Soft drinks
- Highly processed refined carbo-hydrates such as cookies, crackers, and chips

Favor:

- Nuts
- Foods high in omega-3 fatty acids, such as flaxseeds, salmon, and walnuts
- Olive oil
- Organically grown fruits, especially berries, pomegranate, papaya, and cherries

- Organically grown vegetables, especially artichoke, leafy greens, all squashes, avocados, and sweet potatoes
- Spices and herbs: cinnamon, ginger, turmeric, garlic, cumin, holy basil, oregano, mint, rosemary, sage, and thyme
- Green tea

properties that studies show can reduce the risk of many chronic disorders, including arthritis, dementia, heart disease, and certain cancers—especially of the breast, prostate, and colon. They have also been shown to reduce signs of aging in the skin.

The enzyme cyclooxygenase-2 (COX-2) is involved in inflammation. It has also been found to powerfully promote the growth of certain cancers, especially breast, prostate, and colon. There are more than a dozen ways this enzyme promotes tumor growth and helps tumors to metastasize or spread to other areas in the body. COX-2 anti-inflammatories block this enzyme and all of its damaging effects. I don't recommend taking pharmaceutical COX-2 anti-inflammatories, because they have very serious side effects, including increasing the risk of strokes, heart attacks, and death.

Instead, I recommend taking herbal anti-inflammatories. Research shows that they are just as effective and don't have any dangerous side effects.

Some of the best herbal COX-2 anti-inflammatories are turmeric, ginger, holy basil, rosemary, oregano, and green tea. All of these herbs have been extensively studied and found to have profound health benefits, especially reducing the risk of chronic diseases associated with inflammation. When it comes to natural COX-2 inhibitors, none is as powerful as turmeric. A study published in the *Indian Journal of Medical Research* compared the anti-inflammatory effects of oral curcumin (one of the active ingredients in turmeric and the source of its bright yellow-orange color) against two powerful anti-inflammatory medications: cortisone and phenylbutazone. The study found that curcumin was *just as effective* as these two potent anti-inflammatory medications!

Turmeric has three major ways that it reduces inflammation in your body. First, it stimulates your adrenal glands to release the natural, powerful anti-inflammatory substances called "corticosteroids." Second, it prevents the breakdown of cortisol, so more of this natural anti-inflammatory stays in your body. Third, it makes your body's cortisol receptors more sensitive. When the receptors are more sensitive, it only takes a small amount of cortisol to produce big anti-inflammatory effects.

Turmeric can also be used as a topical anti-inflammatory and analgesic (pain reliever). When applied over strained muscles, pulled tendons, and arthritic joints, turmeric can help to reduce swelling and pain. It also depletes substance P, a chemical produced at nerve endings that causes the sensation of irritation and pain.

The best anti-inflammatory herbal supplement I know of is Zyflamend. Made by the company New Chapter, it is available in most health food stores and groceries. Zyflamend contains ten different COX-2 anti-inflammatory herbs, including green tea, turmeric, holy basil, rosemary, ginger, oregano, skullcap, barberry, and the Chinese herbs Hu Zhang and Chinese goldthread. Individually, these herbs have been the subject of thousands of studies that document profound and diverse health benefits. Currently, there are approximately two dozen published studies that have investigated Zyflamend, including studies conducted at the prestigious MD Anderson Cancer Center in Houston, Texas. This herbal product has been found to reduce the risk of cancers of the prostate, pancreas, mouth, and skin (melanoma). It has also been shown to be very beneficial in the treatment of both osteoarthritis and rheumatoid arthritis.

Throwing Life Preservers to Your Telomeres

Certain substances have been shown to increase the lifespan of animals by preserving the length of telomeres on the end of chromosomes. As you may recall, telomere length is strongly associated with aging and survival: The shorter the telomere length, the shorter is the predicted lifespan. Shorter telomere lengths are also associated with certain age-related disorders, including wrinkling and diminished skin elasticity, atherosclerosis, high blood pressure, obesity, cancer, dementia, diabetes, osteoporosis, age-related cataracts, and glaucoma.

The following are a few substances that can be taken as nutritional supplements, which research shows help to preserve telomere length, slow aging, and extend lifespan.

Carnosine

Carnosine is described as an anti-aging compound, because it prevents damage to telomeres and preserves their length. It also has a beneficial influence on a wide range of age-related processes and functions. Composed of two amino acids, beta-alanine and l-histidine, carnosine is found naturally in skeletal muscle. Studies show it slows the aging of mice and increases their lifespan by 20 percent. In human clinical trials, carnosine was also found to improve brain function and memory, help to protect against Alzheimer's disease and Parkinson's disease, and decrease blood pressure. In addition, carnosine offers protection against diabetes due to its ability to regulate blood sugar and to prevent or reverse diabetic complications, such as nephropathy (kidney disease) and ocular damage.

The recommended dose of l-carnosine is 100–300 mg daily. It is preferable that it be taken with other antioxidants.

Omega-3 Fatty Acids

In a 2014 study published in the journal *Nutrition*, the rate of telomere shortening was significantly slower in the patients with mild dementia who were given omega-3 fatty acid supplements compared to those who did not take the supplements. Researchers at the University of California, San Francisco, found a linear relationship between the levels of omega-3s and telomere length. For each one standard deviation in DHA and EPA levels, there was a 32 percent reduction in the odds of telomere shortening. The recommended daily dose of omega-3 fatty acids is 500–1,000 mg.

Antioxidants

Studies show that higher dietary antioxidants are associated with slower aging and longer telomere length. Taking antioxidant supplements, such as CoQ10 and selenium, have also been shown to preserve telomere length and extend lifespan. Research shows that CoQ10, for example, lengthens the lifespan of numerous types of organisms ranging from fruit flies to mice.

Gymnema sylvestre

This *Ayurvedic* herb is traditionally known as an effective natural remedy for diabetes by lowering blood sugar, improving insulin sensitivity, controlling sugar cravings, and promoting regeneration of the pancreas. Research show this herb has a broad range of therapeutic effects. It has strong anti-inflammatory properties and is a diuretic. *Gymnema sylvestre* can improve arthritis, anemia, osteoporosis, hypercholesterolemia, congestive heart failure, asthma, constipation, microbial infections, and indigestion. It has also been shown to extend the lifespan of diabetic rats. The recommended dose is 200–600 mg daily.

Ginkgo biloba

The ancient Chinese recognized thousands of years ago that ginkgo is beneficial for healthy aging. Extracts of ginkgo are rich in flavonoids and terpenoids, which improve blood flow to the nervous system and brain, and enhance the function of platelet and nerve cells. That's why ginkgo is thought to be beneficial in the prevention and treatment of Alzheimer's disease. Studies also indicate that ginkgo may extend lifespan. The recommended dose of ginkgo varies widely based on the condition it is being used to treat or prevent: If you are taking ginkgo supplements for memory impairment, cardiovascular function, or poor circulation, take 120–240 mg per day in two or three divided doses. If you suffer from tension glaucoma, use 40 mg of ginkgo daily for up to four weeks. For peripheral vascular disease, vertigo, or tinnitus, take no more than 120 mg per day in divided doses. It is important to start out with low doses of 120 mg or less to avoid stomach upset.

Turmeric (Curcuma longa)

The most researched herb in the world, turmeric and its major active ingredient curcumin have an extraordinary array of biological activities, which you learned about in the previous chapter. In addition to the long list of health benefits on pages 115–117, turmeric has been found to slow aging and prolong lifespan, according to numerous studies, including one published in the journal *Age* in 2013. Most experts agree that the health benefits of turmeric are so remarkable that everyone should take it every day. The recommended dose of turmeric is at least 1,000 mg per day.

Ginseng

Both American ginseng (*Panax quinquefolius, L.*) and Asian ginseng (*Panax ginseng*) contain strong anti-inflammatories and antioxidants, and have numerous research-proven health benefits. Just of few of them include improving energy; lowering blood sugar and cholesterol; protecting against the harmful effects of stress; promoting relaxation; and improving cognitive function, diabetes, and sexual dysfunction in men. Ginseng has also been found to have strong anticancer effects. Animal studies show it slows aging and can extend lifespan, too.

A 2013 study evaluated another type of ginseng called "Korean red ginseng" for its anti-aging effects and found it also extends lifespan, increases resistance to starvation stress, and prevents weight gain.

According to *The Complete German Commission E Monographs*, 1–2 grams of the crude preparations of the dried root powder can be taken daily for up to three months. In numerous clinical trials, the dosage of crude root has ranged from 0.5–3 grams per day and the dose of extracts has generally ranged from 100–400 mg.

Putting Them Together: A Simple Convenient Option

There are several products on the market made from a combination of plants with known abilities to slow aging and extend lifespan. For example, research shows that KPG-7, a mixture of extracts from thyme, rosemary, curcumin, fennel, grape seed, silk protein, dandelion, and eleuthero extends lifespan in animals.

Another combination supplement, NucleVital®Q10 Complex, shows strong anti-aging benefits in humans. It contains omega-3 fatty acids (1,350 mg/day), CoQ10 (300 mg/day), astaxanthin (15 mg/day), lycopene (45 mg/day), lutein palmitate (30 mg/day), zeaxanthin palmitate (6 mg/day), l-selenomethionine (330 mg/day), vitamin D3 (30 mcg/day), and alpha-tocopherol (a vitamin E isomer, 45 mg/day). An experimental group of sixty-six healthy volunteer women aged thirty-five to fifty-five were given NucleVital®Q10 Complex for twelve weeks. They were found to have a significant increase in antioxidant and anti-aging markers, including an increase expression of the longevity genes SIRT1 and 2, and a 25 percent increase in the level of the enzyme telomerase, whose job is to preserve telomere length.

Hundreds of studies in the medical literature identify other plants that have the ability to extend lifespan of various animals. Some of these plants and plant compounds were presented in the previous chapter including blueberry, acai, oregano, chlorella, quercetin, *Rhodiola rosea*, cocoa, cinnamon, green tea, resveratrol, olive oil, and pomegranate juice.

Remember that even if you eat a diet high in organically grown fruits and vegetables, you still need a few key supplements to get all the vital nutrients needed for extraordinary health and longevity. Nutritional supplements are not a replacement for nutritious foods, but they can give an added boost of vitamins, minerals, and other nutrients that have been shown to improve your health and longevity. I recommend taking supplemental omega-3 fatty acids and antioxidants at the very least. Depending on your specific health needs and intentions, you can add other supplements. Working with an *Ayurvedic* physician or other holistic physician to determine what supplements are best for you is ideal. But all of the herbs and supplements I presented in this chapter are generally safe for you to try on your own. Don't overdo it—you don't need them all! It's hard on your body to take too many supplements. Also, be sure to only buy supplements of good quality. Some of the companies I recommend are listed in the resource section in the back of this book. You can also check on the quality of specific supplements on the Consumer Lab's website, www.consumerlabs.com.

CHAPTER 6

Medicinal Movement

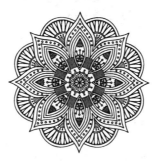

An Elixir for Life

*Those who think they have not time
for bodily exercise, will sooner or later
have to find time for illness.*

~EDWARD STANLEY

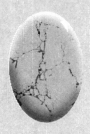

THE SIXTH GEM—TURQUOISE

Turquoise is the sixth gemstone in your breastplate and is a symbol of the extraordinary medicine you can receive from movement. Although it is known to strengthen and align all the chakras, turquoise is most associated with the throat and heart chakras—the center for self-expression and love. When you find an activity that you love and expresses who you are, you will not only gain the physical benefits of exercise, but you will also experience joy and happiness.

The color turquoise is a blend of blue and green, and is cool and calming. It shares many of the same benefits you gain from exercise: It is refreshing, enhances energy, creates emotional balance, is spiritually grounding, and generates joy and tranquility. Like exercise, turquoise is also a master healing stone that can benefit your whole body—emotionally, mentally, and physically.

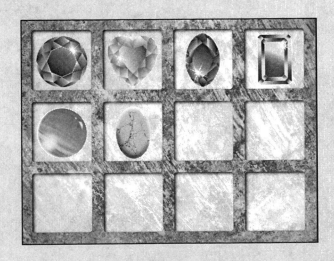

"It is a shame for a man to grow old without seeing the beauty and strength of which his body is capable."

~SOCRATES

t's no secret that regular exercise is essential for good health at every age. But what you may not know is just how powerful keeping fit can be for your health and longevity. The right type of movement, at the right time of day, is an extraordinary elixir for life. It produces a cascade of health-protecting chemicals and hormones that decrease the risk of a multitude of disorders, boosts your mood and appreciation for life, and dramatically slows aging.

Recent research shows that the effects of moving your body—or *not* moving—are more profound than scientists ever imagined. Of all the health practices, regularly exercising seems to have one of the greatest positive impacts. In fact, an extensive review published in December 2010 *International Journal of Clinical Practice* said that apart from not smoking, being physically active is the most powerful lifestyle choice any individual can make to improve his or her health.

Not only can the right type and amount of regular exercise prevent or improve uncomfortable age-related symptoms such as joint pain, sleep problems, and menopausal symptoms, but it also can improve or prevent the most common chronic diseases and add many quality years to your life. The best news yet, it doesn't require a lot of activity to experience tremendous health benefits. In fact, a study published in the *Journal of the American College of Cardiology* in 2014, which followed 55,000 people over fifteen years, found that as little as five minutes a day of jogging at a slow pace lowered the risk of dying from cardiovascular disease by 45 percent!

Fitness and Longevity

Numerous studies show that those who maintain or improve adequate physical fitness reduce their mortality rate considerably—from 29 to 59 percent—compared to those who remain unfit. For example, a 2009 study by Stanford University School of Medicine followed 538 running club members and 423 healthy non-runners who were over fifty years old. After twenty-one years, 34 percent of the non-runners had passed away, while only 15 percent of the club members died during the same period. Those who jogged had fewer deaths from infections, cancers, and heart and neurological diseases.

On the other hand, research shows that low fitness is so detrimental to your health that it reduces your predicted lifespan as much as having diabetes or smoking does! For instance, in a Finnish study published in the *American Journal of Epidemiology* in 1996, sedentary men were almost three times more likely to die of any cause and just under four times more likely to die of cardiovascular disease than the men who were most active.

You were designed to move. If you don't move at all (for instance, if you are bedridden), in very short order your body will begin to break down. If you have ever had your leg or arm in a cast, I'm sure you remembered being shocked at how much smaller and weaker your limb was when the cast was removed.

In general, the more you move—the healthier you will be. Vigorous activity is especially associated with longevity. Yes, it is possible to overexercise. Studies show that running more than 25 miles a week may have detrimental health effects. Marathoners have been found to develop actual damage to their heart muscles causing fibrosis or scarring. However, not exercising enough is a much more significant problem in this country. In fact, an estimated 80 percent of us don't exercise enough.

> *"If we could give every individual the right amount of nourishment and exercise, not too little and not too much, we would have found the safest way to health."*
>
> ~HIPPOCRATES

Ideally, if you want to stack all the odds in your favor of enjoying good health and longevity, you should stay physically fit over your entire lifetime. However, the impact of being fit on your health and longevity is so strong that whenever you decide to get fit, you'll reap tremendous benefits. For instance, in a study published in *JAMA* in 1995, the relationship of changes in physical fitness and all-cause mortality were examined in healthy and unhealthy men. The risk of mortality in those men who had been unfit and then became fit, dropped by 44 percent compared to the men who stayed unfit. In other words, the men who maintained or improved adequate physical fitness were less likely to die during the study from all causes when compared to the men who remained unfit.

In another study, the association of physical activity and mortality was analyzed in postmenopausal women. Those who engaged in regular physical activity were found to have the lowest mortality. If you think that you have to work out strenuously for hours every day to improve your longevity, think again. The study also showed that women who engaged only in moderate activity, such as brisk walking—as little as just *one hour a week*—had a significantly reduced mortality risk.

> *"The sovereign invigorator of the body is exercise,*
> *and of all the exercises walking is the best."*
>
> ~THOMAS JEFFERSON

How Exercise Promotes Longevity

Scientists are now avidly investigating your genes and the effects that various foods and activities, including exercise, have on them. In a study published in 2008 in the *Journal of the American College of Cardiology,* physical exercise was found to lengthen the telomere-regulating proteins in heart muscle. Endurance athletes were found to have the highest amounts of these proteins in their white blood cells and the longest telomere lengths. In another study published in 2009 in the journal *Circulation* exercise was found to increase telomerase—the enzyme that helps to build and preserves your telomere length. Exercise also activates longevity genes called the "sirtuin system" (SIRT). These are the same genes activated by calorie restriction and resveratrol, which were discussed in previous chapters.

Another way that exercise slows aging and improves longevity is by keeping your immune and nervous systems strong. One of the major theories of aging centers on the observation that the function of the immune and nervous systems declines with age, which leads to ill health and eventually death. According to a 2010 study in the journal *Neuroimmunomodulation,* exercise slows aging by improving the function of the immune cells.

In another article published in the *Proceeding of the National Academy of Sciences* in August 2010, exercise was found to also delay aging of the nervous system. According to the researchers, age-related cognitive decline involves deterioration of the "synapses" or the connections between nerve cells; or between nerve cells and the muscles that they control. As nerves age, they shrink in size and lose their connection with muscles. Without stimulation from nerves, muscles begin to shrink and lose much of their volume. Exercise can reverse some of these age-related changes by preventing the loss of volume of nerve cells, which keeps synapses strong and also preserves muscle tone and mass.

More Anti-Aging Effects: Growth Hormone and Stem Cells

Human growth hormone is responsible for many essential functions throughout your life. When you are young, it is required for the growth of your muscles, bones, and collagen. Later in life, it helps to keep your body composition healthier by speeding up fat metabolism, while supporting lean muscle mass. The release of growth hormone is increased by exercise and good-quality sleep. According to a study published in *Sports Medicine* in 2003, resistance training and higher intensity exercise produces the highest amount of growth hormone.

In 2010, researchers from Tel Aviv University Sackler School of Medicine found yet another reason that older people who exercise seem to age more gracefully: Exercise increases the number of muscle stem cells that normally decline with aging. In an animal study, younger mice that ran on a treadmill daily had an average of 20 to 35 percent more stem cells in their muscles. Older rats who exercised reaped an even greater benefit from exercise. Their muscle stem cells increased by 33 to 47 percent.

Healthy and Happy

I'm sure you'll agree that you would only like to live for a long time *if* you are also able to enjoy good health and happiness. Guess what—research shows that moving your body is the most proven and effective way to not only enhance your quality of life, but also your state of happiness. A study published in 2001 by the University of Washington School of Public Health and Community Medicine in Seattle, Washington, found that improved fitness and good nutrition were the key factors contributing to the best quality of life.

Exercise produces a cascade of "feel good" hormones that have been found to be equal to, or even more effective at alleviating depression, than antidepressant drugs. If you are resistant to exercising, you may have simply forgotten how good it feels! Get up from your chair and go for a brisk thirty-minute walk. Then observe what it does to your mood. Chances are you feel significantly better. Just thirty minutes of brisk walking a day can have a profound impact on your health and happiness—and it is free. If you find you can't fit exercise in every day, remember even as little as once a week of participating in invigorating activities can make a difference.

Good for Your Heart

Being physically active is best known for being good for your heart; however, only recently have scientists determined specifically how much exercise is required to make a difference. A 2001 study published in *JAMA* and conducted by Brigham and Women's Hospital in Boston, Massachusetts, not surprisingly found that vigorous activity is associated with a lower risk of cardiovascular disease. But what was unexpected is how little exercise is required to make a significant difference: just one hour a week of moderately paced walking. The researchers found walking one hour a week lowered the risk of cardiovascular disease—even in those who were at high risk because they were overweight, had high cholesterol levels, or were smokers.

Another study from the same institution found that both walking and vigorous exercise caused a similar and substantial reduction in the risk of cardiovascular disease in postmenopausal women. The risk was reduced even further by a more brisk walking pace and fewer hours spent sitting.

A 2008 meta-analysis review study from England found that when it comes to lowering your risk of cardiovascular disease, the pace at which you walk is more important than the distance you cover. For example, walking briskly for a mile lowers your risk by 48 percent, but if you walk slowly for a much longer distance, your risk will lower by only 26 percent.

The Harvard School of Public Health published a study in *JAMA* in 2003 that investigated the effects of different exercise types and intensities on the risk of coronary artery disease (CAD) in men. The researchers found that thirty minutes of brisk walking a day lowered the risk of CAD by 18 percent, weight training for thirty minutes or more per week caused a 23 percent reduction, and running one hour or more per week dropped the risk by 42 percent. As found in the previous study, walking pace had a much greater impact at lowering the risk than did the total time spent walking. According to an earlier study conducted by the same institution and published in the journal *Stroke* in 1998, walking and other moderate-intensity activities also reduces the risk of strokes.

Physical Activity and Diabetes

The incidence of diabetes has doubled in the last twenty years and now affects 25 percent of Americans over the age of sixty-five and is the seventh leading cause of death. Research shows that the risk of this debilitating and deadly disease can be drastically lowered by simply walking at a brisk pace every day. For example, a study published in *Diabetes Care* in 2007 pooled the data from ten prospective studies and found that physical activity of moderate intensity, such as brisk walking, substantially reduces the risk of type 2 diabetes in both men and women.

In 2010, researchers at the University of Michigan discovered one reason why exercise has such a profound protective effect against diabetes. Type 2 diabetes develops as a result of your cells becoming increasingly resistant to the hormone insulin. Glucose—a type of sugar that is used for energy by your cells—can only get into your cells with the help of insulin. When your cells lose much of their ability to use insulin, glucose cannot get into your cells and instead builds up in your blood. Excess glucose sticks to the outside of your cells and eventually converts to a substance called "sorbitol." Sorbitol is extremely damaging to your cells and contributes to many of the terrible complications associated with diabetes, including heart attacks, strokes, blindness, deafness, amputations, brain damage, impotence, and a host of other problems.

The blood test HBA1C measures the amount of glucose, or sugar, coating your red blood cells. If you have diabetes, this test indicates how severe your disease is and how high your risk is of developing complications. A study from the University of Calgary published in the September 2007 issue of the *Annuals of Internal Medicine* found that both aerobic exercise and strength training lower HBA1C by 0.5 percent in diabetics. For those study participants who did both types of exercise, HBA1C levels went down by 1 percent. That does not sound like much, but a 1 percent drop of HBA1C is associated with a 20 percent decrease in the risk of heart attacks and strokes, and a 25 to 40 percent decrease in the risk of diabetes-related eye and kidney disease.

Exercise not only helps to lower your blood sugar levels while you engage in it, but also for a few hours afterward. According to a study published in the *Journal of Applied Physiology* in February 2010, when your muscles contract during exercise, they remove sugar rapidly from your bloodstream without the need of insulin and continue to do so for an additional hour. Another study published in the *American Journal of Clinical Nutrition* in 2008 found that these effects actually continue to taper off for seventeen hours after you finish exercising!

If you exercise in the morning on an empty stomach, you will reap more benefits than if you eat first and exercise later. Three different studies published in the *Journal of Physiology* by Belgium researchers found that exercising before eating in the morning causes the greatest improvement in fat-burning and insulin sensitivity.

Moving Protects Against Neurological Diseases

The National Institute on Aging published a study in 2008, which found that exercise is extremely beneficial for your brain. It improves learning and memory, and prevents or delays the loss of cognitive function and the development of neurodegenerative diseases. The researchers also found that omega-3 fatty acids enhance the neuroprotective effects of exercise. Another study published in 2009 found that the more exercise you do, the lower your risk is of common degenerative neurological diseases, including Alzheimer's disease and other forms of dementia, as well as Parkinson's disease.

There are two specific ways that engaging in invigorating movement protects your nervous system. First, exercise increases the production of a protein called "brain-derived neurotrophic factor" (BDNF), which encourages the growth of neurons and protects, strengthens, and improves their function. Secondly, moving your body causes the blood flow to your brain to increase. Better circulation delays the accumulation of plaques in your brain that can increase your risk of Alzheimer's disease.

Exercise and Academic Performance

If you want your grades to go up, instead of studying more, you might want to consider going for a hike. According to many studies, exercise improves academic performance. For example, a study published in the August 2006 issue of *Medicine & Science in Sport & Exercise* randomly assigned physical education classes to 214 sixth-grade students. Moderate to vigorous activity outside of school was assessed as well. The students who either performed some vigorous activity or met the Healthy People 2010 guidelines for activity had significantly higher grades than students who performed no vigorous activity. Moderate physical activity did not affect grades.

High school students who are interested in improving their test scores might also want to consider chewing gum in their classroom. The teacher might object, but a study presented at the American Society for Nutrition (ASN) Scientific Sessions and Annual Meeting at Experimental Biology in 2009 by Baylor College of Medicine found that "mouth exercises"—chewing gum—in classrooms can boost the academic performance of teenagers. The study examined whether chewing Wrigley sugar-free gum can lead to better academic performance in a "real life" classroom setting. The researchers found that the gum-chewing students had a 3 percent increase in their standardized math test scores, and their final grades were significantly better than those who didn't chew gum.

To achieve the best health and academic performance, regular vigorous aerobic exercise is required—not just gum chewing. Sorry, but gum chewing is not a vigorous aerobic activity—no matter how fast you chew! Research shows the reason gum chewing may help one's grades has nothing to do with aerobic exercise. Rather, it helps to reduce stress, improve alertness, and relieve anxiety—all of which are associated with better test scores.

Physical Activity and Cancer Risk

Staying physically fit can lower your risk of many of the most commonly diagnosed cancers, including cancers of the breast, prostate, colon, and lung. A Canadian study published in 2002 reviewed 170 studies of physical activity and cancer risk. The researcher found strong evidence that physical activity significantly reduced the risk of breast and colon cancers. There was a smaller, but still significant, protective effect against cancers of the prostate, lung, and endometrial cancers associated with staying active.

Another review study by Brigham and Women's Hospital and Harvard Medical School added that active people have a 30 to 40 percent reduction of colon cancer and a 20 to 30 percent decreased risk of breast cancer compared to inactive people. It appears that thirty to sixty minutes of moderate to vigorous intensity physical activity every day is needed to decrease the risk.

Exercise has a number of positive effects that help to protect you from these cancers, including:

- Reducing your body fat and preventing obesity
- Cooling inflammation
- Balancing your hormones
- Improving insulin resistance
- Supporting your immune system
- Activating tumor suppression genes

If you have been diagnosed with cancer, research shows that staying physically active, especially during your treatments, can significantly improve your chances of survival. A 2005 study published in *JAMA* by Brigham and Women's Hospital and Harvard Medical School found that if you are diagnosed with breast cancer and exercise during your treatment, your chances of surviving are twice as high. Just walking at a moderate pace for an average of three to five hours a week can make a significant difference.

Researchers at the Harvard Public School of Health found that vigorous activity also improves survival from prostate cancer. In their study published in the *Journal of Clinical Oncology,* 2,705 men diagnosed with prostate cancer were followed for eighteen years. The researchers found that those who engaged in regular vigorous activity had the lowest risk of dying from prostate cancer—in fact, 61 percent lower. However, both non-vigorous and vigorous activities were found to be beneficial for overall survival. Simply walking at a normal or brisk pace for ninety minutes or more a week lowered the risk of dying from any cause by 46 percent.

Exercise, according to numerous other studies, also has a positive influence on other aspects of the cancer experience, including cancer detection, quality of life, and recovery.

Exercise and the Immune System

If you want to keep your immune system strong, moving your body is essential—but not too much. A study published in the *British Journal of Sports Medicine* in 2010 found that moderate exercise, such as brisk walking just a few times every week, improves your immune system so greatly that your risk of getting a cold is significantly reduced. Whereas, overexercising or exercising too little can weaken your immune system and increase your risk of colds and the flu.

How Much Should You Do?

You might be wondering what types of exercises are best and how much you should do of them to achieve the best state of health. Numerous studies have focused on answering these questions. As you are aware, studies have found that you don't have to engage in a lot of strenuous activity to gain tremendous health benefits. Simply brisk walking for as little as five to ten minutes a day can dramatically improve your cardiovascular health and longevity. However, the American Heart Association stresses that a minimum of thirty minutes a day of aerobic exercise, five times a week, should still be your goal. A 2004 study conducted by the Cooper Institute in Dallas, Texas, concluded that if you did more than thirty minutes of moderate intensity exercise per day, your health benefits would be even greater.

If fitting thirty minutes or more of exercise in a day is tough for you, recent research shows that just twenty minutes a day may be enough. According to a study published in the March 15, 2010, issue of the *Journal of Physiology*, working out for just twenty minutes a day of "high intensity interval" training—short bursts of exercise with rest periods between—may provide the same, or even better, benefits than workouts done in a conventional "long-duration" slower steady-paced style.

Several studies show that high-intensity interval exercise is actually superior to long continuous exercise, such as jogging, brisk walking, or biking, because it burns more fat. For example, one study measured the amount of fat loss in women who exercised twenty minutes, alternating eight-second sprinting on a bike with twelve seconds of exercising lightly. They then compared these women to women who exercised at a regular pace for forty minutes. After exercising three times a week for fifteen weeks, those who did the twenty-minute alternating routine lost three times as much fat as those who exercised twice as long at a regular pace.

Researchers believe the reason interval training causes you to burn more fat is because it causes the release of high amounts of hormones, called "catecholamines." The catecholamine hormones include dopamine, norepinephrine, and epinephrine (or adrenaline)—all three enhance the ability of your body to use fat for fuel.

They are produced by your adrenal glands, which are found on top of the kidneys, and are released into your bloodstream whenever you are under physical or emotional stress. Emotional stress, however, also causes the release of cortisol, which has the opposite effect and encourages belly fat. So keep your emotional stress to a minimum and focus on raising your fat-burning catecholamines with high-intensity interval exercise.

High-intensity exercise causes the release of another beneficial hormone, called "growth hormone" (GH). Growth hormone has many anti-aging effects, including promoting bone density and improving your body composition by not only burning fat, but also by enhancing your muscle tone. You can maximize the fat-burning effects of this type of exercise by helping your GH levels to stay up for several hours after training. The trick to keeping your GH up is to eat only lean protein or to fast for two hours after your workout. If you consume sugar during this time, the production of GH will shut off along with all of its health benefits.

Consuming sugar right after you exercise—for instance, a high-carbohydrate drink, candy bar, or anything with refined sugar—causes your blood glucose levels to spike. In response, your pancreas sends out a blast of insulin. Insulin causes a rise in another hormone called "somatostatin," which also shuts down the production of the growth hormone released by exercise. In other words, if you eat or drink refined carbohydrates within two hours after working out, both the sugar and somatostatin put a lid on growth hormone and wipe out many of the health benefits you could have received.

In addition to aerobic exercise, resistance training and stretching at least twice a week are also important for your overall health and quality of life. These activities help you to maintain lean body mass, improve your muscular strength and endurance, and preserve the function and flexibility of your body.

> *"Too many people confine their exercise to jumping to conclusions, running up bills, stretching the truth, bending over backward, lying down on the job, sidestepping responsibility and pushing their luck."*
>
> ~AUTHOR UNKNOWN

Ancient *Ayurvedic* Wisdom

To achieve extraordinary health and longevity, *Ayurveda* recommends that you engage in the "right" type and amount of "medicinal movements" every day. Either too little or too much exercise can cause detrimental effects. For instance, too much of the wrong kind of exercise for your body type puts a strain on your body and can cause injuries and imbalances that increase you risk of disease. Putting too much force into invigorating activities causes the release of oxygen free radicals, which accelerate aging, weaken your immune system, and promote chronic diseases. Extremely heavy exercise may make your muscles stronger, but it can weaken the overall health of your body.

Ayurvedic Exercise Recommendations

1. **Exercise to 50 percent of your capacity.** For example, if the most weight you can benchpress is 50 pounds for ten reps, do five reps instead. If you

follow this advice, you'll never overstrain your body and will gradually become stronger. You'll be able to exercise every day and won't need to take days off to recover. Moving your body will cause you to feel exhilarated and energized, rather than drained.

2. **Don't strain when your exercise.** Cut back if you start to breathe heavily through your mouth. Research shows that overexercising can actually be detrimental to your health. It depresses your immune system and increases the production of oxygen free radicals. So it's important not to stress yourself too much during exercise. Just like medications, herbs, foods, or anything else that's good for your health, there's a proper amount to take; too much or too little can create imbalances that lead to disease.

3. **Exercise in the morning before 10 a.m.** Different types of energy govern different times of the day. Between 6:00 a.m. and 10:00 a.m. is *kapha* time when your energy tends to be settled and slow. If you exercise during this time, you wash away any sluggishness and charge yourself with energy all day. Incidentally, waking up in *kapha* time can make you feel lethargic for the rest of the day. That's why *Ayurveda* recommends waking up before 6:00 a.m. during *vata* time.

   Between 10:00 a.m. and 2:00 p.m. is *pitta* time. *Pitta* is associated with heat and digestion, and, therefore, *pitta* time is considered the worst time to exercise. When the sun is at its zenith, you can easily become overheated by exercise. This is also the time of day when your digestion is at its peak. Therefore, you should eat your largest meal of the day between 10 a.m. and 2 p.m., and avoid exercise.

   Between 2:00 p.m. and 6:00 p.m. is *vata* time. As you may remember, *Vata* governs movement, so this is an acceptable time to exercise, although the *kapha* morning time is considered best. The cycles then repeat. *Kapha* time is from 6:00 p.m. until 10:00 p.m. Only light exercise, such as walking, is recommended during this time, because you should use this time to slow down and get ready to go to sleep. Vigorous activity during these hours is too stimulating and may cause you to have difficulty falling asleep.

4. **Perform special movements to facilitate the union of your mind/body and breath.** In addition to regular exercise, *Ayurveda* recommends that

you begin your morning with yoga, too. Yoga actually got its start in *Ayurveda*. The word "yoga" means union. The purpose of the exercises is to bring union to the mind and body, create balance, and enhance your body's inner healing intelligence. Yoga also helps to increase and maintain flexibility even as you age. In addition, yoga has been found to reduce anxiety, fatigue, tension, and stress and to improve mental function. Specific poses are prescribed to help restore balance for disease conditions. For example, inversion poses improve blood flow to the neck and can help to restore balance to the thyroid gland.

A Japanese study published in June 2000 in the journal *Perceptual and Motor Skills* examined brainwave activity, as well as the level of the stress hormone cortisol in yoga instructors during their practice of yoga. Researchers found a predominance of alpha brainwaves, which correspond to a state of restful alertness also experienced during the practice of Transcendental Meditation (TM). In addition, researchers found that yoga caused the stress hormone cortisol to decrease.

5. **If you meditate, practice yoga before meditation and participate in conventional exercise afterward.** Yoga helps to center and relax your body and mind and prepare it for meditation. On the other hand, stimulating exercise activates the body and the mind—the opposite of the effect required to foster meditation.

6. **Choose movements that are right for your type.** *Ayurveda* recognizes that each of us is different. Different activities are recommended depending on your body type. Just as there are *vata*, *pitta*, and *kapha* times of the day, there are *vata*, *pitta*, and *kapha* types of people.

Vata people are thin and prone to anxiety and nervousness; they frequently experience the sensation of being cold and they operate on high speed. If this is you, slow-paced light exercises such as swimming, walking, and yoga are recommended.

If you have a medium build, usually feel hot, have a quick temper, and sharp intelligence, you are a *pitta* type. Moderate exercise such as brisk walking, cross-country skiing, swimming, cycling, weightlifting, and tennis are best for you.

If you have a tendency to be overweight and are easygoing and reliable—but, possibly, also a little lazy—you are a *kapha* type. You need to get up and get moving as much as possible. Vigorous exercise, such as jogging, more intense weight lifting, and aerobics are excellent for you.

7. **Wait at least two hours after a full meal to exercise.** It takes two hours for your stomach to empty after a full meal. During this time, blood flow is increased to the digestive tract to facilitate digestion. If you exercise too soon after eating a full meal, you will divert the blood flow from your digestive tract to your muscles and impede the digestive process.

8. **Wait at least thirty minutes after you exercise before you eat.** When you exercise, blood flow increases to your muscles and is shunted away from your digestive tract. Therefore, if you eat while exercising, or too soon afterward, there won't be enough blood available for your digestive tract to function properly. Not only can it decrease the absorption of nutrients, but it can also cause uncomfortable symptoms such as indigestion and cramping. After about thirty minutes of rest, your muscles no longer need additional blood so your digestive tract can get all the blood it needs without any interference.

The Peril of Sitting Too Much

No matter how much you exercise, it is important to not sit too much! A 2013 study published in the *International Journal of Behavioral Nutrition and Physical Activity* found that compared to those who sit fewer than four hours a day, those who sit more than four hours a day are significantly more likely to have a chronic disease, including cancer, diabetes, heart disease, and high blood pressure. The University of Sydney, Sydney School of Public Health followed 200,000 adults ages forty-five and older for three years. Those who sat eleven hours or more a day were 40 percent more likely to die during the study than people who sat fewer than four hours.

In another study published in the journal *Cancer Epidemiology, Biomarkers & Prevention,* in 2015 women who spent the most time sitting were found to have a 10 percent higher risk of cancers of the breast, ovary, and blood (multiple myeloma).

10 TIPS TO KEEP MOVING

Ideally you want to stay in motion as much as possible during each day. Here are ten tips that can help you get enough exercise in every day even if you don't think you have the time:

1. If you work at a desk, get up every thirty minutes and move.

2. Park your car in the spot that is furthest away from your destination.

3. Take the stairs whenever you can.

4. Don't aim to exercise; play a sport instead.

5. Find an exercise buddy.

6. Chose a variety of activities to keep you from getting bored—for example, tennis, dancing, classes at the gym, biking, hiking, or brisk walking.

7 Use a pedometer to make sure you are getting the recommended 10,000 steps a day.

8. Don't sit to watch TV—walk on a treadmill or do stretching exercises instead.

9. Stand up or walk when you talk on the telephone—don't stayed glued to your chair.

10. Dance! In a ballroom or in your living room, it's a great way to have fun while burning calories.

Finding Your Own Movement

If you have never experienced a form of movement that expresses your soul, keep looking; you'll find it. You were designed to enjoy moving with vigor and dynamism. Nature created special neuropeptides to reward you with bliss when you dance and move to the individual expression of your soul. These magical molecules of movement create a feeling of exhilaration and make you naturally high on life.

There are so many different ways to express yourself in movement. No matter what your personal preferences are, or what physical condition you are in, you can find something that resonates with you. Consider biking, jogging, or brisk walking; you can do these activities solo or with a friend. If you like to have company when you exercise, find a partner for a two-person sport such as tennis, racquetball, or one-on-one basketball. Or you may simply want to find a buddy to work out with at the gym. If you discover that you enjoy working out at a gym, but need a more structured format to keep you motivated, make a series of appointments with a personal trainer. Last, if you like to be part of a group that meets regularly, then it would be a great idea to take an exercise class. You can find a class for just about anything: aerobics, cycling, kickboxing, martial arts, dancing, rowing—you name it.

Even if you are obese and haven't exercised in years, it's never too late to start. However, be sure to speak with your doctor before you begin any exercise program. Walking is a great activity for just about anyone who wants to begin exercising. Each day, choose a destination that's a little farther away or simply pick up the pace at which you walk. Beginner's yoga is another good starting point. Try different activities to find the ones that are fun for you and suit you best.

CHAPTER 7

Ambrosias of the Night

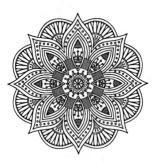

The Healing Tonic of Sleep

A good laugh and a long sleep
are the best cures in the doctor's book.

~IRISH PROVERB

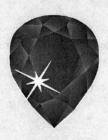

THE SEVENTH GEM—BLACK ONYX

The profound balancing, restorative, and rejuvenating effects of optimal sleep are represented by black onyx—the seventh gemstone in your breastplate.

The color black symbolizes the night—the ideal time for sleep. It also reminds you to keep your room as dark as possible to enhance your sleep hormone, melatonin. Black also represents mystery and the unknown. When you sleep, you experience all sorts of mysterious states of consciousness without being aware of them. Completely unknown to you during the night, your body produces a miraculous cascade of biological processes that purify and rejuvenate you.

Onyx is said to encourage happiness and good fortune. It is thought to protect you from negative energy by absorbing it, while at the same time helping you to take in all the energies you need from the universe —also some of the profound benefits of a good night's rest. Additionally, onyx further enhances your sleep by reducing stress.

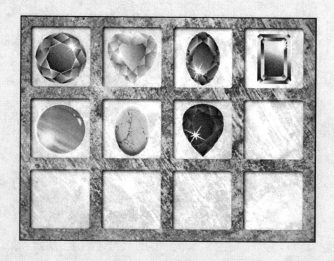

hink about a time when you found yourself yawning in the early evening. Instead of fighting your fatigue, you decided to surrender to your body's desire for rest. Just after dusk, you melted into your bed and drifted into a peaceful rejuvenating night of sleep. The next morning, you awoke before dawn feeling fresh and unusually full of energy and optimism. When you looked in the mirror, the youthful and radiant face looking back at you took you by surprise. That radiant glow—the gift of luxurious sleep—is the end result of a multitude of biological processes designed by Nature to keep you healthy. When you follow the laws of Nature, these are the results you can expect to achieve.

It's a timeless *Ayurvedic* principle that *proper sleep and rest are fundamental to health and longevity. Activity must be balanced with rest.* Modern science couldn't agree more. Research confirms that the right amount of sleep and rest, at the right times, are of supreme importance when it comes to supporting your health, strength, vitality, and beauty. What could be a bigger gift from Nature than knowing that one of the most important keys to your good health and radiant beauty requires you to do nothing but rest.

> *"Sleep is that golden chain that ties health*
> *and our bodies together."*
>
> ~THOMAS DEKKER

The Medicine of Melatonin

When we sleep, the body repairs and purifies itself. The process is stimulated through the release of critically important hormones that are essential for maintaining health and promoting longevity. One of the hormones of greatest significance is *melatonin*—our "sleep" hormone. Melatonin is also referred to as the "hormone of darkness" because when darkness falls, the pineal gland in your brain increases its production of melatonin.

As the level of this hormone rises, you start to feel sleepy. The moment you fall asleep, its flow intensifies. If you go to bed around 10 p.m., the unimpeded current of melatonin surges forth. It flows faster and faster as you sleep until it becomes a raging river of healing ambrosia, cresting around midnight to 1 a.m. This spike in melatonin is crucial for good

171

health. If you consistently stay up late, you stunt its surge; instead the melatonin river barely rises—the consequences of this drought can be broad and
destructive.

Not Just a Sleep Hormone

Melatonin is not just our "sleep" hormone. It has many other functions,
one of the most notable being that it is a very potent antioxidant. Antioxidants, as you know, are powerful defenders against the attack of oxygen
free radicals, which can damage your DNA and increase your risk of cancer,
fuel chronic degenerative diseases, and accelerate aging.

Melatonin has numerous crafty ways that it deters the growth of certain
cancers. For example, it lowers the risk of breast cancer by slowing down
the production of estrogen in your body, preventing its overproduction, and
suppressing its stimulatory effect on breast cells. It also blocks two other
threats that can increase cell division in the breast—the hormone prolactin
and the growth factor known as "epidermal growth factor." In addition,
melatonin enhances the tumor-fighting power of vitamin D, causing it to
be twenty to a hundred times stronger. Moreover, it gives a major boost to
the immune system, which helps to protect you from foreign invaders such
as bacteria, viruses, and cancer cells.

This multitasking hormone is great for your brain, too. Researchers at
the University of Illinois found that it is important for learning and memory. It may also help reduce the risk of Alzheimer's disease by deterring the
aggregation of abnormal proteins called "amyloid beta" that are a hallmark
of the disease and by preventing the death of neurons or brain cells.

Melatonin supplementation has been shown to be beneficial for
menopausal women in three different ways: it improves thyroid function,
helps to restore fertility, and prevents depression. Melatonin is also effective
at improving another type of depression called "seasonal affective disorder,"
which is caused by the lack of light in wintertime.

If you suffer from migraine headaches, you'll be happy to know that melatonin has also been shown to be useful in their prevention and treatment.

Melatonin may also help you if you occasionally have discomfort due
to gallbladder issues. Several studies show that it helps to reduce the formation of gallstones.

According to a study published in 2000 in the journal *Endocrinology,* melatonin is involved in energy metabolism, and when it is given as a daily supplement, it helps to reduce body weight and abdominal fat in middle-aged animals. But before you run out to buy melatonin supplements to help you reduce your middle, be aware that scientists don't know if melatonin is helpful in fighting obesity in human beings, because clinical trials have not yet been done.

With our attention recently drawn to the real and dangerous health consequences of radioactive fallout after the meltdown of the reactors at the Fukushima Daiichi Nuclear Power Plant in Japan, you may think that realistically there is little you can do to shield yourself. However, both animal and several human studies conducted by the University of Texas Health Science Center in San Antonio show that melatonin is potentially very protective against ionizing radiation. Most of the damage from ionizing radiation is believed to be due to oxygen free radicals. Researchers credit melatonin's major radioprotective effects to its powerful antioxidant capacity.

Lastly, melatonin shows significant anti-aging properties. Studies have found that it plays a noteworthy part in the aging process and that taking supplemental melatonin may slow and even reverse some of the changes. For instance, an animal study conducted by the University of California, Irvine, found twenty-five genes that substantially change with age—nine of which code for inflammation. When older animals were given supplemental melatonin for eight weeks, thirteen of the twenty-five genes that alter with age were found to revert back to their more youthful form, or in scientific terms, a more "youthful expression." Another animal study found that because melatonin counteracts oxidative damage and reduces inflammation, it slows down some of the damage to your nervous system caused by the normal wear and tear associated with aging. In this study, melatonin also improved longevity.

On the other hand, if natural melatonin levels are chronically low, due to too many late nights or a variety of other factors discussed in the next section, research shows it significantly increases your risk of poor health and accelerates aging. Specifically, it increases your risk of obesity and many common chronic diseases, especially high blood pressure, heart disease, diabetes, and cancers of the breast, prostate, and colon.

Other Factors That Disrupt Melatonin Production

There are many other factors that can suppress your melatonin levels. A study published in October 2001 in the *American Journal of Epidemiology* found that light, being overweight, consuming alcohol, and taking certain medications can dampen melatonin. The melatonin-disrupting medications include two classes of heart medications: beta-blockers and calcium channel blockers; and specific types of psychiatric drugs that alter mood or behavior.

Of all these factors, light seems to have the most influence on melatonin. Just like Count Dracula, melatonin is nocturnal and shuns the light. The more light in the environment, the lower the production of melatonin is. Conversely, the darker the environment, the more melatonin levels rise. Even though you don't consciously *see* when you sleep, your eyes still perceive light. Any light at night—a soft nightlight or the numbers on an electric clock—can inhibit your melatonin levels from rising to their full potential. Researchers believe one of the major reasons why cancer rates are higher in cities is due to the melatonin-suppressing effects of the bright lights that flood the night skies

When it comes to alcohol and melatonin levels, one glass of wine appears to be okay, but if you indulge in more than one, it will restrict its flow. In a study from the University of Connecticut, published in *Epidemiology* in November 2000, researchers found that the more alcohol a woman consumed in a twenty-four-hour period, the lower her melatonin level was. One alcoholic drink didn't have any effect, but two drinks caused a 9 percent reduction in melatonin, and three drinks dropped it by 15 percent.

Electromagnetic frequencies emitted from electrical devices—even seemingly small amounts like those created by the wires and appliances in your home—can also disturb your melatonin levels. Researchers have found that residential 60-HZ magnetic fields caused by normal electrical wiring in the home and equipment (such as clock radios, electric blankets, and televisions) depress melatonin. That's why it is recommended to keep all electrical devices far away from where you sleep. Shut off your cell phone, Wi-Fi, and any other electrical devices in or near the room where you sleep. Use a battery-operated alarm clock instead of an electrically powered clock radio.

Not Too Little—Not Too Much

As a general rule in life, either too much indulgence or too much restriction of virtually anything that is considered "good"—even essential—for life usually leads to problems. Whereas, temperance is usually the ideal choice: the middle way, or the amount that Goldilocks so wisely exclaimed was not too big and not too small, but "just right." Sleep is a perfect example.

Sleeping too few hours, or sleeping too many hours, can have a serious negative impact on your health. These less than optimal sleeping times are associated with premature aging, increased mortality, and a higher incidence of diseases including diabetes, obesity, high blood pressure, cardiovascular disease, and cancer. The magic number of hours for sleep appears to be seven to eight hours. In a study published in the journal *Sleep* in August 2010 and conducted by researchers at the West Virginia University's faculty of medicine, study participants who slept fewer than five hours a day, including naps, had more than double the risk of angina, coronary artery disease, heart attacks, and strokes. Those who slept more than seven hours also had an increased risk of cardiovascular disease. The participates who slept nine hours or longer were one-and-a-half times more likely than seven-hour sleepers to develop the disease.

A review study published in the *Journal of Sleep Research* in 2009, which looked at the associations between sleep duration and all-cause and cause-specific mortality, found a statistically significant increase in all-cause mortality, especially of cardiovascular disease and cancer in those who slept either too many or too few hours. In another study conducted by the University of California, San Diego, and published in 2002, researchers found a 15 percent increased risk of mortality in those who slept more than eight and a half hours or less than four and a half hours.

If you want your brain firing on all cylinders, getting the proper amount of sleep is essential. The Whitehall II study enrolled 1,459 women and 3,972 men ages forty-five to sixty-nine and then followed them for an average of just over five years. At the beginning of the study and then again five years later at the end of the study, participants reported how many hours of sleep they got on an average weeknight. They also took cognitive-function tests on both occasions. Those who either fell short of the recommended six to eight hours of sleep or who got more than eight hours had the lowest scores. In fact, both the short sleepers and the long sleepers had scores that were on a par to someone many years older.

"Even where sleep is concerned, too much is a bad thing."

~HOMER

Too Little Is Too Big of a Problem

How big of a problem is disrupted sleep in America? According to a study published in 2006, 50 to 70 million Americans chronically suffer from sleep disorders that hinder daily functioning and adversely affect health and longevity. The National Sleep Foundation conducted a poll of Americans and the majority (63%) said they do not get the recommended seven to eight hours of sleep. Nearly one-third (31%) reported sleeping less than seven hours a night. One in five adults stated that they were so sleepy during the day that it interfered with their daily activities. Seven in ten adults (69%) said they experience frequent sleep problems.

Chronic Disease and Accelerated Aging

A Harvard University study published in 2010 followed 56,000 American adults and found that sleeping fewer than seven hours a night increases the risk of obesity, diabetes, high blood pressure, and heart disease. Another study published in the journal *Lancet* in October 1999 found several biological signs of "accelerated" aging in healthy young men after they slept only four hours per night for one week. Those signs included changes in their glucose and stress hormone (cortisol) levels to that which is typically seen in middle age. According to the researchers, the physiological changes observed in the sleep-deprived young men could predispose them to diabetes, high blood pressure, obesity, and memory loss.

Reaction Times and Mental Functions

Sleep deprivation hinders you both mentally and physically. It interferes with perception, vision, speech, reaction times, athletic performance, and the ability to concentrate and learn. It also results in poor memory and clouded thinking, which can lead to wrong decisions. A study published in 2009 from the Sleep Disorder Center at the University of Michigan found that sleep problems in children caused a wide range of behavioral, cognitive, and mood impairments, including hyperactivity, slow learning, lower school grades, and depression. David Dinges, Ph.D., from the University of Pennsylvania found that sleeping six hours or less a night for two weeks had the same negative effect on attention span and reaction times as two nights of total sleep deprivation.

With all the mental and physical impairments associated with the fatigue from less than optimal sleep, it's not surprising that the risk of on-the-job errors and accidents is much higher in tired workers. Worker fatigue is credited for such major accidents as the Chernobyl nuclear meltdown and the Exxon Valdez oil spill. Research shows that 60 percent of road accidents are caused by fatigue due to lack of sleep.

In a Polish study published in 2010, test subjects who stayed awake continuously for twenty to twenty-five hours were found to have impaired performance comparable to being legally drunk. In another study, drivers who stayed awake for more than seventeen hours had significantly impaired coordination, reaction time, and judgment. Even more frightening, these sleep-deprived drivers were found to be *more* severely impaired than drivers who are legally drunk!

Emotional Disturbances

If you are not getting enough shut-eye, there's a good chance you might feel a bit down in the dumps or out of sorts. Emotional disturbances such as poor relationship skills, depression, anxiety, and increased aggressiveness are common symptoms of chronic poor sleep. For example, a study from the University of Arkansas, published in September 2010, tested the effects of sleep deprivation on eighty-eight physically and psychologically healthy adults. The researchers found that the subjects reported general distress with an increase in anxiety and depression.

Insomnia often precedes the onset of a mood disorder, especially depression. According to a Canadian study from the Department of Psychiatry at the University of British Columbia, Vancouver, BC, in 2008, the association between sleep disturbances and depression has long been recognized. The researchers stated that early recognition and treatment of sleep disturbances may therefore be important for the treatment and prevention of recurrent depression.

Immune and Hormonal Responses

Poor sleep also has a serious deleterious effect on your hormones and immune system. German researchers found that hormones produced by the pituitary gland (prolactin and growth hormone) and adrenal glands (cortisol) are profoundly regulated by sleep. These hormones are also known to be involved in the regulation of the immune response. Researchers at the Pennsylvania State University College of Medicine discovered that cortisol levels and IL-6 (a pro-inflammatory cytokine) increase with nocturnal wake time and daytime sleepiness. In other words, if you often stay up late at night, your body will have a stress response and produce inflammation—both of which contribute to every type of chronic disorder and accelerate aging.

Sleep deprivation weakens your immune system in another way—it decreases the number of circulating immune cells, particularly natural killer cells. These cells have the important role of seeking out and destroying foreign invaders, such as bacteria and cancer cells. Your immune system appears to need at least seven hours to adequately recharge. According to a 2009 study published in the *Archives of Internal Medicine,* people who sleep fewer than seven hours a night are three times more likely to develop respiratory infections than those who sleep eight hours.

Obesity and Diabetes

According to a study published in 2007 from the University of Chicago, one contributing factor to the ever-growing obesity and diabetes epidemics may be that too many of us are not getting enough sleep. In this investigation, healthy young volunteers were experimentally sleep deprived—all of them complained of increased hunger. Blood samples showed that the increased hunger they experienced was caused by a drop in the hormone leptin (which is responsible for decreasing hunger) and a rise in the hormone ghrelin (which causes hunger to increase). Because the sleep-deprived subjects were hungry, they ate more—especially at night—and took in more daily calories than needed. Their glucose sensitivity also became worse, which is an early warning sign of type 2 diabetes.

British researchers conducted a meta-analysis of studies from around the world regarding the relationship between short sleep duration and obesity. They found a consistent increased risk of obesity among short sleepers in both children and adults. Finally, a study by Columbia University researchers found that people between the ages of thirty-two and fifty-nine, who slept only four hours, were 73 percent more likely to become obese than those who slept seven to nine hours. Even shaving off one valuable hour a night made a significant difference, because those who slept six hours a night were 23 percent more likely to be become obese.

If you are trying to lose weight, cutting your sleep short can sabotage your efforts. A 2010 study from the University of Chicago reported that overweight adults on a moderate diet who slept eight and a half hours a night lost 56 percent more body fat than those who slept only five and a half hours. Just one night of sleep deprivation can wreak havoc with your metabolism, according to a 2011 study published in the *American Journal of Clinical Nutrition*. This study found that just one shortened night of sleep acutely reduced the energy expenditure in healthy men by decreasing their metabolic rate and the number of calories that they burned.

Catch-up Sleep

There is good news for those who tend to be chronically sleep deprived during the work week. Several studies show that you can "catch up" a bit on your sleep. In other words, if you sleep less than the ideal seven to eight hours during the work week, but sleep in on the weekend—for example, you sleep ten hours a night on Friday and Saturday—you can "reset" your physiological markers. In a study conducted by David Dinges, Ph.D., who heads the sleep and chronobiology unit at the University of Pennsylvania School of Medicine, those subjects who were sleep deprived during the week had slower reaction times and more difficulty focusing. But, if they had an additional hour or two of sleep over the weekend, their alertness improved. Likewise in a 1999 study, young men who were sleep-deprived for one week turned their accelerated age-clock back to their right age after twelve hours in bed for several nights. But, since older people or those who are chronically sleep-deprived were not included in the study, it is unknown if these individuals can recover like the young men did.

A follow-up study published in the journal *Sleep* by the same researchers at the University of Pennsylvania found that a night of ten hours of recovery sleep greatly improved test scores, but it was not enough to make up for the lost sleep. In this study, 142 adults with severely restricted sleep—just four hours of sleep from 4 a.m. to 8 a.m.—were given a series of tests every two hours after awakening. Not surprisingly, the sleep-deprived individuals suffered slower reaction times and had more trouble focusing. The volunteers still scored poorly on attention span and reaction times after one ten-hour night of sleep. Several nights of extra sleep were required to make up for the severe sleep deficit and return test scores back to normal.

SLEEPY OR NOT?

A number of studies show that after chronic sleep deprivation, the area of our brains that controls our circadian rhythms—a portion of the hypothalamus—gets so disrupted that we no longer recognize how "sleepy" we are. Subjects who were sleep-deprived believed that they felt reasonably "normal"; however, when they were tested for performance, their scores were poor. Being unaware that you are sleep-deprived is somewhat similar to the state of consciousness you experience when you unaware that you are impaired from having had a bit too much to drink.

Sleeping at the Right Times

As important as the number of hours you sleep is to your health and longevity, the *exact times* that you go to sleep and wake up is equally important. Staying up late even if you get seven or eight hours of sleep, or working the night shift, has a significant deleterious effect on various hormone levels and inflammatory markers. Sleeping at the "wrong" times increases your risk of the same chronic diseases associated with sleeping too few hours: Diabetes, obesity, cardiovascular disease, gastrointestinal disorders, depression, and cancer—especially breast, prostate, endometrial, and colorectal cancers. For example, a study published in the journal *Cell Metabolism* in August 2010 found that staying up until 2 a.m. upset the body's internal clock and caused triglycerides, fatty acids in the blood, to become abnormally high. High triglycerides are known to increase the risk of heart disease.

In another study, researchers at the University of Texas Health Science Center at San Antonia, Texas, reported that epidemiological studies find an increase of breast, prostate, endometrial, and colon cancers in individuals who work at night or whose circadian rhythms had been disrupted for other reasons. Disruption of the normal circadian rhythms has also been associated with poor pregnancy outcomes. In contrast, going to bed before 10 p.m. and getting up by 6 a.m. can reduce your risk of all of these conditions by as much as 50 percent.

> *"And if tonight my soul may find her peace in sleep,*
> *and sink in good oblivion, and in the morning wake*
> *like a new-opened flower then I have been dipped*
> *again in God, and new-created."*
>
> ~D. H. LAWRENCE

Getting a Good Night's Sleep

Of all the thousands of natural laws governing your health, there are three that *Ayurveda* considers to be the most important. As mentioned earlier, they are described as the "three pillars" of *Ayurveda*. Proper sleep is one of those pillars. The other two are proper diet and lifestyle. Unfortunately, our fast-paced world is out of balance with the natural laws that govern us. Therefore, many of us suffer from sleep disorders.

Ayurveda recognizes three distinct types of sleep disorders that correspond to imbalances in the three different *doshas* introduced in chapter 1: *vata, pitta,* and *kapha.* Generally these disorders come from imbalances due to improper diet, daily routine, and behavioral patterns. If you have trouble falling asleep, you may have a *vata* disorder. If you are able to fall asleep, but tend to wake up in the middle of the night, then your *pitta* may be aggravated. A *kapha*-related problem may be what's ailing you if you sleep heavily through the night and have difficulty waking up and feel heavy, or wake up tired, achy, and your mind is lethargic. The corrections of these disorders are based on restoring balance through diet and lifestyle measures that help to pacify the specific *dosha* that is out of balance. They are briefly discussed in chapter 1.

AYURVEDIC TIPS FOR A GOOD NIGHT'S SLEEP

1. Eat three nutritious meals a day. The evening meal should be light and early.

2. Exercise regularly, preferably early in the day. If you exercise in the late evening, it may keep you up.

3. Go to bed by 10 p.m.

4. Eliminate or severely restrict stimulants such as caffeine and alcohol.

5. Wear comfortable clothing to bed.

6. Avoid hot, spicy foods at dinner.

7. Do not bring work-related material into the bedroom and turn off the TV.

8. Keep your bedroom dark.

9. A gentle massage of your hands, feet, and neck before bed can aid relaxation.

10. Stress can definitely interfere with your sleep. So practicing an effective stress-reducing technique such as Transcendental Meditation, qigong, or yoga can be very beneficial. For example, a study of sixty-nine men and women over age sixty who had sleep problems were divided into three groups: The first group participated in an hour of yoga practices six days a week, the second group took an *Ayurvedic* herbal tonic, and the third made no change to their routine. The groups were then followed for six months. Overall, those in the yoga group experienced the best improvement in sleep. Relaxation is the key. Doing something as simple as taking long, deep, easy breaths, and letting your mind and body settle down when you first go to bed can do wonders.

Maharishi Ayurveda Products International (www.mapi.com, use the code "radianthealth" for a 10% discount) offers teas and aromas to balance the *doshas* and help with sleep. There are also herbal sleep aids that can be taken if your *vata or pitta dosha* are out of balance. Each includes a variety of herbs that are gentle and non-habit forming. If you have *vata* sleep issues, take Blissful Sleep; for *pitta* disturbances take Deep Rest. *Kapha* sleep disturbances are best treated with purification techniques, diet, and lifestyle changes.

> *"I love sleep. My life has a tendency to fall apart*
> *when I'm awake, you know?"*
>
> ~ERNEST HEMINGWAY

Here are a few more suggestions for a good night's sleep:

- **Make sure your room is dark:** If you can't get it completely dark, wear a comfortable eye mask. It can also be helpful to have your room be quiet and cool.

- **Exercise in the morning:** According to a study done at the Fred Hutchinson Cancer Research Center in Seattle, women ages fifty to seventy-five who started taking brisk thirty-minute walks each morning improved their ability to fall asleep by 70 percent. However, those who exercised in the evening—within three hours of bedtime—had trouble falling asleep. The researchers felt this could be due to the fact that physical activity inhibits the natural drop in temperature that helps you to doze off.

- **Avoid alcohol:** Alcohol interferes with melatonin levels. It may help you fall asleep, but it can also cause you to wake up in the middle of night.

- **Listen to soothing music in bed:** According to a 2005 study conducted by Marion Good, Ph.D., R.N., at Case Western Reserve University, listening to soothing music for forty-five minutes in bed improved subjects sleep quality by an average of 35 percent over three weeks.

- **Take a warm bath in the evening:** Several studies show that a warm bath one or two hours before going to bed can help you to fall asleep. For instance, a 1999 study published in the *European Journal of Applied Physiology* found that a ten-minute evening bath helps the elderly to sleep better.

- **Avoid EMFs:** EMFs, as mentioned previously, can disrupt the flow of melatonin. Remember that you can significantly reduce the amount of

EMFs in your bedroom by turning off your cell phone, Wi-Fi, and any other electrical devices in or near the room where you sleep. Don't use an electric blanket. Choose a battery-operated alarm clock instead of an electrically powered clock radio.

• **Create a bedroom that is soothing:** Feng shui experts say that you should paint your bedroom in warm flesh tones, tan, gold, and chocolate colors to create a nurturing, peaceful ambiance. Avoid bright colors as they are stimulating, especially yellow. Studies show that bright yellow increases feelings of irritation and aggression. Keep your bedroom neat and free of clutter. Clutter is also known to increase agitation. Make sure you can shut out ambient light as much as possible—use window shades and/or opaque curtains. Do not watch television, use your computer, or use your bedroom for any activities other than sleeping. It trains your mind and body to associate your bedroom only with peaceful sleep.

Slumber-Enhancing Supplements, Herbs, and Scents

Sometimes, after following the previous suggestions, you may find that you still need some help in getting a good night's sleep. That's when certain nutritional supplements and herbs may be of great help. Everyone is different, so what may work for your friend, for example, may not have the same effect on you. I recommend trying one, such as melatonin first. Give it a fair try—a week or two—to see if it works for you. If not, try the next one listed in this section and so on, until you discover what consistently gives you a peaceful night of rest.

Another good approach is to start with a product that is formulated with a combination of several different sleep enhancing herbs, such as Blissful Sleep and Deep Rest available on www.mapi.com (use the code "radiant health" for a 10% discount).

Supplements

Melatonin: Our natural sleep hormone taken as a supplement has been found to be very helpful for achieving a peaceful night of sleep without causing daytime drowsiness. Higher doses can sometimes cause strange dreams. Dosage: 5–10 mg at least an hour before bed.

5-HTP: This supplement increases the production of the neurotransmitter, serotonin, which is effective for alleviating sleep disturbances. It increases the amount of REM sleep (the time in which you dream) and improves depression. Dosage: 100 mg, thirty minutes before bed.

Calcium and magnesium: These minerals are natural relaxants. Dosage: Take 1,000–1,200 mg of calcium if you are premenopausal and 1,500 mg if you are postmenopausal. 500 mg of magnesium should be taken with every 1,000 mg of calcium. Magnesium is also helpful for "restless leg syndrome," which can disturb sleep.

Vitamin B12: This vitamin helps to reset the circadian clock by helping reestablish a healthy melatonin rhythm. Dosage: 2–3 mg per day.

Taurine: An amino acid that has a calming effect and when taken with another amino acid, l-tryptophan (see below), can be helpful for promoting sleep. Dosage: 1,000–2,000 mg daily before sleep. You can repeat the dose if you wake up at night to help you get back to sleep.

L-tryptophan: Another type of amino acid that causes a hypnotic type of effect and helps promote sleep. It's found in turkey meat and credited for why eating turkey can make you sleepy. Dosage: Take 500–3,000 mg before sleep. Begin with 500 mg and increase every third day by 500 mg as needed. If you wake up at night, take half your nighttime dose.

Herbs

Valerian: This herb, which has been used for hundreds of years, is a sedative and a relaxant. It relieves anxiety, insomnia, and muscle spasms. It has also been shown to improve sleep quality. Dosage: 500-mg capsules. Take one or two capsules before bed.

Passion flower: Native to southern U.S., this climbing vine has sedative and tranquilizing qualities and, therefore, helps insomnia and disturbed sleep patterns. Passion flower is also great for anxiety, tension, and irritability. It has mild, non-addictive effects that are similar to valerian. Dosage: Take as instructed on the bottle, as brands vary.

Hops: Known best for its use in beer, this grain is a sedative and relieves anxiety, tension, irritability, and stress. Dosage: taken best as a tincture (a small amount dissolved in alcohol); put 10 drops or up to a maximum of 40 drops in a small amount of water and drink it before bed.

Kava kava: This Polynesian vine is revered for its ability to effectively reduce anxiety and stress, and to encourage sleep. Dosage: As a tincture, put 30 drops in water and drink it three times a day.

Skullcap: A member of the mint family, the root of this plant has been used in Traditional Chinese Medicine for centuries to relieve stress, anxiety, and insomnia. Dosage: 200-mg capsules two times daily.

Lemon balm: Another member of the mint family, the leaves of lemon balm are good for reducing anxiety, irritability, and restlessness. Dosage: As a tincture, take one-half teaspoon with water three times a day. You can also add lemon balm to salads and drink it as a tea.

Chamomile tea: A daisy-like plant that decreases tension and irritation, chamomile also helps to induce sleep, especially in children. Dosage: Drink one cup of tea at night. It can also be added to an evening bath. Put 4 teaspoons of dried herb in 2 cups of water and strain it into your bathtub.

Aromatherapy

Poppies are infamous for being a source of the natural narcotic opium, but simply smelling them will not intoxicate you to sleep like it did for Dorothy in *The Wizard of Oz*. There are, however, several essential oils used in aromatherapy that research shows can help to calm you and improve mild insomnia, including jasmine and lavender. According to a 2005 Japanese study, both jasmine tea and lavender odors cause a significant decrease in heart rate and calm the mood.

Jasmine: Brain chemicals, called "neurotransmitters," influence the brain in a variety of ways. GABA is one type of brain chemical that calms the mind and helps you to sleep. Researchers have tested hundreds of fragrances to determine their effect on GABA receptors in humans and mice. A study conducted in 2010 by German researchers found that two fragrances associated with jasmine—vertacetal-coeur (VC) and the chemical variation (PI24513)—had the strongest GABA effect. These jasmine-derived chemicals increased the activation of GABA receptors by more than five times—which is as strong as any of the known drugs.

Lavender: Many studies show that lavender aromatherapy is relaxing and can help you to fall asleep. For example, a single-blinded, randomized British study from 2005 found that lavender aroma is a good treatment for mild insomnia. Another study from the University of Miami in 2008 showed that lavender baths help young infants to sleep.

Maximizing the Medicine of Sleep

Just like exercise and an excellent plant-based diet, the medicinal effects of proper sleep are so profound that if drug companies could make a pill that contained all its benefits, it would be the best-selling drug of all time. Here is one fundamental aspect of health that is free, requires no special equipment (although a comfortable, nontoxic bed is preferable), and requires no special skills, trainers, or support buddies. Best of all, unlike exercise, it requires *no effort* and for most people is incredibly enjoyable.

The medicine of sleep is so strong and powerful that you don't want to ever cut it short if at all possible. If you have been a night owl and don't think you can ever fall asleep before 10 p.m., try this: go to bed fifteen minutes earlier every week. Eventually, you will have backed yourself up to 10 p.m. and trained your body to go to bed at this most health-supporting time.

If you have trouble sleeping, please try all the gentle, natural approaches presented above rather than using pharmaceutical medications, which can disrupt the full medicine available in sleep. You may also want to create a ritual that is most relaxing for you—one that best prepares you to ease into this extraordinarily powerful, health-promoting, sublime activity. Soothing music, warm baths, gentle massages, perhaps reading an uplifting book or hearing the calming voice on an enjoyable audiobook, or simply being in quiet meditation or prayer, you may find is the perfect approach that consistently and magically lulls you to sleep. Find what works for you. Make it a nightly ritual or habit so that your mind/body will learn to anticipate this glorious restorative state and will quickly and effortlessly drop into its pool of tranquility. Sweet dreams.

CHAPTER 8

Detoxification

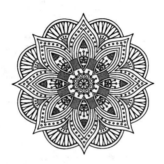

Removing the Blocks to Your Healing Intelligence

Because we cannot scrub our inner body we need to learn a few skills to help cleanse our tissues, organs, and mind. This is the art of Ayurveda.

~SEBASTIAN POLE

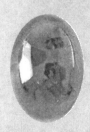

THE EIGHTH GEM—AMBER

The ability to detoxify and purify your body is embodied by amber, the eighth stone in your breastplate. Amber is a fossilized resin that traps insects and debris within it, just as your body traps toxins.

Amber is said to transmute negative energy into positive energy. When toxins are removed from your body, their negative energy goes with them too, which causes your energy to rise and become cleaner and brighter. Amber has a sunny, bright, soothing energy that calms your nerves—which is exactly how you'll feel after the impurities that have been aggravating and dragging down your body have been removed.

Amber is said to help purify your body, mind, and spirit—the ultimate goal of an effective cleansing program, especially *Ayurveda*'s *panchakarma*.

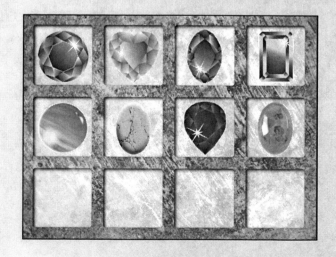

*W*hen you hear the word "detoxification," you might think it would involve unpleasant, even painful, procedures. But the ancient *Ayurvedic* technique for detoxification and rebalancing, called *panchakarma*, is quite the opposite. Imagine lying on a comfortable table with warm soothing oil being gentle poured onto your body. Now imagine two therapists simultaneously massaging the oil into both sides of your body in synchronized motions. The sensation is so soothing, your body melts into relaxation, and your mind drops into a pool of tranquility and pleasure. This is just one of the many treatments prescribed in *panchakarma*.

Panchakarma involves a series of relaxing treatments over several days, done in a spa-like setting with medical supervision. The treatments are gentle and deceptively simple, but their effects are remarkably powerful. The intelligence in the body is given such a boost through the techniques of *panchakarma* that it is capable of triggering phenomenal purification and healing.

Dislodging Impurities and Toxins

Panchakarma is especially effective at dislodging impurities and toxins that are stored in your fat cells and flushing them from your body. A study published by Dr. Bob Herron and Dr. John Fagen in 2002 in the journal *Alternative Therapies, Health, & Medicine* found that the levels of polychlorinated biphenyls (PCBs) and pesticides, including DDT, dropped by 50 percent in test subjects after just one five-day series of treatments. These researchers also tested the toxin levels in the fat cells of individuals who had undergone at least five days of *panchakarma*, an average of twice a year, for more than nine consecutive years. They found that the toxin levels were so low in all of these individuals that they were undetectable. The researchers concluded that regular *panchakarma* treatments are highly effective at removing toxins from your body and keeping your toxin load extremely low. In fact, research shows that *panchakarma* is the *only* proven therapy that effectively rids body fat of toxic chemicals.

Toxins are unavoidable. They are ubiquitous in the environment and in your food. When a toxin gets into your body, it concentrates and stores in your fat cells. You also accumulate impurities from the waste products that are created by normal cellular metabolism. Intense unpleasant emotions also create toxic molecules that have negative effects in your body, such as increasing inflammation and weakening your immune system.

According to *Ayurveda*, all toxins in the body form a white sticky substance called *ama*. Too much *ama* can clog your system, decrease its ability to function well, and create imbalances that lead to disease. For instance, atherosclerotic plaques are a form of *ama* that can block your arteries and cause a heart attack or stroke. Stones that form in your gallbladder and kidney are also a type of *ama*. The ancient *Ayurvedic* texts state that one of the main purposes of *panchakarma* is to get the *ama* out.

Panchakarma also profoundly balances the mind/body and prevents or reverses the development of disease. Preliminary research indicates that it may slow the aging process, too. The first time I went through this series of gentle but powerful techniques, within forty-eight hours, I looked ten years younger and had never felt better in my life! This experience made me a believer in the power of *Ayurveda*.

The 5 Steps of Panchakarma

1. Home Prep

The majority of *panchakarma* is done in a medical spa-like setting over a period of time from several days to several weeks. For the best results, you should go for a minimum of three days; however, five to seven days is considered ideal. In India, *panchakarma* is recognized as essential for good health. It is standard practice for employers to give their employees up to thirty days off work to do *panchakarma!*

Before you arrive at the *panchakarma* spa, you will need to prepare for a few days by doing some specific steps at home, called "home prep." The home prep is designed to begin the process of softening impurities and toxins, and mobilizing them from your fat. It is technically called "internal oleation," meaning saturating the inside of your body with oils. The most common oil recommended in home prep is *ghee*, or clarified butter. *Ghee* is made by boiling butter until all the milk solids precipitate out (always use organic, unsalted butter). In other words, butter without milk solids and water is *ghee*. The spa you choose will give you the specifics on how to make ghee, how much to take, and when to take it.

Ghee has very different properties from butter. First, it stays solid at room temperature and never needs to be refrigerated. Second, it lasts virtually forever without going bad. In India, you can purchase 100-year-old *ghee*. Third, unlike butter, *ghee* doesn't raise your cholesterol or promote hardening of the arteries. *Ayurveda* considers *ghee* to be an extraordinarily powerful medicine that, according to ancient texts, soothes all the *doshas* (properties found in all living things: *vata* governs movement; *pitta*, metabolism and transformation; and *kapha*, structure). *Ghee* is also said to improve memory and mental function, strengthen the body, promote longevity and beauty, and protect the body from various diseases. You can purchase organic *ghee* in most health food stores, or prepare it yourself by simply melting unsalted organic butter in a pan and boiling it until the milk solids precipitate to the bottom. Cool the ghee and then pour it through cheese cloth into a sterile jar. Refrigerate until solid, and then you can leave it at room temperature.

During home prep, *ghee* is taken in increasing amounts every day for four days. The *panchakarma* facility will instruct you on how much to take based on your individual needs. Instead of drinking melted ghee straight, which can be a bit challenging, mixing it with one-quarter cup of heated organic soy, almond, or rice milk will make it much more palatable. The purpose of drinking *ghee* is to raise the level of fat or lipids in your blood to form a "concentration gradient" between the stored toxins in the fat cells in your body and the pure fat (*ghee*) in your blood.

You may recall from high school biology that a concentration gradient is produced anytime there is more of a particular substance on one side of a semi-permeable membrane than on the other. A law of physics dictates that the concentration of molecules on one side of a semipermeable membrane must equal the other. So, molecules on the side with the higher concentration will pass through the membrane to the side with the lower concentration until the amounts are equal on both sides of the membrane.

Here's how *panchakarma* uses the concentration gradient to get toxins out: During the home-prep portion of *panchakarma*, you also consume a low-calorie, plant-based diet of easily digestible lightly cooked fruits, vegetable, and grains. The recommendation is to eat to three-quarters of your capacity. In other words, stop eating *before* you feel full. The fat stored in your fat cells is used for energy. Your fat cells become smaller as more fat is used. The amount of space for toxins in your fat cells lessens, so the toxins become more concentrated. The pure organic *ghee* you consume contains no toxins. By introducing large amounts of toxin-free fat into the blood, you create a concentration gradient between the toxin-filled fat in the body and toxin-free fat in the blood—a physiological condition that isn't normally present. The concentrated toxins will flow out of your fat cells into the pure ghee in your blood until the concentration of toxins is equal in your fat cells and in your blood. According to physics, a 50 percent reduction in the amount of toxins in your body would be expected. That is exactly what Bob Herron's research, which was presented at the beginning of this chapter, showed.

For some individuals, *ghee* might be contraindicated and another type of oil, such as flax oil, or another preparation may be prescribed. You'll need to check with the physician at the *panchakarma* clinic to determine the best home-prep program for your individual needs.

After the internal-oleation phase of *panchakarma* is complete, a twenty-minute hot bath is recommended. The heat increases blood flow and speeds up the delivery of toxins to the intestines. Due to the relatively large amount of ghee that is ingested during home prep, not all of it will be digested. The undigested *ghee* stays in the intestines. This again sets up a concentration gradient, and toxins and impurities are drawn into the intestines. Following the bath, a mild laxative such as castor oil, senna tea, or a special herbal mixture prescribed by the *panchakarma* clinic is taken to eliminate the toxins from the intestines.

2. Pulse Diagnosis: Detecting Imbalances

After completing the first phase of *panchakarma*, you are ready for the relaxing and enjoyable part: the in-residence treatments at an *Ayurvedic* medical spa. When you arrive at the clinic, an *Ayurvedic* physician, or *vaidya*, takes your pulse and asks you a series of questions. The *vaidya* picks up a lot more information from your pulse than just your heart rate, as is described in chapter 1. As you may recall, an expert in pulse diagnosis can feel, with remarkable precision and accuracy, the state of balance and imbalance in all your body systems and tissues.

Based on all the information from the pulse, the *vaidya* prescribes a specific series of *panchakarma* treatments customized to your current state of health. The *vaidya* has many treatments from which to choose, each with its own special benefits and purposes, but all with the ultimate purpose of restoring balance.

3. Massage: Moving the Toxins and Inducing Balance

The prescribed series of *panchakarma* treatments usually begins with a special type of massage called *abhyanga*. *Abhyanga* is performed by two technicians who apply warm sesame oil simultaneously to each side of your body using synchronized movements. The massage technique is designed to facilitate getting the toxins out and, at the same time, soothing and balancing the nervous system. No deep tissue pressure is applied. Rather, the pressure that is used is generally soft, and the movements are extremely relaxing.

When both sides of your body are stimulated in the same way at the exact same time, the brainwaves in the two hemispheres of your brain will synchronize. This brainwave phenomenon is also seen during the practice of Transcendental Meditation. Not surprisingly, people who practice this highly effective form of meditation report the experience of "transcending" during *abhyanga*.

Researchers have also observed that there is a strong correlation between the synchronicity of brainwaves and depression. Depression is characterized by very asynchronous brainwave patterns, meaning that the brainwave patterns emitted by one hemisphere of the brain are very different from those emitted by the other side. Significant relief of depression is associated with the brainwave patterns becoming more synchronized. Researchers believe that one of the main reasons *abhyanga* has been found to be so effective at easing depression is because it causes brainwaves to become more synchronized.

Sesame oil is the most penetrating of all the oils, and for that reason, it is the preferred type of oil used for *abhyanga*, as well as for many other techniques in *panchakarma*. Sesame oil absorbs so quickly through the skin that it appears in the blood within minutes. For those who have naturally high amounts of the *pitta dosha*, oil that is cooling, such as organic coconut oil, may be prescribed instead. The oils applied to the skin during *panchakarma* are also designed to contribute to the blood-lipid/body-fat concentration gradient, which helps to flush additional toxins out of the body.

Usually, finely ground herbs with special medicinal properties are added to the oil. In classical *panchakarma*, up to seventy-five different herbs may be selected. The oil acts as a carrier to transport medicinal herbs into the body. Delivering medicinal herbs through the skin may seem like an unusual practice, but it's not. Western pharmaceutical companies use this route, too, for many types of medications. There are medications, for example, that are administered topically in patches such as nicotine, nitroglycerin, and estrogen. Just like the herbs in the oils used in *panchakarma*, these medications are absorbed through the skin. A network of blood vessels under the skin picks up these substances and transports them to the rest of the body.

Research has found that sesame oil also has several other beneficial effects, including anticancer properties. It can inhibit the growth of melanoma and colon cancer cells. It also contains antioxidants. Interestingly, researchers discovered that heating the oil—as is routinely done in *panchakarma*—causes the antioxidant activity to increase.

There are other types of whole-body massage techniques in *panchakarma* that may also be prescribed based on a person's specific health needs. Two examples are *udvartana* and *garshan,* both of which help to promote weight loss. *Udvartana* is performed using a paste made of ground grains. *Garshan* is performed using raw silk or wool gloves. Both techniques clean the skin and create friction, thus stimulating circulation, which helps to promote weight loss.

Panchakarma also includes two techniques that focus on the head: *nasya* and *shirodhara*. Although both are soothing to the mind and nervous system, *shirodhara* is principally prescribed for this purpose, and *nasya* is usually recommended for its other health benefits.

Nasya—This technique is designed to purify and powerfully balance and enhance your five senses. *Nasya* also improves mental clarity and stabilizes the mind. It's especially good for people with sinus problems and headaches. The technique of *nasya* begins with a luxurious head and shoulder massage while you sit in a chair. Following the massage, the technician will have you gently inhale herbalized steam. Then, he or she will have you will lie down on a bed with your head slightly tilted back and place a series of drops of herbalized sesame oil in your nose, which soothes your sinuses and helps to facilitate the release of any congestion.

Shirodhara—*Shirodhara* is a technique that involves lying on a table while a gentle stream of warm herbalized oil is applied to your forehead. This procedure is actually considered a cooling treatment and is designed to relax your mind, soothe and nourish your nervous system, and detoxify your body. The technician begins by covering your eyes with cotton balls and a washcloth, and placing a soft roll under your neck to tilt your head slightly backward. Then he or she very slowly applies a stream of sesame oil to your forehead in an infinity (or figure-eight) pattern. Within a short time, you will feel your mind settle down and become deeply relaxed. Many people report experiencing a blissful, expanded state of consciousness.

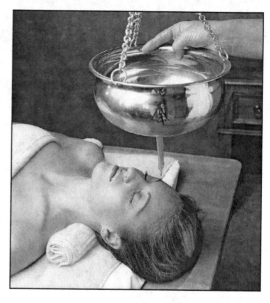

Shirodhara is particularly good for stabilizing the mind and alleviating anxiety, insomnia, nervousness, and worry. It also improves malaise and is good for your skin, too. Many people notice a distinct glow to their complexion following a soothing, relaxing, peaceful session of *shirodhara*.

4. Heat Treatments: Melting the Impurities

The next major step of *panchakarma* uses a group of heat treatments to dilate the channels in your body and increase circulation, which facilitates the flow of toxins and impurities to your intestines for elimination. Toxins are also removed from your body as you sweat. There are three main heat treatments in *panchakarma: swedana, pizzichilli,* and *pinda swedana.*

Swedana—*Swedana* is a traditional herbalized steam treatment. It's like a steam sauna, but with a few important differences. Instead of sitting completely inside a sauna, you lie on your back or sit up in a cedar cabinet with your head *outside* the cabinet, because *Ayurveda* advises against overheating your head. To help keep your head cool and comfortable during the treat-

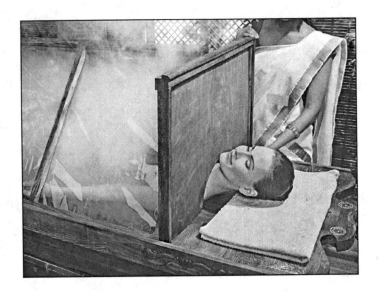

ment, the technician may also apply a remarkably refreshing cool cloth or a frozen cube of coconut oil to your head and face. In addition, you are given frequent sips of cool water, so that you can stay well hydrated.

Pizzichilli—This is my personal favorite of all the treatments. It's considered a royal treatment, and it's easy to understand why. Imagine lying on a table while two technicians massage your body as they use a hose to continuously pour thick streams of soothingly warm sesame oil over you. The first time I experienced the sensation of the warm oil cascading in waves over my body, I actually moaned out loud. It felt like warm melting butterscotch. After the treatment, I felt deeply relaxed and I glowed from head to toe. *Pizzichilli* is excellent for soothing sore muscles and joints.

Pinda Swedana—The third heat treatment, *pinda swedana*, is performed by two technicians who massage your body using quick long strokes with boluses of precooked herbs and hot medicated oils in soft, smooth cloth packs. *Pinda swedana* is designed to soothe any kind of musculoskeletal problems, especially arthritis. It's also noted to nourish the body, enhancing its vitality.

5. Cleansing: The Final Stage

External oleation and heat treatments are performed each day to help lift the impurities and toxins out of the tissues and transport them into the intestines. Once in the intestines, it's very important to get them out. This is facilitated by a simple procedure called a *basti*, which is a gentle internal cleansing of the colon with either herbalized water or lubricating oils. The oil-based *basti* and the water-based *basti* are administered on alternating days. You can think of a *basti* as a very gentle herbalized colonic. Getting the toxins out of the colon quickly is powerful medicine, so some people find it to be a little uncomfortable. *Ayurveda* says that the *basti* treatment is so important that it alone could cure 50 percent of illnesses.

Many Immediate and Long-Term Benefits

After completing *panchakarma*, people report having greater energy, clarity of mind, and a sense of well-being. They also report relief of symptoms and improvements in disorders of both the mind and body. *Panchakarma* restores balance to the physiology and significantly reduces oxygen free radicals according to numerous studies. Oxygen free radicals increase your risk of cancer and other degenerative disorders and accelerate aging. In the *Journal of Research and Education in Indian Medicine* (1993), H. Sharma, M.D., documented that patients doing *panchakarma* had an initial rise in lipid peroxidase, an enzyme that goes up in the presence of oxygen free radicals. Yet, following therapy, lipid-peroxidase levels fell way below pre-treatment levels. These findings correspond to the rise of toxins in the blood as they are mobilized during treatment and the fall of toxins after they are eliminated from the body.

Researchers have also found psychological improvements in patients following *panchakarma*. Standard psychological tests show that people are less anxious, less depressed, less distressed, and less fatigued. In 1988, researcher Rainer Waldschütz used the Freiburg Personality Inventory, a standardized test that measures twelve different personality scales, to evaluate patients who had just finished *panchakarma* treatments. These post-*panchakarma* patients showed improvements in six of the twelve scales: decreased body complaints, reduced irritability, less bodily strain, fewer psychological inhibitions, more openness and greater emotional stability.

Panchakarma also significantly improves several cardiac risk factors. Blood samples taken from patients shortly after they completed *panchakarma* showed many beneficial changes. For example, vasoactive intestinal peptide (VIP)—a substance that dilates coronary arteries—increased by 80 percent. The "good" kind of cholesterol (high-density lipoproteins; HDL) increased by 75 percent, and total serum cholesterol decreased.

Nothing is more powerful than this special series of techniques for eliminating the impurities that obstruct your full strength; nothing surpasses the balancing and healing effects; nothing centers you more; and nothing recharges you more. After a week of *panchakarma*, the unobstructed flow of your healing intelligence becomes so powerful and so intense that most people positively glow with self-luminescence and beauty.

(Pages 192–200 adapted from *Waking the Warrior Goddess* by Christine Horner, M.D., used with permission of Basic Health Publications.)

Home Detoxifying Programs

If you cannot go to a *panchakarma* clinic, you can detoxify at home. Although home detoxification programs are not as powerful as *panchakarma*, they can effectively remove some toxins.

Toxins are eliminated mainly through your liver, kidneys, colon, and skin. There are specific detox programs that target one or more of these elimination pathways. For instance, you could do a modified *panchakarma*-like program by beginning with the home-prep program. Then for two weeks following the prep, take herbs that detoxify the liver, kidneys, and colon. For example, milk thistle, dandelion, and turmeric help purify the liver and boost liver enzymes. Licorice root, psyllium seed, alfalfa, yucca root, violet leaf, cascara sagrada, and marshmallow root act as colon-cleansing agents. Horsetail, uva ursi, and nettles help to flush toxins from your kidneys. You could work with a knowledgeable herbalist to determine which herbs to take and at what dosages, or you can purchase a detoxification kit from your local health shop, which includes standard doses of colon and liver herbs, such as Whole Body Cleanse made by Enzymatic Therapy.

Another convenient approach I highly recommend is to simply use three excellent detoxification herbal formulas made by Maharishi Ayurvedic Products International (www.mapi.com, use the code "radiant health" for a 10% discount). To cleanse the bowel, take two to five tablets of Digest Tone or two to four tablets of Herbal Cleanse before going to bed each night. Take two tablets of Elim-Tox morning and evening to cleanse the liver, blood, sweat glands, and the elimination system. Or take Elim-Tox-O if you have any symptoms of reactive toxins such as skin breakouts or other inflammatory symptoms. Finally, to purify the urinary tract and assist the removal of toxins, take two tablets of Genitrac in the morning and evening.

During the cleanse it is very important to follow a pure diet consisting of lightly cooked fresh organic fruits, vegetables, and whole grains. Be sure to avoid alcohol, sugar, chocolate, cold foods, dairy, meat, drugs, cigarettes, and canned, preserved, and/or processed foods. You can boost the results by also giving yourself a sesame seed oil massage every morning. If you have access to an infrared or dry sauna, give yourself the oil massage first and then sit in the sauna for twenty minutes or so several times a week. The heat treatment will enhance the absorption of the sesame oil and speed up the movement of toxins out of your body.

Other Detox Programs

There are a variety of other home-based programs that are also effective in helping to get toxins out of the body. They range from very simple, gentle programs, to more aggressive programs that should only be done if your health is generally strong. You might want to work under the supervision of a naturopath or other holistic health practitioner if you have any health concerns.

First, let's start with the simplest. Because your body naturally detoxifies itself, you can work with that natural ability without having to go anywhere or do anything exotic, time consuming, or expensive. Simply stop pouring in the toxins, drink plenty of pure clean water, and get some exercise—as easy as fast-paced walking will do the trick. It's amazing to me to hear that many people don't drink water. Instead, their fluid intake each day comes primarily from coffee, sodas, and beer. No kidding! So if you happen to be one of those folks whose dietary habits are unhealthy—for example, if you eat lots of fast foods and sugar, and drink very little water—a great way for you to help your body to begin to gently detox is to eliminate red meat, sugar, coffee, and preserved and processed foods. You'll notice that every detox program always includes eliminating major sources of toxins. Fill your plate instead with fresh, organically grown vegetables, fruits, and whole grains. Lightly cooked foods are easier to digest, and research has shown light cooking actually enhances the availability of certain nutrients, especially antioxidants.

Fresh vegetable-based juices are wonderful to consume daily. Every time I make a commitment to juice every day, within just a week or so, my skin takes on a self-luminous glow. Comments like, "What are you doing? You look amazing! Your skin looks radiant!" come from nearly everyone I encounter. There's nothing more affirming and encouraging than having the evidence of your efforts toward a better state of health radiantly displayed on your face! I haven't found any published research specifically measuring what happens when a person consumes a glass of fresh organic vegetable-based juice each day. But it's only logical that more nutrients and antioxidants are absorbed in the body, compared to those from eating solid food, which requires a lot of digestion.

However, there is a study that sheds some light on what contributes to a healthy "glow." Published in the December 2010 journal *Evolution and Human Behavior*, researchers at the University of St. Andrews in Scotland found that individuals with a greater intake of carotenoids—antioxidant compounds found in fruits and vegetables—have an increased yellow skin tone, which makes one look healthier and more attractive. In this study, volunteers judged the appearance of Caucasian and African faces for attractiveness. Those who had the golden color associated with carotenoids were judged to be "healthier" and more attractive. When it came to attractiveness, the rich carotenoid color scored higher than a suntan. So, if you are interested in looking good *and* feeling great, nix that tanning bed and head to the juice bar instead. There is nothing better than beauty that radiates from true health.

The Importance of Pure Water

Our bodies may look solid; however, they are composed mostly of water. Estimates of how much water each of us hold range from 70 to 90 percent. The exact amount doesn't matter—what's important is to understand that our bodies are composed mostly of water. That's why it is so important for

us to *drink* water. Consuming at least eight 8-ounce glasses a day is recommended, and much more if you are active and perspiring. Tragically, we
are now challenged by the fact that much of our water is contaminated. I
know, I know, it seems like another catch-22 situation. You need to drink
water, but most sources of water are contaminated with health-destroying
toxins.

Municipal tap water, for instance, commonly contains dangerous con-
taminants like chlorine, heavy metals, pesticides, pharmaceutical drugs,
and much more. Bottled water isn't a great alternative for many reasons.
First, most of it comes in plastic bottles, which have estrogen-mimicking
molecules, including BPA and phthalates, that can leach into it. Next,
there's no regulation on bottled water and an estimated 40 percent is merely
tap water! The Environmental Working Group (www.ewg.org) analyzed
173 different varieties of bottle water to determine if companies disclosed
their source of water, how the water was treated, and if they tested their
water for purity—and if so, what the results of those tests were. More than
half of the manufacturers would not disclose this basic information: almost
20 percent wouldn't reveal the source of their water, and 32 percent
wouldn't discuss the purity of the water or how it was treated. In 2009, the
Environmental Working Group tested ten different brands of bottled water
and found an average of eight toxic chemicals in each. If you would like to
read these reports, they can be found on www.ewg.org.

Another critical issue about bottled water is its severe negative environmental impact. During the processing of the bottles, toxins are released
into the environment. Far worse, however, is the massive amount of plastic
waste material that is produced. In 2007 in the U.S. alone, 8.8 billion gal-
lons of bottled water were consumed. This translates into the use of roughly
63.4 billion plastic bottles per year or about 2 million bottles every five
minutes. Every one of these bottles need to be disposed of in some way.
Only about 10 percent of plastic bottles are recycled. The process of recycling, unfortunately, isn't without its problems: only a small percentage of
recycled plastic is actually recycled, and the recycling process involves
adding even more plastic.

The plastic bottles that are not recycled end up in landfills, on road-
sides, and in bodies of water—rivers, lakes, and oceans. The chemicals
within plastic have nowhere to go and leach into our ground water and

oceans. Tragically, our oceans have become filled with plastic. Huge floating islands of plastic bottles are being discovered worldwide. One of the most infamous of these islands is in the north Pacific. It is estimated to be twice the size of Texas!

The major problem with plastic is that it is non-biodegradable. In other words, it can't break down. It will always stay in our environment. It can, however, break up into smaller and smaller particles. But that's not a good thing, because these small particles have filled our oceans. Charles Moore, captain of an oceanographic research vessel, states in a video posted on savetheocean.wordpress.com/2010/10/08/world-biggest-garbage-dump-plastic-in-the-ocean that he became alarmed at the increasing amount of plastic he saw in the oceans. He and his coresearchers devised a series of experiments to test just how many plastic particles are in the ocean. Normally, the ocean's surface is filled with plankton, tiny sea creatures, which is a major source of food for fish and birds. Disturbingly, the surface of the ocean is not only filled with plankton, but now is also filled with plastic particles. Wildlife, therefore, is consuming large amounts of plastic along with the plankton and many are dying because of it. Significant amounts of plastic particles were found in every location that the researchers tested in the Pacific Ocean. Shockingly, in one of the more polluted areas, the amount of plastic particles outnumbered the plankton six to one. Please visit www.savetheocean.wordpress.com to learn more.

So, what form of water is safe to drink that won't harm the environment? Drinking filtered tap water is thought to be the best solution by most experts. Ideally, you should have a whole-house water-filtration system installed. The next best option is to use a system, such as a reverse osmosis system, that fits under your sinks and/or place filters directly on your faucets and showerhead. You can also filter your water with separate filtration systems such as Brita water filters. Fill stainless steel bottles with filtered water to take to the gym, or wherever you go.

You can help the plastic problem in our environment further by:

- Avoiding using plastic as much as possible.

- Recycling all the plastic you can. The only types that can be recycled are labeled with #1 or #2 in a triangle embossed usually on the bottom of the container.

- Picking up plastic bottles whenever you find them in the environment, especially if you are at the beach, and make an effort to recycle them.

Remember, we are all in this together and all of us need to do our part to help save our planet.

Liver Cleanses

One of the principal functions of your liver is to help process the toxins in your body. You can help your liver a lot by decreasing the load of toxins that it has to process. This means consciously avoiding all the common sources of toxins, which include conventionally processed foods, excess dietary "bad" fats such as saturated animal fats and *trans* fats, refined carbohydrates, sugar, and alcohol. You should also avoid over-the-counter medications and drugs. Next, there are varieties of ways that you can improve the function of your liver by promoting the exit of toxin-carrying bile and improving its level of enzymes—specialized proteins that function to facilitate the breakdown of toxins.

Ann Louise Gittleman, a nationally respected nutritionist and author, describes an excellent and effective "Fast Track Liver Detox" diet that helps to improve liver function and promote elimination of toxins through the colon. It is divided into a three-stage process and is simple to work into your normal life. The first stage is a "Seven-Day Prequel," which consists of eating lots of foods that are great for your liver. These foods include cruciferous vegetables (broccoli, cauliflower, cabbage, and Brussels sprouts); leafy greens (parsley, kale, chard, cilantro, and dandelion greens); citrus fruits (oranges, lemons, and limes); sulfur-rich foods (garlic, onions, eggs, and daikon radish); and liver health-promoting foods (artichokes, asparagus, beets, celery, dandelion-root tea, whey, and nutritional yeast flakes). She also recommends drinking half your weight in ounces of filtered or purified water, and consuming 1 to 2 tablespoons of healthy oil, such as flax oil or olive oil, each day. The second stage is a one-day "fast" that involves drinking filtered water (a minimum total of 72 ounces) alternating with a mixture you prepare (a total of eight cups for the day) of cranberry juice, water, freshly squeezed orange and lemon juice, and a variety of delicious spices—specifically, cinnamon, nutmeg, and ground ginger. A colon-cleansing supplement, either psyllium husks or ground flaxseeds, is taken at the beginning and the end of the day. Light exercise, such as a twenty-minute walk, is also recommended. The third stage is a three-day sequel, which involves the same diet as the prequel, along with probiotic foods that promote "good" intestinal bacteria. Examples of these foods include sauerkraut and yogurt, and a hydrochloric acid formula. Volunteers who completed this program had several laboratory tests done, including a caffeine clearance test and a urinary sulfate/creatinine ratio, which found that this program did, in fact, improve liver function by 23 to 47 percent.

Another, much more aggressive liver cleanse requires drinking apple juice for several days followed by a dose of olive oil, Epsom salts, and the juice from either a fresh lemon or grapefruit. This regimen causes the liver and gall bladder to release stones—or congealed bile—which can obstruct the optimal function of the liver. A juice fast consisting of fresh carrot and celery juice is recommended for the final two days. This cleanse should be done only if your health is good. It's far more challenging to do, and the process of releasing the stones can cause you to feel nauseated and exhausted. You won't be able to work that day. Plan to spend the day resting.

Colon Cleanses

There are many different types of colon cleanses designed to help facilitate removing toxins from your body. They range from mild cleanses done at home with herbal laxatives to colon irrigations done with large volumes of water administered by a certified colon hydrotherapist. The colonic machine uses a low-pressure gravity-driven pump to deliver water through a tube, which has been inserted into the rectum. After an appropriate amount of water has been administered, the therapist then flushes out the water and waste matter through the tube. The process is repeated until the therapist determines that the colon has been adequately cleansed. The contraindications to this procedure include inflammatory bowel diseases such as diverticulitis, ulcerative colitis, and Crohn's disease, as well as severe hemorrhoids, colorectal tumors, or having had recent surgery.

Colon cleansing goes back thousands of years. *Ayurveda* has considered it an important part of achieving and maintaining health for 5,000 years, and the Greeks recognized its value in ancient times as well. Despite the large number of certified colon hydrotherapists, the thousands of colonics performed every year, and a myriad of available colon-cleansing programs, there has been virtually no research nor have there been clinical trials focused on this technique. The medical literature has a few studies, but none explore clinical health benefits. One study reports that colon irrigation causes white blood cell movement from gut-associated lymphatic tissue to the peripheral blood, which may improve colon and immune function. The others report on rare complications of colon hydrotherapy, such as infection and perforation. Given the fact that thousands of these procedures are performed in this country and around the world every year, the incidence of reported complications is extraordinarily rare.

Physicians who believe that colon cleanses are unnecessary or pure hype say that the colon naturally cleanses itself of stool and, therefore, needs no assistance. They argue that mechanical irrigation simply washes out both good and bad bacteria. However, *Ayurveda* views the colon not in a purely mechanical paradigm, but principally from a physiologic and energetic model. In chapter 1, you were introduced to *Ayurveda* and the concept of the *doshas*. *Ayurveda* states that the "seat" of the *vata dosha* is in the colon. Disturbances in this *dosha*—which are the most common *doshic* disturbances seen—can be corrected most powerfully by carefully prescribed *bastis*. The improvements are confirmed by changes in the pulse. In addition, flushing the colon sets up a concentration gradient, which helps to draw toxins out of the body and into the colon where they can be eliminated. Quality research on *panchakarma* reported in the first part of this chapter demonstrates the effective elimination of fat-soluble toxins using this technique.

The mistaken logic that Western-trained doctors use to discredit colon cleanses is based on thinking that the effect of these cleanses is purely mechanical. Rather, the benefits come from physiological effects. Clearly, there is a need for good research that measures the proper factors, including the physiological changes, so that the health benefits of colon cleanses can be accurately known.

Sweating Out Toxins

Most of us are aware that the sweat our body produces isn't just water; it also contains salt. All of us have experienced the salty taste of sweat and felt it crust on our skin. But what many people may not be aware of is that sweat also contains many other trace minerals, heavy metals, and toxins. Therefore, your sweat provides another channel for the elimination of toxins—which is why heat treatments are an important part of *panchakarma* treatments, especially *swedena*.

The heat causes several beneficial physiological effects. First, it increases heart rate and blood flow, which helps mobilize toxins into the organs of elimination including the colon, kidneys, and skin. Next, it causes your skin to release sweat in an effort to cool the body and, as a side benefit, also releases toxins. Surprisingly, there haven't been many studies analyzing what's in your sweat. The only published studies are from the late 1970s and 1980s, which looked at the trace element concentration in human sweat. Researchers found that there was considerable variation from individual to individual. Concentrations of elements were found to vary in different body locations and between genders. The researchers consistently found that heavy metals, including copper, lead, cadmium, nickel, and zinc, were released in sweat. A study published in the *Annals of Clinical Laboratory Science* in 1978 found that the concentrations of nickel and cadmium were higher in sweat than in urine.

Researchers at the University of Southern California published a study in *Archives of Environmental Health* in 1989 of firemen who were exposed to PCBs and the byproducts generated from a transformer fire and explosion. The firemen were treated with a two- to three-week detoxification program consisting of a medically supervised diet, sauna treatments, and exercise. The major symptom displayed by all of the firemen was significant memory impairment. After the detoxification program, every fireman showed marked improvement of memory based on the results of three different types of memory tests.

As you may recall, the *panchakarma* sweat treatment, *swedena,* is done with the body in a steam sauna box, but the head remains out to avoid too much heat. However, most facilities and home saunas are not designed this way. *Ayurveda* cautions that sauna durations should not be over twenty minutes to avoid excessive heat in the head. The most common types of saunas are steam, dry, and far-infrared saunas. Far-infrared saunas have been shown to help several health conditions, including improving cancer treatments by synergistically increasing the tumor-killing effects of chemotherapy and radiation. It lowers blood pressure in patients with high blood pressure, treats congestive heart failure, reduces chronic pain, and possibly improves chronic fatigue syndrome, fibromyalgia, and multiple chemical sensitivities. It also aids weight loss.

You should not go into a sauna if you have unstable angina, have had a recent heart attack, or suffer from severe aortic stenosis. Never drink alcohol before you go into a sauna. It increases the risk of a dangerous drop of your blood pressure and can cause cardiac arrhythmias or sudden death.

The Life Vessel

A new technology called the Life Vessel, an extraordinary "quantum" device, is a cozy, relaxing chamber that uses light, sound, frequency, and vibration to balance and detoxify the body. The results for a variety of ailments have been nothing short of miraculous. Invented by Barry McNew in Cottonwood, Arizona, the "Life Vessel" improves certain physiological measures so effectively that it was certified by the FDA in 2006. Treatments are administered in four one-hour sessions over the course of three days. Heavy metals, petroleum products, and a variety of other toxins are mobilized and released by the treatments.

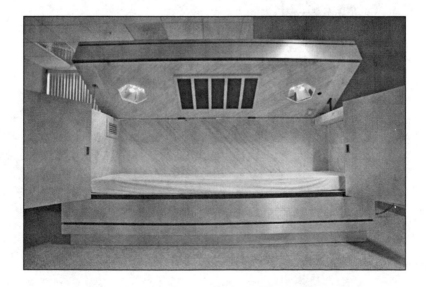

The detoxification has been found to be significantly improved by drinking lots of pure water—a recommended one gallon a day—along with infrared sauna sessions, followed by colon hydrotherapy. Life Vessel Centers can be found in numerous cities in the U.S., including Colorado Springs, CO; Davenport, IA; Denver, CO; Fort Wayne, IN; Hutchinson, KS; Scottsdale, AZ; Santa Fe, NM; San Juan Capistrano, CA; Santa Barbara, CA; Santa Rosa, CA; and Wilmington, NC. For more information go to www.lifevessel.com.

A buildup of toxins in your body clogs its channels and decreases the ability of your organs to function well. Over time, these toxins can cause imbalances and damage that can lead to chronic diseases. They also make your skin dull and can cause it to become inflamed with acne or cysts. Keep in mind that most of these chemicals can be removed with effective detoxification techniques. Because it is impossible to avoid exposures to potentially harmful chemicals no matter how hard you may try, it is important to make regular detoxification a part of your health routine. *Ayurveda* recommends for optimum health that you do *panchakarma* at least two or three times a year, ideally at the change of seasons.

There's nothing that boosts radiant health and beauty quite like a week or two of a good detoxification program. It's a quick and very effective way to not only remove toxins, but also to achieve a better state of balance, enhance your inner healing intelligence, improve your appearance, and charge your enthusiasm for life!

CHAPTER 9

Leaning into Longevity

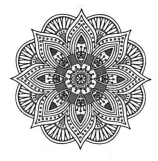

Why Keeping Your Weight Ideal Is So Important

To lengthen your life, shorten your meals.

~PROVERB

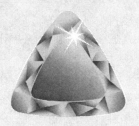

THE NINTH GEM—CITRINE

The ninth gemstone in your breastplate is citrine and reflects your ability to keep your body at its ideal weight. A citrine is one of only two stones that doesn't hold or accumulate negative energy, such as the negative energy and toxins that can store in excess fat. It enhances your solar plexus chakra—the center of your personal power and creativity. So, it can help you come up with creative ways to powerfully keep your body lean, healthy, and primed for extraordinary longevity.

A citrine is said to help dispel anger and fear, and bring emotional balance. Overcoming emotional issues is fundamentally important for anyone, including you, to successfully lose excess weight and keep it off. This gemstone is also recognized for aiding digestion and improving thyroid function—two extremely important factors to support a healthy metabolism and your ability to stay lean.

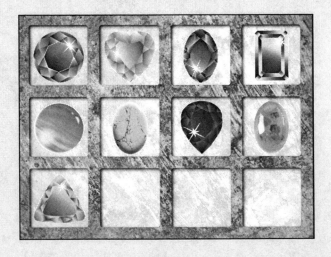

"He who lives with his senses well controlled, moderate in his food and drink, he will not be overthrown, any more than the wind throws down a rocky mountain."

~BUDDHA

When it comes to your good health and longevity, research shows that staying in an "ideal" weight range—weighing neither too much *nor* too little—is extremely important. In fact, being either considerably underweight or overweight is one of the greatest risk factors for poor health and a shortened lifespan.

It's no secret in this country that carrying too much weight is a far more common problem than carrying too little. Obesity is now an epidemic in the industrialized world. More than two-thirds of American adults and one-third of children are now considered overweight or obese. Consuming too many calories, especially from nutrient-depleted high carbohydrate foods such as sugary drinks, along with too little exercise are mostly to blame. Scientists believe there may also be other contributing factors—for example, toxins in your food. Studies show that being excessively overweight is one of the most serious risk factors for poor health. It increases many chronic diseases, including heart disease, diabetes, gall bladder disease, arthritis, dementia, and cancer—each of which contributes to an early death.

"Your body is a temple, not a drive-through."

~AUTHOR UNKNOWN

What Is the Purpose of Fat?

You may wish you didn't have it, but fat is essential for your body. It stores energy as lipids; stockpiles the essential fat-soluble vitamins A, D, E, and K for later use; insulates your body from the heat and cold; and cushions it from trauma. Fat is also necessary for milk production. Scientifically called "adipose tissue," you may not realize that fat is a major endocrine organ, producing several different hormones. After menopause, fat becomes the primary site for estrogen production. Fat also manufactures leptin—the hormones that stimulates hunger, as well as a cancer-fighting substance called "tumor necrosis factor-alpha" (TNF-[alpha]).

There are two categories of body fat: essential fat and storage fat. As its name implies, essential fat is necessary for the normal, healthy functioning of your body. It is stored in small amounts in your bone marrow, organs, central nervous system, and muscles. In men, essential fat makes up approximately 3 percent of body weight. Women, however, have a higher percentage of essential fat—about 12 percent. The additional amount of essential fat, found primarily in the breasts, pelvis, hips, and thighs, is believed to be critical for normal reproductive function. By contrast, men tend to store fat in their bellies due to the influence of different sex-specific hormones.

> *"No diet will remove all the fat from your body because the*
> *brain is entirely fat. Without a brain, you might look good,*
> *but all you could do is run for public office."*
>
> ~GEORGE BERNARD SHAW

Why Excess Belly Fat Is Dangerous

Where your excess fat is located is even more important than the total amount you have. Recent studies have shown that if you carry your extra fat around your waist, you are at a higher risk for developing the diseases mentioned earlier than if you carry the same amount of extra fat in your thighs and buttocks. When you have too much fat inside your abdomen, called "visceral fat" or "belly fat," it will cause your abdomen to protrude excessively, as it does in pregnancy.

Genetics, gender, and diet all play a role in causing belly fat. Men who consumes high-calorie, high-carbohydrate meals have the highest risk for developing belly fat. Drinking too much beer is also known to contribute— hence, the name "beer belly." Another major contributor is chronic stress. Chronic stress causes your cortisol levels to go up and stay up. Chronically high cortisol has many undesirable side effects, including causing your cells to become more resistant to insulin and encouraging the accumulation of fat in your abdomen.

Excess belly fat produces a variety of hormones, which increase your risk of chronic diseases. For instance, resistin is a hormone manufactured by belly fat, which causes your cells to become more insulin-resistant and, therefore, increases your risk of type 2 diabetes. Other hormones increase inflammation, so they raise your risk of inflammatory diseases, such as arthritis and dementia, as well as other obesity-related diseases. Belly fat also produces interleukin-6 (IL-6), a substance in your immune system that fuels chronic inflammation and cancer.

HEALTHY RANGE OF BODY FAT

AGE	FEMALE	MALE
18–39	21–32%	8–19%
40–59	23–33%	11–21%
60–79	24–35%	13–24%

The Importance of Lean Body Mass

Lean body mass is a term that describes all the muscles in your body, including your heart muscle, as well as the tissues of your other internal organs and your bones. It also includes all the water in your body. This is the part of your body you want to maintain or increase.

How much lean body mass you have is the most important factor in determining your metabolism (the rate at which you burn the calories). The more lean body mass you have, the higher your metabolic rate will be and the more calories you will burn when you are at rest. A higher metabolic rate makes it easier to maintain your weight. Strength training—also known as resistance training—is one of the best ways to increase your lean body mass.

What Happens When You Gain Weight?

When you gain weight as an adult, the volume of your lean body mass and fat both increase. The amount of fat you gain usually far exceeds the increase of your lean body mass. On average, the extra weight you gain is approximately 60 to 80 percent fat and 20 to 40 percent lean body mass.

Therefore, if you gained ten pounds, about six to eight pounds would be fat and two to four pounds would be lean body mass. There are exceptions to this rule, especially when you intentionally gain weight while participating in a training program specifically aimed at increasing your muscle mass, such as body building.

"Your stomach shouldn't be a waist basket."

~UNKNOWN

What Happens When You Lose Weight?

When you lose weight, you lose lean body mass, fat, and water. It is important to replace the water you lose by drinking plenty of purified water every day. The healthiest way to lose weight and maintain your metabolic rate is to preserve as much lean body mass as possible as you reduce your body fat. The best way to do this is to include strength training and to eat adequate amounts of lean protein.

BMI and Mortality

Studies throughout the world have examined the relationship between body mass index (BMI) and mortality in different age groups. Each of these studies has found the same pattern: Either being excessively underweight or overweight significantly increases your risk of early death. For example, a Norwegian study published in the *European Journal of Epidemiology* enrolled 5,653 individuals of various ages from 1965 to 1971 and then followed them until 2007. During that time, 66 percent of the study participants died. In the elderly, between the ages of sixty-five and seventy-five, the risk of death followed a U-shaped curve that was associated with their BMI. In other words, the more underweight or overweight a person was, the higher was his or her risk of dying. Interestingly, the highest mortality was seen in those who were the most underweight.

In another study, Chinese researchers also found a U-shaped curve for mortality in relationship to BMI for the middle aged and elderly. The lowest mortality occurred in those with a BMI between 23.6 and 26.2.

The National Cancer Institute published a meta-analysis in the December 2010 issue of the *New England Journal of Medicine,* which pooled the data from nineteen studies that focused on the relationship of BMI and mortality. The study was considered very large and, therefore, significant because it included a total of 1.46 million people. The researchers found that the healthiest BMI falls between 22.5 and 24.9. All-cause mortality was about 10 percent higher for those who were overweight compared to those who were normal weight. Morbid obesity—defined as a BMI of 40 or greater—was associated with a mortality rate that was 250 percent higher than those who were a healthy weight. Being underweight—a BMI less than 20—was also associated with higher mortality.

Defining Obesity—Body Mass Index (BMI)

Researchers use very specific measures to define a body as being overweight or obese. The measures include the BMI and the percentage of body fat. Your BMI is traditionally calculated by dividing your weight in kilograms by your height in meters squared. It can also be calculated by dividing your weight in pounds by your height in inches. Then, that number is divided by your height in inches again, and the result is multiplied by 703. The National Heart, Lung, and Blood Institute has a BMI calculator on its website (www.nhlbisupport.com/bmi/bmicalc.htm), so you don't have to do the math yourself. If you don't know how to convert your weight and height to metric measurements, that's okay; this website can calculate your BMI using standard American measurements.

Ideally, your BMI should be in the range of 18.5 to 24.9. If your BMI is greater than 25, you're considered overweight. If it's greater than 30, you're classified as obese. BMI, however, is not the best measure to determine if you're overweight or obese because it doesn't take body composition into account. Muscle weighs more than fat. For example, bodybuilders may weigh a lot for their height, but their above-normal weight is usually due to their large muscle mass, not excess fat. These toned athletes may have a BMI greater than 30, but they are certainly not obese.

Even more important than BMI is the measurement of waist circumference (WC) and waist-to-hip ratio. Both measure abdominal obesity, which research shows is associated with a higher mortality independent of BMI.

In a study 2010 published in the *Archives of Internal Medicine* by researchers at the American Cancer Society, 48,500 men and 56,343 women fifty years old and older were followed in the Cancer Prevention II Nutrition Cohort Study from 1997 to 2006. During that time, 9,315 men and 5,332 women died. Those who had very high waist circumferences—more than 47 inches in men and 43 inches for women—had a two times higher risk of mortality regardless of the BMI.

Percent Body Fat

A better way to determine whether you are overweight, obese, or just "solid" is to measure your percent body fat. This measurement is an assessment of your body composition. It evaluates how much of your weight is lean body mass (muscle, bones, and so on) and how much of it is actually fat. There are several different ways to get this measurement. The most accurate way involves completely submerging your body into a tank of water. This fairly expensive test measures the amount of water you displace in the tank and compares it to your height and weight. Fat is lighter than muscle. So pound for pound, fat takes up much more space than muscle. The more water you displace for your height and weight, the higher your percent of body fat.

Body fat can also be calculated by the method known as "bioelectrical impedance." This test is performed by passing a small, low-amp electrical current through your body and measuring the speed at which the current flows through you. Fat doesn't conduct electricity very well, but muscle does. So, the more fat tissue you have, the slower the current travels.

The simplest and least expensive way to measure percent body fat is to use a series of skin-fold measurements. However, calculating body fat using this technique has some limitations and is a lot less accurate than the other methods. The accuracy of this approach very much depends on the skill of the person doing the evaluation. Also, skin-fold measurements are unreliable for estimating the amount of body fat on people who are either extremely thin or very obese.

To calculate percent body fat using this technique, a caliper is used to measure the thickness of skin folds in several very specific areas of the body. The skin and the underlying fat are pinched into the caliper—a device that looks and feels a lot like a vise. Yes, sometimes it hurts a little bit. The thickness of each skin fold is read from the numbers on the caliper. After all the measurements are taken, they are added up and divided by the person's body weight. That number is then multiplied by a conversion factor to obtain the estimated percent body fat. Certified personal trainers are taught how to take these measurements as part of their certification training. Most gyms and fitness clubs have a personal trainer who can do these measurements for you. You can also make a rough approximation by yourself.

(Pages 217–219 adapted from *Waking the Warrior Goddess* by Christine Horner, M.D., used with permission of Basic Health Publications.)

CALCULATING A ROUGH ESTIMATE OF BODY FAT

There's a quick way that you can get a rough estimate of your percent body fat without using any fancy or expensive tests, and you can do it by yourself. It's not as accurate as the other techniques, but it will give you a ballpark figure. It involves a lot of simple measurements.

First, weigh yourself (in pounds) in the nude, and then multiply your total weight by 0.732. Take that number, and add 8.987. This number is your weight factor.

(your weight in pounds x 0.732) + 8.987 = weight factor

Then, measure your wrist in inches, and divide it by 3.140. This number is your wrist factor.

wrist measurement in inches / 3.140 = wrist factor

Next, measure your waist in inches at the navel, and multiply it by 0.157. This number is your waist factor.

waist measurement in inches x 0.157 = waist factor

Now, measure your hips, and multiply that number by 0.249. This number is your hip factor.

hips measurement in inches x 0.249 = hip factor

Measure the distance around your forearm, and multiply it by 0.434. This is your forearm factor.

forearm measurement in inches x 0.434 = forearm factor

Now, to calculate:

1. Take your weight factor, and add your wrist factor.
2. From that number, subtract your waist factor.
3. Take that number, and subtract your hip factor.
4. To that number, add your forearm factor. This number is your lean body mass.

**weight factor + wrist factor – waist factor – hip factor
+ forearm factor = lean body mass**

Next, take your total weight and subtract your lean body mass to get your amount of fat in pounds.

weight in pounds – lean body mass = fat in pounds

Now, multiply your fat in pounds by 100, and divide by your total body weight. This number is your percent BF.

(fat in pounds x 100) / weight in pounds = percent body fat

Adapted from *Dynamic Nutrition for Maximum Performance* by Daniel Gastelu and Dr. Frederick C. Hatfield (Avery Publishing Group, 1997) with permission.

"I never worry about diets. The only carrots that interest me are the number of carats in a diamond."

~MAE WEST

Chronic Diseases and Obesity

The reason carrying too much weight can shorten your life is that it is a major risk factor for a variety of chronic diseases, which are responsible for the majority of early deaths in this country. These diseases include all the top killers: cardiovascular diseases, which cause heart attacks and strokes;

type 2 diabetes; and cancers of the esophagus, uterus, breast, prostate, kidney, and colon. Obesity also increases the risk of gall bladder disease, dementia, osteoporosis, osteoarthritis, and macular degeneration (the leading cause of adult-onset blindness).

Cardiovascular Disease (CVD)

Researchers at the British Heart Foundation Glasgow Cardiovascular Research Centre followed 6,000 middle-aged men with high cholesterol, but no history of diabetes or cardiovascular disease for fifteen to twenty years. The results showed that the more a man weighed, the higher was his likelihood of having risk factors for cardiovascular disease. The risk of death was significantly elevated in men who were obese—defined as a BMI between 30 and 40.

According to a 2010 study by the Mayo Clinic, a weight gain as little as nine pounds can cause changes to the endothelial cells lining the arteries, which increase the risk of cardiovascular disease and mortality—even in those who are young and healthy.

When it comes to life expectancy, being overweight is just as detrimental as smoking. The Framingham Study found that nonsmokers who were overweight (BMI 25–30) at age forty lost three years to their life expectancy. Those men and women who were obese (BMI>30) lost seven years. Smoking causes a similar reduction in life expectancy. Individuals who are overweight and smoke lose thirteen to fourteen years of life compared to healthy-weight nonsmokers.

Researchers from Dublin, Ireland, discovered one reason why obesity can shorten your life. They found that excess weight causes a reduction in the number and function of natural killer (NK) cells. NK cells provide a major defense against cancer and pathogens, such as bacteria and viruses. Smoking also debilitates your NK cells. If you are obese and smoke, your diet and lifestyle choices cause your immune function to be so compromised that your life expectancy drops by fourteen years.

Another reason obesity shortens your lifespan is that the vast majority of those who are obese live a sedentary lifestyle and, as a consequence, also have a low level of fitness. Low fitness significantly increases your risk of cardiovascular disease and all-cause mortality. Researchers at the Cooper Institute for Aerobic Research in Dallas, Texas, published a study in the

Journal of the American Medical Association in 1999, which followed 25,714 men for twenty years. They found that 50 percent of the obese men in the study also had low fitness, which caused their risk of cardiovascular disease mortality to increase by 39 percent and to increase from all causes by 44 percent.

Cancer

Numerous studies show a clear correlation between obesity and cancer, including a November 2010 report by the American Institute of Cancer Research. In fact, obesity is thought to contribute to more than 100,000 cancer cases in the U.S. every year. Researchers point out that obesity causes low-grade inflammation, as well as increased production of hormones and insulin resistance—all of which are associated with an increased risk of cancer.

A 2006 study on mice found yet another reason why obesity increases the risk of cancer: Fat may decrease the body's ability to kill off cancer. Rutgers University scientists found that fat cells may secrete substances that block one of the body's main antitumor defenses—apoptosis. Apoptosis is a process where cancer cells autodestruct. When apoptosis is blocked, cancer cells can continue to grow unimpeded.

Type 2 Diabetes

The link between obesity and type 2 diabetes is very strong. Of all the people diagnosed with type 2 diabetes, about 80 to 90 percent are overweight. Being overweight causes several physiological changes that increase your risk of diabetes. First, it causes your cells to become more resistant to insulin, which raises your blood glucose levels. Next, excess fat—especially around your abdomen—is known to increase the production of inflammatory proteins, and inflammation is a major contributor to diabetes. Lastly, excess calories are thought to damage the cells in the pancreas, which produce insulin, adding to your risk of developing diabetes.

Dementia

Obesity, especially abdominal obesity, during middle age is associated with a high risk of developing dementia. A large French Study found that older people with larger waist lines, high blood pressure, and other risk factors associated with metabolic syndrome were 20 percent more likely to have cognitive decline on a memory test. In another study conducted by researchers at Boston University School of Medicine in 2010, excess abdominal fat was found to cause otherwise healthy middle-aged people to be at higher risk for dementia later in life. The researchers found an inverse association between BMI and brain volumes. In other words, as your weight increases, the size of your brain shrinks. The smaller your brain becomes, the higher will be your risk of dementia. Abdominal obesity increases your risk of dementia and Alzheimer's disease even more than your BMI does.

Weight Loss and Longevity

You would probably think that losing your extra weight would help you to live longer. Surprisingly, studies show it may not. However, losing excess weight can tremendously improve and even cure many chronic diseases, such as high blood pressure or diabetes. If you are overweight, the best way to improve your chances for a long, healthy life is not weight loss, but rather exercising and achieving a state of good cardiorespiratory fitness—the subject of chapter 6—as well as eating a healthy diet.

Obesity: Not Just About Calories

You might assume that obesity is simply the result of eating too many calories and not getting enough activity. But researchers are finding that there are a variety of factors that may also contribute significantly to the condition—from biology, physiology, psychology, genetics, and the environment. In a study published in the February 2011 issue of *Journal of Obesity,* Italian researchers found that regularly eating at restaurants, sleeping too few hours, and keeping your house at a higher temperature also contributed to obesity.

The genes that make you prone to drug addictions may also cause you to overeat. According to a study published in 2011, rich food activates the same pleasure centers of the brain as heroine or cocaine. Other studies show that these pleasure centers become "tolerant" to food just as they do to drugs. Just as an addict over time requires higher doses of drugs to stimulate the same amount of pleasure, overeaters require increasing amounts of food to feel the same amount of emotional satisfaction. Another gene—NRXN3—plays a role in substance abuse and has also been associated with obesity.

Adding to the difficulty of obesity are the hormones and neurotransmitters that not only contribute this condition but also can cause depression. If you struggle with obesity, studies show that the chances are very high that you may frequently feel sadness, self-loathing, disgust, and frustration. All of these emotions can make it much more difficult for you to successfully lose weight.

Your friends and family might also be adding to your weight issues. According to studies, the more obese friends you have, the more likely you are to become obese. A 2010 Harvard study found that if you have four obese friends, your chances of becoming obese are twice as high when compared to someone who has no obese friends. The influence of having just one friend, sibling, or a spouse who is obese is so significant that, according to an earlier Harvard study, your chances of becoming overweight greatly increase.

When it comes to bedtime, early to bed and early to rise may not only help you to be healthy, wealthy, and wise, but it can also help your waistline. Staying up too late at night can lead to significant weight gain and obesity. Research shows there are a variety of factors caused by staying up too late at night that contribute to obesity. For example, one of the most significant factors has to do with the timing of your meals. In an October 2010 study published in the *Proceedings of the National Academy of Science*, researchers at Ohio State University found that light at night increased the body mass of animals by shifting the time of food intake to the nighttime.

If you eat at a time when you should be sleeping instead, your body does not metabolize your food calories the same way it does during the day. That's because your hormone levels begin to shift significantly after 10 p.m., which encourage your cells to shut down to rest and detoxify. During the night, your cells give their full attention to these essential nocturnal rejuvenating processes. They aren't distracted with other tasks that they do during the day, particularly the function of bringing in glucose and converting it to energy. To avoid this daytime task during the night, your cells become resistant to insulin. If you eat when your cells are resistant to insulin, it causes your blood glucose and insulin levels to rise. So instead of being used for energy, the calories you consume at night go straight to fat. Not only does your risk of obesity increase, but high glucose and insulin levels also increase your risk of diabetes.

When it comes to weight loss, the total number of hours you sleep is also very important. A study published in the *International Journal of Obesity* in 2011 followed 470 patients in a weight-loss program at Kaiser Permanente Center for Health Research in Portland, Oregon, for six months. The researchers found that those who slept between six and eight hours a night had less stress, were less depressed, and were more successful at weight loss.

Toxins—Not Calories

If you are active and you don't overeat, yet you are still overweight, a slow metabolism may not be the only explanation. In an article published in the *Journal of Complementary and Alternative Medicine* in 2002, author Paula Baillie-Hamilton presented a new theory about the epidemic of obesity. She said that the amount of obesity that exists in the world today can't be explained by increased calories and sedentary lives alone. She contends that toxins in the environment and in the food you eat may play a significant role in disrupting your body's weight-control mechanisms.

Toxins block the intelligence of your body in many ways. The intelligence that manages weight control seems to be particularly vulnerable to toxins. Growth promoters and hormones are given to animals to fatten them up and to increase the amount of milk they produce. When you eat these animals or drink their milk, you also consume the growth promoters. If these substances put weight on animals, you can be sure that they also put weight on you.

In addition, a variety of synthetic pharmaceutical drugs, including certain antidepressants, anticonvulsants, antihistamines, nonsteroidal anti-inflammatories, antipsychotics, and hormones have been found to cause weight gain. Moreover, studies show that pesticides may cause abnormal weight gain; in fact, animals exposed to pesticides can have *huge* weight gains. In one study, despite no increase in their caloric intake, the body weight of the animals that were given pesticides doubled! Researchers cut the calories in half for other animals that were fed pesticides, and they still gained weight! Numerous studies have shown that animals exposed to environmental estrogens in utero have a higher incidence of reproductive problems and obesity later in life. Epidemiological studies support that exposure to these toxins while in the womb has the same effects in humans.

At low concentrations, all the chemicals listed below have been shown to powerfully promote weight gain:

- Carbamates (a type of insecticide)
- Heavy metals (such as cadmium and lead)
- Pesticides (organochlorines, DDT, lindane, endrin, and hexachlorobenzene)
- Plastics (phthalates and bisphenol A)
- Polybrominated biphenyls (used as a fire retardant)
- Polychlorinated biphenyls (PCBs)
- Solvents (octachlorostyrene, decalin, benzene, toluene, 1,1,1-trichloroethane, and trichloroethylene benzene)

A study conducted at Boston University in 2010 published in the *International Journal of Andrology* found an association between endocrine-disrupting chemicals and obesity. The researchers found that as the level of phthalates (endocrine-disrupting chemicals commonly found in plastics) increased in adult test subjects, especially men, so did their BMI and waist circumference.

Certain food additives, such as MSG, can also increase your risk of obesity. In a 2008 study conducted by the University of North Carolina Gillings School of Global Public Health, reported in the journal *Obesity,* researchers found that those who use MSG as a flavor enhancer are more likely to be overweight and obese than those who don't use it—even though they have the same amount of physical activity and total caloric intake. The study analyzed 750 Chinese men and women, aged forty to fifty-nine. About 82 percent used MSG in their foods. Those who used the most MSG were nearly three times more likely to be overweight when compared to the non-users.

You can reduce the level of toxins in your body by avoiding them. Always choose organically grown and produced foods, as well as nontoxic cleaning agents and personal-care products, and don't store or microwave your foods in plastic. Regular detoxification, which was discussed in the previous chapter, can help to get these toxins out.

How Metabolism Effects Weight

Metabolism refers to the chemical process that your body employs to extract the calories and nutrients it needs to function from your food. It involves a myriad of enzymes that break down proteins, carbohydrates, and fats. Your metabolic rate refers to how fast you burn the calories from your food. The same factors that influence your weight—for example, genetics, diet, digestion, lifestyle, quality of sleep, toxins, relationships, and stress—also influence your metabolism. They can either stoke the fires of your metabolism or throw retardant on it.

Your metabolism is also influenced by your age and gender. As you age, your metabolic rate slows down. Around age twenty-five, the average person's metabolism begins to decline by 5 to 10 percent per decade—which means you will lose between 20 percent and 40 percent of your metabolic power over the course of your adult lifespan. After age thirty, one of the main reasons that your metabolism slows down is due to the decrease of your muscle mass. Muscle burns more calories than fat. Most people lose 3 to 8 percent of their muscle mass per decade. So, as you age, to maintain a stable weight, you must lower your caloric intake and continue or increase physical activity—especially aerobics and strength training.

Even if you have a genetic predisposition to obesity, one of the best tools to keep your weight down is to move your body. A 2010 study tracked the physical activity levels of 20,430 people in Great Britain with twelve genetic variants known to increase the risk of obesity. The researchers found that physical activity—just thirty minutes a day of brisk walking—reduced the genetic tendency toward obesity by 40 percent.

The average man's metabolism is about 10 to 15 percent higher than a woman's, mainly because of his greater muscle mass. A woman's body also has a higher percent of low-calorie-burning body fat, the purpose of which is to support a healthy pregnancy. That's why, in general, men have the seemingly unfair advantage of being able to eat more than most women and can lose weight faster. If you are obese, biological changes can occur that affect your metabolism and can make it much harder for you to lose weight.

What Is the Best Method to Lose Weight?

The greatest success for weight loss comes from combining a healthy low-calorie diet with exercise. You'll be disappointed with your results if you only do one approach without the other. The best programs for losing weight also help you to lose the highest percentage of fat you can, while at the same time preserving your lean body mass. A balanced healthy diet with portion control combined with physical activity that includes aerobics and strength training to build or preserve muscle is considered ideal.

The average amount of weight loss should be no more than two pounds a week. If the calories you eat are too low and you lose weight too fast, you will lose a greater percentage of lean body mass than is desirable. This, in turn, will lower your metabolic rate and conflict with your goal. Some dietary strategies may allow you to lose pounds faster; however, they promote the loss of both lean body mass and body water. Therefore, even though the number of pounds you lose may be higher, you will be losing the wrong type of weight.

Not only does a program that combines diet and exercise help you to lose weight, but according to a study published in *New England Journal of Medicine* in 2011, it will also significantly improve your overall physical function, balance, strength, and quality of life.

> *"The biggest seller is cookbooks and the second*
> *is diet books—how not to eat what you've*
> *just learned how to cook."*
>
> ~ANDY ROONEY

The following are 55 healthy tips and tricks to help you lose weight:

1. **Eat your main meal at noon.** Your "digestive fires" are at their peak from 10 a.m. to 2 p.m. That means you are able to digest the food you eat better in the middle of the day than you can early in the morning or late at night. Shoot for consuming 50 percent of your daily calories with your noon meal.

2. **Eat sitting down.** When you eat standing up, you tend to eat faster, chew less, and become distracted—all of which are not good for digestion. Blood flow to your stomach and intestines, which is essential for good digestion, is better when sitting.

3. **Eat in a calm environment.** When your environment is loud, aggravating, or chaotic, stress hormones are released that impede your digestion. Soothing music, delightful conversations, and a beautiful setting have the opposite effect.

4. **Eat to three-quarters of your capacity.** This great rule of thumb keeps you from eating too much. You cannot digest well when you've packed too much in. Excess calories are a major cause of obesity, diabetes, heart disease, and many types of cancer.

5. **Chew well.** Chewing is the first stage of digestion. Your saliva contains enzymes that begin to break down your food. The better you chew your food, the easier it is for the rest of your digestive tract to do its job.

6. **Eat slowly (set a timer for 20 minutes).** Research shows that you eat less and digest your food better when you take more time to eat. The tricks: savoring each bite, chewing your food thoroughly, putting your fork down between bites, and taking a rest.

7. **Nix iced drinks.** Chilly fluids put out your digestive fires and freeze the power of your enzymes. Avoid drinking too much fluid with meals; it dilutes the strength of the enzymes in your stomach. Limit your liquids to small sips—room temperature or warm is best.

8. **Wait at least three hours between meals.** Give your previous meal plenty of time to digest. Eating again too soon stresses your system. If you are tempted to reach for food before three hours after your last meal—go for a walk, get up and dance, or drink a glass of water instead.

9. **Favor lightly cooked foods.** Lightly cooking your food breaks it down, making it easier to digest. In a study comparing the amount of nutrients absorbed, this method came out on top when compared to eating

raw foods. Don't overcook! Excess cooking destroys important vitamins and antioxidants, and creates toxic substances.

10. **Favor fresh organically grown plants.** Fresh organic vegetables, fruits, whole grains, nuts, and seeds are packed with vitamins, minerals, and essential nutrients, making them powerful natural plant-medicines. They also contain lots of fiber, which is crucial for good digestion, absorption, and elimination.

11. **Put your full attention on your meal.** At mealtime, focus on your food. Don't watch TV, read, or text your friends. The more you pay attention to what and how you eat, the less you are likely to eat too much and the easier your food will digest.

12. **Avoid pesticides and toxins in foods and household products.** Studies show that certain toxins found in your food, environment, and home cause you to gain weight. Mice exposed to toxins gained twice as much weight eating half the amount of food. Eat only organic foods—it's worth the extra cost. Make sure all the products you bring into your home are nontoxic, especially household cleaners and personal-care products.

13. **Eat with the seasons.** You were designed to flow with the rhythms of nature: daily, monthly, and seasonally. Your body works best if you consume the foods that grow locally and naturally in each season. Best place to find them: your own garden or your local farmer's market. In the spring, favor asparagus, baby greens, morel mushrooms, and strawberries. In the heat of the summer, add zucchini, tomatoes, cucumbers, avocados, peaches, plums, and blueberries. As the leaves begin to turn and the nights become cooler, favor beets, broccoli, Brussels sprouts, cabbage, sweet potatoes, apples, and grapes. When the days become shorter and the air cold and crisp, keep warm and energized with hearty bean soups, winter squash, and kale.

14. **Get the toxins out.** Your body accumulates toxins from your food and environment. It also clogs up with debris from poorly digested foods, stress, inactivity, and staying up too late. For your body to hum, it's important to get those toxins out, flush your system, and open all the

channels. To kick start your body's own detox systems, veto the meat, chips, and alcohol. Instead, sip warm water and herbal teas throughout the day; favor fresh, organic, lightly cooked plants; move your body; and go to bed by 10 p.m. For a super cleanse, take a week or so to go to a purification spa. You won't believe how great you will look and feel!

15. **Sip hot water throughout the day.** Deceptively simple, but enormously powerful, frequent sips of hot water keeps your digestive tract moving and helps to flush out toxins. Instead of plain water, make your own detox tea with a half teaspoon each of the whole seeds of cumin, coriander, and fennel. Boil the seeds for five minutes in four to five cups of purified water, strain, and put in a Thermos. Many have been surprised to find pounds shedding, skin brightening, and digestion improving in no time.

16. **Go to bed by 10 p.m. and get up by 6 a.m.** Recommended by *Ayurveda* for 5,000 years, research confirms that these are the optimal hours to sleep. Your body rests and purifies during the night. Those who stay up too late and cut their sleep short obstruct this essential process. The risk of life-threatening illnesses, including heart disease, diabetes, obesity, and cancer, nearly doubles in those who stay up past midnight!

17. **Move your body every day.** Eighty percent of us do not get enough exercise for optimum health. Your body is designed to move. Regular exercise—even brisk walking—is extraordinary medicine. Not only does it help you to lose weight by burning more calories and sparking your metabolism, research shows it strengthens your organs and activates genes that help keep you healthy and encourage longevity. Just thirty minutes of activity a day can boost your mood, improve sleep, and lower your risk of chronic diseases, such as heart disease, dementia, and cancer.

18. **Spice up your life.** Spices aren't just for flavoring. Each one contains special medicines, including those that help you to lose weight by balancing fat and sugar metabolism while curbing carb cravings. Gymnema, fennel, cinnamon, and cardamom are good examples. Rev up your digestion by cooking with asafoetida (hing), black pepper, and turmeric.

19. **Avoid sugar, corn syrup, and fructose.** Dense in empty calories, these sweeteners pack on the pounds and fuel inflammation. In a meta-analysis published in 2008, researchers reviewed hundreds of studies, pooled all the data, and concluded that "high blood glucose is a universal mechanism for chronic disease progression." In other words, eating too many refined carbs and sugars fuels the progression of *every* chronic disease!

20. **Whack out whites.** Eliminate white rice, white bread, white pasta, white fries, and processed foods using white flour and sugar (pastries, cookies, and crackers). These refined carbohydrates are metabolized exactly as sugar and share all of its dangerous health effects.

21. **Avoid processed foods, junk foods, and foods that are deep fried or frozen.** These foods are nutrient depleted, calorie rich, laden with potentially dangerous additives, and lifeless. Fresh organic vegetables, fruits, whole grains, nuts, and seeds have the opposite qualities, which your body craves: nutrient dense, calorie light, no harmful chemicals, and filled with life-sustaining energy.

22. **Include all six tastes in each meal.** *Ayurveda* says a balance in the six tastes—sweet, salty, pungent, sour, astringent, and bitter—creates balance in your body and enhances your body's inner healing intelligence. Consuming mostly sweet and salty—an American diet faux pas—causes imbalances and obstructs the flow of intelligence, making you more prone to ill health.

23. **Massage yourself using a raw silk glove.** This *Ayurvedic* technique, called *garshan*, is prescribed to help with weight loss. The friction of the gloves stimulates circulation, lymphatic flow, and the release of weight-promoting toxins.

24. **Protect against stress.** Chronic stress causes the release of cortisol, which has dangerous side effects, including weight gain, high blood pressure, and diabetes. Research shows that you can minimize the release of stress hormones with the daily practice of an effective stress-reducing technique such as meditation, breathing exercises, yoga, or tai chi. A study in 1996 found that practicing Transcendental Medita-

tion (a specific type of meditation discussed earlier) just twenty minutes, twice a day, cuts the risk of most chronic diseases by more than 50 percent and cardiovascular disease by 87 percent!

25. **Get out in nature.** A walk in nature is a great way to alleviate stress and burn more calories. The color green in grass, trees, and plants has been shown to lessen depression, anxiety, and nervousness.

26. **Keep a regular routine.** Your body loves a schedule. If you wake up, eat, exercise, and go to bed around the same time every day, your body will learn to anticipate those activities. It sets up a wave you can ride to glide through each activity with the greatest of ease and the least amount of stress.

27. **Discover your triggers.** Anxiety, boredom, and depression are common triggers for "emotional" eating—which usually involves high-calorie "comfort" foods. Notice which emotions send you to the chip bag or the cookie jar. Next time that emotion causes the urge to snack—choose a healthier non-caloric approach. Call a friend, go for a walk, take a nap, drink a cup of soothing herbal tea, or turn on your favorite music and dance.

28. **Invite good bugs.** There are good guys and bad guys—microbes—that live in your intestines and profoundly influence your health. Supporting the good guys and discouraging the bad guys is crucial for good health. Healthy bacteria have many functions, including supporting your metabolism and helping you to lose excess weight. A 2012 study found that obese individuals given probiotics to increase the amount of healthy bacteria in their colons experienced weight loss and improved metabolism.

29. **Fill up with fiber.** Consuming plenty of fiber—at least 25 grams per day for women and 38 grams for men—curbs hunger, favors beneficial gut bacteria, slows the absorption of sugar, keeps things moving through your system, and improves digestion and fat metabolism. Here's the secret: Fiber is only found in plants. Another reason to eat your fruits, vegetables, whole grains, nuts, and seeds!

30. **Practice portion control.** Supersize meals will turn you into a super-size! The French are famously thinner due to one major factor: Their portions are routinely smaller than the usual American's. Always order the smallest size in restaurants. At home, use a smaller plate, measure your portions, and serve your meal on a single plate. Don't serve from a bowl on the table where second and third helpings are hard to resist.

31. **Keep a notepad with you.** Write down everything you eat, when you eat, what you eat, and how you are feeling. Most people can't remember everything they eat throughout the day. If you can't understand why you aren't losing weight, it may be because you are eating more calories a day than you think. By writing down everything you eat, you can become more conscious of what you eat. You might be surprised at how much you "unconsciously" snack.

32. **Eat five to six small meals a day.** Smaller meals keep your blood sugar stable and prevent excess hunger that can lead to overeating. Weight lifters use this trick to decrease their body fat and build or keep lean muscle.

33. **Park your car as far away as possible.** Finding simple ways to get more exercise and burn more calories each day adds up. Take the stairs at work several times a day. Clean your own house. Walk during your lunch hour.

34. **Don't sit too long.** Get up every hour. Not only do you burn fewer calories when sitting, but research shows that sitting for too long causes a variety of health problems. Sitting more than five hours on a regular basis—even if you exercise every day—is so damaging to your health that it can shorten your life!

35. **Pump some iron.** Strengthening and building your muscles by weight lifting can boost your metabolism and promote weight loss at the same time. Muscle burns four times more calories than fat. Lift weights at least three times a week for the best results.

36. **Get a buddy.** Research shows that exercise and weight loss programs are far more successful if you buddy up. It's easy to talk yourself out of walking or going to your exercise class. But if you have a buddy, the

chances are great you will show up even if you don't feel like it. Checking in with a buddy online about your weight-loss progress has been shown to make a difference.

37. **Wear a pedometer.** Ideally you want to walk 10,000 steps per day—which is equivalent to about four to five miles. A pedometer is a great way to keep track and to let you know when you need to take an extra lap around the block before you settle in for the evening.

38. **Color your plates red.** Swiss researchers found in a 2012 study that participants drank less from a red-labeled cup than from a blue-labeled cup, and ate less snack food from a red plate than from a blue or white plate. The researchers concluded that, "The color red causes people to eat and drink less because it functions as a subtle stop signal."

39. **Eat water-rich vegetables at beginning of a meal.** Vegetables with high water content such as cucumbers, tomatoes, lettuce, and celery are low in calories and can fill you up. Eat a fresh salad or vegetable-broth based soup before your main course to curb your appetite.

40. **Switch from fancy coffee to ordinary coffee.** A Frappuccino with whipped cream might be your favorite coffee drink, but the calorie count is many times greater than a cup of plain Joe. Switching back to the low-calorie variety will help your pocketbook and your waistline.

41. **Watch hidden calories.** Condiments—particularly mayonnaise, sour cream, and salad dressing—are a hidden source of calories. Instead, use mustard or place silken tofu in a blender for a delicious mayo substitute. Make your own salad dressing vinaigrette with healthy ingredients, such as balsamic vinegar and olive oil. Add some zip with low-calorie salsa and hot sauce.

42. **Eat whole fruit instead of fruit juice.** Whole fruit contains fiber, which slows down the absorption of the natural sugars found in fruits and, at the same time, fills you up. Fruit juices tend to be high in calories because it takes a lot of fruit to make a cup of juice, and sugar is added to most commercial fruit juices. Because juice doesn't contain fiber, the sugar it contains rapidly absorbs into your blood and stores as fat.

43. **Limit alcohol.** Alcohol has more calories than carbohydrates. One gram of alcohol has seven calories and one gram of carbs contains only four. Alcoholic fruit drinks are packed with sugar and calories. A twelve-ounce piña colada, for example, typically has over 500 calories!

44. **Walk before dinner.** A trip around the block can triple your metabolic rate. This boost continues after you stop moving and may help to curb your appetite.

45. **Plan your meals.** Selecting exactly what you will eat for a meal stops you from grabbing for high-calorie snacks when you get hungry. Make a list when you go to the grocery store. Make sure you have just eaten so that you aren't hungry when you shop. Walking into a store while you are hungry makes everything look too good and too tempting!

46. **Don't keep unhealthy snacks in the house.** Plan your snacks too. Keep cut fresh veggies or a serving of nuts, such as almonds, in a snack bag.

47. **Stay hydrated.** Sometimes you feel hungry when what you really need is more hydration. Try drinking a cup of water when hungry between meals.

48. **Take an omega-3 fatty acid supplement daily.** According to researchers at the University of Ontario, omega-3's dramatically boost your metabolism—by as much as 400 calories a day. Make sure to take a high-quality organic supplement, such as Barlean's Omega Swirls.

49. **Make love!** It's great exercise, reduces stress, decreases hunger, and boosts your immune system and your mood.

50. **Weigh yourself once a week.** Studies show that those who check their weight regularly tend to lose more and maintain a healthier weight.

51. **Get enough vitamin D.** The sunshine vitamin controls hundreds of functions in your body. Low levels raise your risk of dozens of diseases, including cancer, dementia, and multiple sclerosis. According to a 2013 study, lower levels of vitamin D are also a potential risk factor for obesity and type 2 diabetes. Russian researchers found that low vitamin D levels correlated with excessive body fat, high glucose levels, and decreased insulin sensitivity. Most experts say healthy people need at least 2,000 IU per day. If you are sick, you may need more.

52. **Buy a fabulous outfit that is slightly too small.** It's great incentive. Give away your fat clothes. You'll be more motivated to keep the weight off if gaining the weight back means you'll have to buy a whole new wardrobe!

53. **Don't skip meals or fast for long periods.** Starvation diets never work in the long run. Researchers at Appalachian State University in Boone, North Carolina, found that metabolism falls by 15 to 20 percent when you drop your calories to only 400–800 per day. Eating fewer than 900 calories a day also prompts your body to burn muscle tissue as well as fat, which lowers your metabolic rate even more. Stick with 1,200–1,500 calories a day to slim down and keep your metabolism up.

54. **Get the help you need.** Changing your diet and lifestyle isn't easy—especially when you are trying to do it alone. Don't be afraid to get help. Hire a personal trainer. See a therapist to help you with emotional issues that might be obstructing your weight-loss success.

55. **Track and celebrate your success.** Measuring your progress and tracking your success with pictures and journal can help keep you motivated. Reward yourself for every step. Get a massage or a pedicure, buy a new workout outfit, get a makeover, and throw a party!

If you are overweight or obese, it is very important to lose the extra weight so that you can lower your risk of debilitating chronic diseases. Losing weight can also give you more energy and vitality, and increase your chances of living a long, healthy life. Most people find that they are able to lose weight more effectively and keep it off if they use a variety of tips listed above. Enrolling your significant other, family, and friends to help you or to help each other is another great way to ensure your success.

Remember that the most important factors for losing weight are your diet and exercise. Doing one without the other won't work. You can run a marathon and still not burn off all the calories you may have consumed in a supersized meal. Portion control and nutrient-dense, low-calorie fresh foods, along with daily exercise are the essential keys for achieving and maintain a healthy weight.

Try as many of these tips as possible and track your success. You might be surprised at how easy it is to speed up your metabolism, drop those extra pounds, and feel energized. Soon you'll find that you're wearing the clothes you never thought you'd get back into, while feeling and looking better than ever.

CHAPTER 10

Good Vibrations

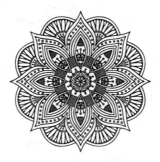

The Electrical Body and Energy Medicine

In every culture and in every medical tradition before ours, healing was accomplished by moving energy.

~ALBERT SZENT-GYÖRGYI, NOBEL LAUREATE IN MEDICINE

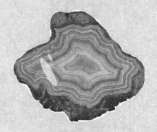

THE TENTH GEM—AGATE

An agate is a stone that can help stabilize your aura, or energetic biofield, which is why it is the tenth stone in your breastplate. In essence, it is a form of subtle energy medicine that can help to balance your physical, mental, and emotional energy.

An agate is said to smooth dysfunctional energy, and transform and eliminate negative energy. When negative energy is removed from your biofield, it can correct energetic abnormalities that can lead to disease. During times of physical "biorhythmic lows," an agate can be helpful in bringing your physical energy into a balanced and steady state, which is the goal of all subtle energy techniques.

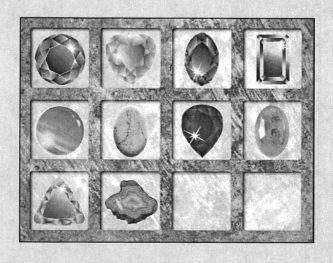

"I think that energy and the use of energy healing will be the biggest frontier in medicine over the next decade."

~DR. MEHMET OZ, CARDIOVASCULAR SURGEON
AND TELEVISION HOST

*E*nergy medicine involves the use of subtle energy techniques to rebalance your body, mind, and emotions, and strengthen your body's ability to heal itself. Because the techniques use only subtle energy, the influence they may have might logically seem small. But quite the contrary is often true. Their effects can be profound. These techniques may seem mysterious given that the way they work is invisible. However, with the aid of a variety of devices, their unseen influence can be made clearly visible and measured.

You actually are already very aware of the electrical nature of your body because of commonly prescribed Western medical tests. When you think of an EKG of your heart, what does it measure? The electrical activity of your heart. An EEG? The electrical activity of your brain.

Energy medicine can be easily understood through simple explanations that are based in physics. Your body is "bioelectric," which means it uses biochemistry *and* electricity to function. Research has focused mainly on the biochemical nature of your body, yet scientists have discovered that your body is governed just as much by its electric nature. Electricity conducted through nerve impulses can carry messages to all the cells in your body and influence their behavior, including those in your immune system. It can even directly affect your DNA and the messages your genes send out.

In addition, the cells in your body have polarities in their cell membranes that create electromagnetism. They are constantly taking in energy and releasing energy. This energy exchange creates oscillations, frequencies, and wave forms, which produce a measurable field, called a "bioelectric field" around your body. This energetic field also produces light. Throughout recorded history, there have been references to the observance of light emitting from the human body. In fact, a significant number of people alive today have the "gift" of being able to see the light of the energetic fields around others.

For the majority of us who do not have this gift, devices have been

241

invented to allow us to see it. The very first photograph of light emissions from the human body was taken in England in 1910 with a colored glass filter. In 1940 in Germany, De La Mar built the first "radionics recorder," which was able to measure the energy released by living tissue. Colored pictures of the energetic field were developed in Russia in 1939, called "Kirlian photography." These images document fluctuations of the energetic field in size, strength, and color that correspond to different emotional states.

In a laboratory at UCLA in the 1960s, Professor Valerie Hunt, Ph.D., used instruments similar to those used to record brain, heart, and muscle waves of astronauts in space to record, for the first time, the electromagnetic vibration emitted from the human body. In the 1970s, she helped to develop a more sophisticated high-frequency device known as the Aura-Meter to measure the human electric field. She continued her research for decades on what she described as, "the relationship between energy field disturbances, disease, emotional pathologies, human field communication and the energy spectrum of consciousness."

Her research revealed that specific fluctuations in human energy fields occur with different emotions, diseases, and the experience of pain. If you are in a state of ordinary consciousness, the energy coming from your brain and nervous system is in the lower frequency range up to 250 Hz. If you are in an altered state, such as hypnotic, or in a meditative or metaphysical reality, the frequency you emit may be as high as 400 Hz or even higher. Those individuals who are considered "mystics" because they have a profound spiritual connection, extraordinary insights, and wisdom, as well as a "non-ordinary reality" (commonly referred to as "psychic" capabilities), were found to emit frequencies that were as high as the machines were capable of measuring—1,000 times higher than those in ordinary reality. Researchers report that they, as well as others, are able to see or sense a powerful white light emanating from these individuals.

You might think that the higher the frequency you emit, the better it might be for your physical, mental, emotional, and spiritual health. But, interestingly, Dr. Hunt found that for optimal health, you have to be able to express the full spectrum of frequencies. In an interview by Larry Triv posted on the Wordpress website "Health on the Edge," Dr. Hunt explained:

"First, for optimal health to exist, the field has to be very broad-spectrum and adaptive. Some of the people we test have electromagnetic energy that is in the middle of the spectrum and is truncated there. They can't go very high, and they can't go very low. They seem to dribble through life and struggle. Then there are the people, such as those who practice certain types of meditation, whose frequencies are extremely high, so that if something happens in the world, they don't respond on the middle or lower branches. They respond on the upper branches. They have a certain kind of peace, yet they often die of hypotension (low blood pressure) or cancer, because they don't have enough vital energy. And then there are some people who are in the lower ranges, which means they don't have the high frequencies, but they have a heck of a lot of energy. They can do things that the rest of us can't physically do even if we push ourselves to exercise and build more strength. These are the people who have difficulty with hypertension, skin conditions, anything that is hyper or excessive in terms of imbalances. The ideal field is one that has the low frequencies, the middle frequencies, the higher frequencies, and no major break in between any of them, so that they can play the total range of the piano, as it were.

The next parameter is power. Power is a quantitative measurement. You may have the complete frequency range, but the only place you have power is in certain aspects of that range. That's where you operate from because that's where you've got power. If you have power in the lower ranges, you will be physically active, and have vital dynamic life. I'm 85 and nobody knows it. I have lower frequencies and this keeps cells and organs working and keeps me looking younger. If you have great frequency in the middle ranges, you can easily handle intellectual issues and can solve problems. If you have power in the upper ranges, you can go into higher states of consciousness, find wisdom and have levels of thought, which are conceptual. But the ideal is to have power within the entire spectrum of frequencies."

(*Source: http://bit.ly/1MkTyxO*)

Dr. Hunt died twelve years after this interview in 2014 at the age of ninety-seven.

Frequency Medicine

Your energy field can be manipulated through a variety of different techniques and devices to help restore it back to normal. All the techniques and devices that work with the energy in your body to help you heal fall under "Frequency Medicine." When the abnormalities in your energy field are corrected, the receptors on your cells will fire optimally, which causes your immune system to become stronger and your genetic code to send messages for good health. It also triggers your unhealthy cells to begin to oscillate at a healthier frequency, which helps to restore them to normal function.

A variety of computerized devices have been developed, which can record the energy patterns in your body. Like a lie detector, the machine sends out questions to your body as energetic wave forms. All the possible wave forms that are associated with imbalances of your organs and emotions can be sent from the computer into your body. Waveforms can also be sent for various toxins, unfriendly bacteria, and viruses. Each time an abnormality is found, the computer is able to determine what it is and what remedy pattern will neutralize or correct it. All the energy disturbances are recorded along with the recommended remedies to correct them. For example, if an emotional issue is found, a Bach Flower Remedy may be recommended to correct it. Or if a weakness in your liver is revealed, milk thistle or dandelion root may be recommended.

Some devices have the ability to send out frequencies or wave-form patterns that act as tuning forks to correct the disturbed energetic patterns. One such device is the Asyra Pro. Used by the Mayo Clinic, it is the first device of its kind to be registered with the FDA as a Class II Medical Device. A study published in 2006 examined the effectiveness of the Asyra Pro in assessing low thyroid levels in women thirty-five to sixty-five years of age. The Asyra Pro found abnormalities in 99.5 percent of the patients with low thyroid function on laboratory tests. You can learn more about the Asyra Pro at www.asyra.com.

The Life Vessel

The Life Vessel, introduced in chapter 8, is another type of device that works through frequency, as well as sound, light, and vibration. Research shows it balances your sympathetic and parasympathetic nervous systems—or your autonomic nervous system. When your autonomic system goes out of balance, it causes the electrical signals in your body to go out of balance and contributes to disease. When brought back into balance, the corrected electrical signals in your body work to improve many functions, including the performance of your cell membranes and the expressions of your genes in your DNA.

Frequency Medicine Performed by Practitioners

Certain energy techniques require no special equipment; only the hands of the practitioner and his or her conscious intention is needed. The most well-known and well-researched techniques are Healing Touch, Therapeutic Touch, qigong, and Reiki. It may not look as if much is going on when practitioners hold their hands lightly on or above a patient and work in their energy field, but over twenty years of research shows that these techniques are very effective in relieving anxiety, accelerating wound healing, and decreasing post-

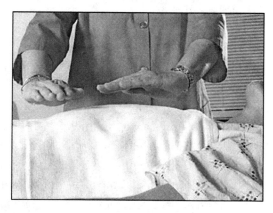

operative complications, such as pain, nausea, inflammation, and fever.

Ancient cultures and systems of medicine recognized the human energy field thousands of years ago. They described it as "that which gives life" or the "life force." It is called *prana* in India, *qi* or *chi* in China, and *ki* in Japan. Pythagoras called it "vital energy." Janet Mentgen, a nurse from Colorado, developed Healing Touch, and Dolores Kreiger is credited for creating the sister system of Therapeutic Touch. Reiki was conceived in Japan around the turn of the century by Mikao Usui (1865–1926) and simplified by one of his students, Chujiro Hayashi, into a practical healing technique that could be taught around the world. Qigong is practiced using movements, similar to tai chi, along with breathing techniques.

You probably have seen images of large groups of people practicing qigong together in China such as this one. But the techniques of qigong can also be administered from a trained expert to a patient. When a practi-

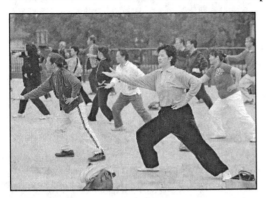

tioner uses qigong to treat a patient, it is called "applied qi." His or her hands are either placed on or above your body similar to Therapeutic Touch or Reiki. Then the practitioner uses his or her breath to direct "universal life force" on you with the intention to help you heal.

Research on these techniques has been conducted for over two decades. All of these techniques cause signs of relaxation, such as slowed breathing and heart rate. They have also been shown to decrease headache pain; ease breathing in asthmatics; decrease fever and inflammation; speed up wound healing; and reduce postoperative pain and complications, including fever, inflammation, and anxiety. For example, a study published in 1992 by researcher D. Wirth, forty-four healthy male volunteers had a punch biopsy on their arms to create a full thickness wound. Half of the men were treated with Healing Touch and half were not (the control group). On the sixteenth day, twelve of the twenty-three treated with Healing Touch had completely healed, whereas none of those in the control group had healed.

Several studies were done at the University of Connecticut in 2008 on the effects of Therapeutic Touch on human cells grown in the laboratory. One study published in the *Journal of Alternative and Complementary Medicine* found that Therapeutic Touch caused accelerated growth of several different types of cells, specifically fibroblasts, which help to create connective tissue and heal wounds; tendon cells, called "tenocytes"; and bone cells, called "osteoblasts." In another fascinating study published in the *Journal of Orthopaedic Research*, Therapeutic Touch stimulated a significant increase in the replication of DNA in human osteoblast cells, caused the cells to mature, and promoted bone formation. Therapeutic Touch also slowed down the growth of osteosarcoma-derived cells—a type of bone cancer.

Many hospitals have nurses and practitioners trained in one of these energy techniques and offer it as an option for their patients. Dr. Mehmet

Oz brought Julie Motz, a Reiki Master, into his operating room to use energy work on his patients during open heart surgery in the mid-1990s. The patients who received the therapy had a much lower complication rate and their hospital stays were shorter. I recommend that you read *Hands of Life* by Julie Motz if you are interested in learning more about her work.

When I was practicing as a plastic surgeon in Cincinnati, Ohio, one of the hospitals employed a team of Healing Touch nurses, who worked on my patients both in the operating room and postoperatively. I found that my patients who received these treatments experienced decreased post-operative pain, anxiety, and nausea compared to my patients who did not.

The following is a link to a YouTube video that covers information on Dr. Oz's experience with Reiki in the operating room, as well as the energy work administered at a UCLA pain-management clinic: www.youtube.com/watch?v=HJ5eajLCzu0.

Homeopathy

Homeopathy is another type of energy medicine that uses remedies to stimulate the body to heal itself. Using the concept of "likes" treating "likes," homeopathic remedies use infinitesimal dilutions of substances that, in higher doses, would cause the same symptoms the patient is currently experiencing. Somewhat like a vaccine, the homeopathic remedies stimulate the body to boost its self-healing power through energetic stimulation by the remedy.

When you meet with a practitioner of homeopathy, he or she will take an inventory of all of your symptoms. Unlike Western medicinal doctors who try to suppress symptoms, a homeopath encourages them because they are understood to be the way your body is trying to heal itself. For instance, if you have a cough, the homeopathic remedy that may best stimulate your recovery may be one that causes a cough in a healthy person.

Homeopathy was developed by Samuel Hahnemann more than 200 years ago in Germany. It was brought to the United States in 1825 by several doctors who had traveled to Europe and learned the system. Around 1900, there were twenty-two homeopathic colleges in the U.S., and one in five doctors in this country used homeopathy in their practice. But, then, the Western model of medicine became dominant and the American Medical

Association made a concerted effort to discredit homeopathy, as well as all other alternative systems of healing. The schools began to close, and by the late 1940s, no courses in homeopathy were available in this country.

Homeopathy has made a comeback in the last several decades due to a growing body of research showing that the remedies are effective for a variety of conditions. For example, a comprehensive review study published in the *Lancet* in 1997 of eighty-nine double-blind, placebo-controlled studies on homeopathy concluded that those patients given homeopathic remedies were 2.45 times more likely to experience a therapeutic benefit compared to those patients given a placebo.

Homeopathic remedies have been found to be helpful for many different ailments, including upper respiratory tract infections in children, allergic reactions, postsurgical swelling and bruising, fibromyalgia and chronic fatigue syndrome, and depression. They have also been found to improve the quality of life of cancer patients.

Flower Remedies

Bach Flower Remedies, developed by Dr. Edward Bach in the 1930s, are based on the essences of thirty-seven different types of flowers and are used for the treatment of primarily emotional and spiritual conditions, such as depression, anxiety, and stress. Like homeopathic remedies, Bach Flower Remedies are created by diluting the components of the flower in an alcohol solution until only infinitesimal amounts are present. Rescue Remedy is the most well-known remedy and is composed of a combination of Rock Rose, Impatiens, Clematis, Star of Bethlehem, and Cherry Plum remedies. When you are under stress and feeling anxious, research shows that Rescue Remedy may be helpful for calming your nerves. A double-blind, placebo-controlled study conducted by the University of Miami and published in *Complementary Health Practice Review* in 2007, found Rescue Remedy caused a statistically significant improvement in those who had high levels of situational anxiety.

Alicia Sirkin is a coauthor of this study and an internationally registered Bach Remedy practitioner. She offers regular training courses in her program, "Live Balanced and Bold: 5 Steps to Change Your Life," which includes the use of Bach Flower Remedies. If you are interested in learning more, her website is a great resource: www.sirkincreativeliving.com.

Gem Therapy

As you are already aware from the metaphor used in this book, gemstones are another form of frequency medicine. Gemstones have been used for thousands of years for healing due to their energetic qualities, including their color. Although it might seem like superstition, quantum physics recognizes that all matter—including gems—produces energy, which can have a measurable influence on your physiology. Thousands of years ago, *Ayurveda* incorporated into its teachings that metals, gems, and stones held energetic qualities that could be used to counteract imbalances in the body.

In his book *Ayurveda: The Science of Self-Healing,* Dr. Vasant Lad, one of the most renowned *Ayurvedic* physicians in the world said, "Gems give off as well as draw in energy through their negative and positive vibrations," and can be used for physical, mental, and emotional healing. For example, lapis lazuli, which has a deep blue color, is said to be good for eye problems, as well as for sensitizing you to higher states of spiritual vibration.

Although gemstone therapy is relatively unknown in the U.S., it is well accepted in other countries. For instance, a study published in the *BMC Journal of Complementary and Alternative Medicine* in 2009, reported on a survey taken at a teaching hospital in Pakistan. More than half of the sample population was aware of the use of the gemstones for their various effects, and over one-third currently used gemstone therapy.

Sound Therapy

The healing influence of music and sound has been recognized for millennia. Thousands of studies in the last several decades unquestionably show that certain sounds and music profoundly induce balance and promote health, not just in humans, but also in animals and plants. Conversely, certain sounds or music can have the opposite effects. For example, more than forty years ago, modern scientists rediscovered the powerful effects of music on plants. In the 1970s, classical music was found to cause plants to grow faster and stronger, whereas hard rock-and-roll caused them to droop and wilt.

The Mozart Effect

Researchers at the University of Wisconsin in 1993 found that normal subjects who listened to Mozart's *Sonata for Two Pianos* (k448) for ten minutes had significantly better spatial reasoning skills for ten to fifteen minutes afterward compared to after periods of silence or after listening to relaxing instructions designed to lower blood pressure. They called this phenomenon the "Mozart Effect." These same researchers found that animals also had a similar reaction to Mozart's music. They played Mozart's *Sonata* (k.448) to rats while they were developing in-utero and continued for sixty days after their births. The researchers found that these rats learned maze running more quickly and made fewer errors compared to those animals that listened to other types of music, white noise, or just silence.

Brain researchers discovered that listening to Mozart causes brainwave activity to become more synchronized. The two hemispheres of your brain normally have brainwave activity that is different from each other, or "unsynchronized." When you are in a state of deep relaxation or meditation, your brain waves characteristically become more synchronized. Not only does Mozart's music cause your hemispheres to become more synchronized, but so does classical music by other composers, particularly certain compositions written by Bach.

The benefits of the Mozart Effect are most impressive in patients with epilepsy. Numerous studies, including a frequently cited study from the University of Illinois, show that classical music drastically reduces the incidence of seizures in patients who have frequent and uncontrolled seizures. Interestingly, researchers have found that the anticonvulsant effect of the music even works in patients who are unconscious. When Mozart was played to patients in a coma, their incidence of seizures significantly reduced.

"He who sings scares away his woes."

~Cervantes

Music Therapy

Music can calm your mind and emotions, and decrease your blood pressure and heart rate. It can also reduce muscle tension and stress hormone levels, boost your immune system, and increase the natural pain reliever chemicals, called "opiates," in your body. In fact, a medical center in Austin, Texas, reported that 50 percent of women who listened to pleasant music during childbirth didn't need anesthesia.

Music can help improve physical coordination, motor movements, and athletic performance. It has also been shown to sharpen mental acuity, improving the ability to think, solve problems, learn, and remember. Listening to music you like can make you more productive. Depending on the music, it can make you feel up, down, romantic, invigorated, or calm; it can bring you to tears or send you off to sleep.

Music therapists use music interventions to promote wellness and to treat certain physical, mental, and emotional conditions. The interventions range from passive listening to actual music lessons, music performance, song writing, and imagery. A certified music therapist evaluates a patient for their emotional well-being, physical health, social functioning, communication abilities, and cognitive skills. He or she then designs a program based on the individual's specific needs and goals.

The first music therapy degree program in the world was offered at Michigan State University in 1944. Today, more than seventy colleges in the U.S. offer bachelor degrees in music therapy and several have Ph.D. programs. Music therapy has become a well-established specialty in healthcare, and approved treatments are covered by many private insurance companies, as well as by Medicare and Medicaid. Certified professionals are required to have a bachelor's degree in the specialty, complete one year of internship, and then pass a certification exam offered by the Certification Board for Music Therapists. The American Music Therapy Association, the largest professional association, reported having more than 5,000 members in 2011.

Research shows that music therapy can be beneficial for children, adolescents, adults, and the elderly with any of the following conditions:

- Mental health needs, especially mood disorders, including depression and anxiety
- Developmental and learning disabilities
- ADD and autism
- Alzheimer's disease and other forms of dementia

- Parkinson's disease

- Brain injuries, strokes

- Substance abuse

- Physical disabilities

- Acute and chronic pain

- Cancer

- Stress

Dr. Valerie Hunt, introduced at the beginning of this chapter, developed a series of music and sound tapes using auric field sounds that were harmonically correlated with music. In other words, she combined the electromagnetic frequencies found in your bioelectric field with the music that matches each frequency. She explained in an interview by Larry Triv published by Wordpress:

"The red, orange, amber frequency spectrum, for example, goes with contemporary African music with a strong beat, and can be used to revitalize the physical body and activate spontaneous emotions. The yellow, green, and gold frequency is a waltz wave. Listening to this music fine tunes sensation and perception, improves the efficiency of the nervous system, and creatively activates the mind. Then you have the blue, violet, and mauve spectrum, which correlates to the great classical music repertory, and encourages a contemplative state of peace, tranquility, and higher consciousness. Then we come into the white and gold spectrum, which correlates to spiritual a cappella choral singing, and elevates thoughts and emotions to a broader worldview of richer beauty and deeper wisdom. Or you can listen to the Rainbow tape, which progresses through all the frequencies to stabilize the field and encourage expanded awareness."

*"Stretch your body to beautiful music and discover
a new way of feeling the positive vibrations of life."*

~J. J. GOLDWAG

Ayurveda and Sound Therapy

Ayurveda contains a very detailed, sophisticated knowledge of the use of sounds to restore balance and create optimal health. Instead of classical music, *Ayurveda* prescribes specific sounds, called "primordial sounds." Examples include chants in Sanskrit called *Rig Veda* and *Sama Veda*, and music called *Gandharva Veda*. There are many types of *Gandharva Veda* music, which are designed to help balance you during specific hours of the day.

Precise types of sounds are also prescribed for various health conditions. A technique called Maharishi Vedic Vibration Technology (MVVT) uses specific *Vedic* sounds or vibrations to correct imbalances, usually stemming from improper diet and lifestyle choices, which are the source of the health condition. A practitioner quietly whispers or silently *thinks* of the prescribed sound while blowing on the affected area of the patient. *Ayurvedic* physicians view the technique as delivering "the missing intelligence" back into your body after it has been lost. Quantum physics confirms that impulses of consciousness are able to produce profound changes in disease states. Research shows that patients with a variety of ailments— mental, emotional, and/or physical—can experience benefits from this technique. The results can be instantaneous or evolve over several days, and they can be significant and long lasting.

A study published in 2003 reported the results of 213 individuals with chronic illnesses who were treated with MVVT. After three treatment sessions, the average self-reported improvement in chronic disease symptoms was 40.97 percent. Conditions related to neck pain improved the most (51.25%), followed by respiratory ailments (48%), digestive problems (46.9%), mental health including anxiety and depression (46.34%), arthritis (41.57%), insomnia (37.38%), back pain (36.32%), headache (35.83%), cardiovascular conditions (22.31%), and eye problems (21.19%). There was also a significant reduction in complaints of pain.

In a double-blind, randomized study published in the *Frontiers of Bioscience* in 2001, 176 patients with arthritis were treated with MVVT. According to the researchers, the results were unprecedented in modern medical science. Sixty-four patients experienced 100 percent *immediate* relief in pain, forty-two reported an 80 percent reduction, and twenty-one had a 60 percent reduction, eighteen had 40 percent relief, and thirty-one said they had less than a 40 percent degree of relief.

For more information on MVVT and to find a location near you where you can receive these treatments, go to www.vedicvibration.com/.

"Everything in life is vibration."

~Albert Einstein

Electromagnetic Frequencies in the Environment

Because you are bioelectrical, electrical fields from electrical devices and the environment can interact with your own electrical fields. Certain types of electricity can have negative effects on your body, especially electrical magnetic energy (EMFs) from electrical devices, such as cell phones, cordless phones, and your computer. For instance, they can cause your immune system to be less effective, disrupt the communication between your cells, and even cause damage to your DNA. They can also cause your genes to start sending messages that contain instructions for poor health.

All electrical devices, both wired and wireless, produce EMFs. Indoors, this includes household appliances, such as microwaves, and personal items, including computers, cell phones, cordless phones, hair dryers, and Wi-Fi. Outdoors, dangers of EMFs are found in power lines, transformers, cell phone towers, and broadcast towers.

Research shows that EMFs interfere with your body in many ways, including:

- Injuring your cell membranes
- Disrupting cell-to-cell communication
- Stimulating oncogenes (genes that promote the growth of cancer)
- Causing injuries to your DNA
- Inducing cell stress
- Increasing oxygen free radicals
- Killing neurons in your brain

- Promoting premature aging

- Causing stress and the release of "heat shock" proteins

In August of 2006, fourteen scientists and experts from around the world collaborated on a major document called the *BioInitiative Report* (www.bioinitiative.org), which reported on all the known health detriments associated with EMFs. The experts found a clear link between EMFs and an increased incidence of:

- Numerous cancers, including childhood leukemia, brain tumors, acoustic neuromas, melanoma of the eye, and breast cancer

- Alzheimer's disease

- Parkinson's disease

- Amyotrophic lateral sclerosis (ALS; Lou Gehrig's disease)

- Immune system disorders

Ann Louise Gittleman, author of more than thirty health books, offers these recommendations from her book about electromagnetic frequency called *Zapped*, and I agree with all of them:

- Text, don't talk, whenever possible—but don't text while driving!

- Use speaker mode to keep your phone as far away from your head as possible.

- Go offline—turn off your cell phone when you're not using it and shut off your wireless router at night. (You'll be amazed by how much more soundly you'll sleep.)

- Get your phone out of your pocket; men who carry their cell phone in their pockets have lower sperm counts than those who don't carry a cell phone.

- Avoid tight spaces (buses, elevators, trains, and subways) where your phone has to work harder to get a signal out through metal.

- Choose a phone with a low SAR (specific absorption rate) number.

- Replace your cordless phones with corded landline phones.

- Don't cradle your laptop—putting it on your lap exposes your reproductive organs to EMFs.

- Most important of all, *restrict cell and cordless phone use during pregnancy.* Heavy phone use then has been linked to increased risk of miscarriage and birth defects. A 2008 survey of more than 13,000 children found that those whose mothers used a cell phone during pregnancy were more likely to have behavior problems, including hyperactivity and emotional outbursts.

Another approach that offers excellent protection against the damaging effects of EMFs is to use devices that alter how your body responds to them. For example, the company GIA Wellness (formally known as BioPro) (www.giawellness.com/2/) produces a variety of devices that research shows have been found to be highly protective against electropollution. These devices range from ones that you wear, to chips that you place on your cell phone and appliances, to "home harmonizers" that you plug in to the walls in your home, to nutritional supplements.

There have been amazing case reports of improved symptoms after using these devices, revealing that EMFs may play a significant role in many health problems. For instance, symptoms including headaches and pain associated with fibromyalgia have resolved. Most impressively, a health provider in Tennessee who specializes in helping autistic children has observed tremendous improvement in her patients using these protective devices. One child began speaking for the first time after using the devices for several weeks! When I started using these devices, I experienced a profound difference in the fatigue and stress I felt, especially while working at the computer.

If you would like more information on these devices or would like to review the research conducted on them, please log on to my website www.drchristinehorner.com.

The Energy of Buildings and Your Health

Have you ever walked into a building and immediately felt closed in, anxious, or so disturbed that you wanted to immediately run out? Perhaps you suddenly got a mild headache, couldn't think clearly, or found it hard to breathe? The moment you got out of the building, you immediately felt better, your body relaxed, and you felt like you could breathe again. What you experienced was a not-so-subtle example of how much the buildings we live or work in can affect us. Sometimes the effect has to do with toxic materials that were used, creating what has been termed "sick building syndrome." Other times, the effect actually has to do with the design of the building, the orientation of the space, or the color of the room. In other words, the design of buildings can have either a positive or negative impact on your energy fields.

Ancient cultures, especially the Chinese and *Vedic* cultures, recognized that the structures we live and work in have a profound influence on our lives and health. The Chinese created a system of architecture, which has gained a lot of popularity today, called *feng shui* and the lesser known *Vedic* civilization's system is known as *Sthapatya Veda*. Both of these systems can be considered "quantum-mechanical" sciences because they are based on the understanding that all things are interconnected and influence one another.

The characteristics of the land a building is on, its slope, orientation, and other special features, in addition to the direction that a building faces, the dimensions of and layout of its rooms, the thickness of the walls, the materials used for its construction—all have predictable influence on our success, happiness, and health. *Sthapatya Veda* buildings are designed to create optimal harmony between the individual and all things in Nature, enhancing human physiology and everything in the surrounding area. In other words, these two systems are designed to make a person feel comfortable in their environment and give them a sense of peace and strength. Their basic purpose is to make everything feel better and work better. You can read more about *Sthapatya Veda* at www.sthapatyaveda.com.

Decluttering

For *Sthapatya Veda* or *feng shui* to work, you have to remove all of the blocks that can be in its way. You can think of it as clearing spaces to prime you for success. When there is clutter, it can distract you, break your attention, and make it difficult to concentrate. Decluttering is a process that requires getting rid of everything you don't need or use, and then organizing all the things you do. You can't take any shortcuts like gathering all your "stuff" and throwing it in your closet or drawers because *feng shui* sees through everything. Here's a helpful way to think about it: If your closets and drawers are a mess, then every day you have to go through the frustration of trying to find things. That can put you in a bad mood that affects your whole day.

Professional "declutterers" recognize that clutter is purely emotional. Hanging on to things we no longer need all stems from an emotional need to "feel safe." We drag things from our past with us out of fear or "in case we might need it someday." But all this "stuff" weighs us down, blocks the flow of energy, invites fear in, and allows no space to invite the future in. Unless the emotional issues that lead to the clutter are addressed, decluttering won't last very long. The space will soon return to its original state. Therefore, decluttering is a process that may take up to a year to complete; there is no quick fix. In order for the changes be permanent, you must work with your head and get at the root of what is emotionally driving you to hang on to too much stuff.

It's normal to feel embarrassed, humiliated, and at a loss about what to do if you are surrounded by clutter. A good declutterer understands this and should be able to work with you without making you feel bad. One declutterer I interviewed said that after just ten minutes of starting the decluttering process with a client, most exclaim, "Oh my God, I feel so much better!" The energy shifts almost immediately. Something in their soul feels lighter.

Good Vibrations

The most important concept to remember is that your body is "bioelectric." It is composed of energy and vibrations that reflect and affect your state of health. Be sure to minimize your exposure to bad vibrations caused by the electromagnetic frequencies produced from electrical devices, poor architecture, and the energy of negative people! Instead, be aware of all the ways you can help to balance your electrical field. If you haven't tried any of the frequency medicine therapies described in this chapter, I suggest you do. It will be an eye-opening experience for you to realize how effective these subtle energy techniques can be.

CHAPTER 11

Spiritual Healing

Surrendering to and Receiving the Infinite Power

If you wish for light, be ready to receive light.

~RUMI

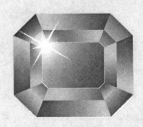

THE ELEVENTH GEM—AMETHYST

The stone of spirituality and contentment is a deep purple amethyst, and the eleventh stone in your breastplate. It helps to facilitate a clear connection to the spirit world—the ultimate source of your healing.

The color purple is associated with your sixth chakra, or third eye, which is the center for spirituality, the sacred, and your higher self. Purple helps to take low energy and convert it to high spiritual energy. It has a variety of effects on your mind and body, including uplifting your spirits, calming your mind and nerves, enhancing feelings of spirituality, and encouraging imagination and creativity. An amethyst is said to assist you in going through a complete metamorphosis, just as a spiritual awakening does, and gives you stability, strength, and peace.

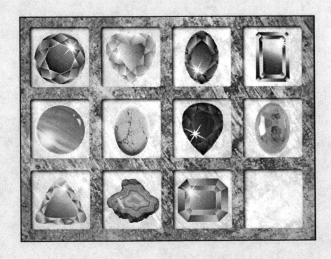

*"Healing does not mean going back to the way
things were before, but rather allowing what
is now to move us closer to God."*

~RAM DASS

hroughout this book, you have read about all the research-proven factors that influence your health and longevity. From the diet and lifestyle choices that you should either avoid or favor to the powerful influence of your emotions and relationships. There are, however, aspects of your life that play an equally important role that scientists can't quantify and measure. Your personal relationship with a higher power, for example, is impossible to accurately measure, but can have a profound influence on your health, quality of life, happiness, and the number of days you walk this Earth. I'm not talking about a religion, but a personal relationship— your relationship with whatever name you prefer for that power: God, Allah, Spirit, Source, Creator, or the Divine; it doesn't matter. I will use a variety of terms to refer to the higher power, but you can translate my words into the one that works best for you.

Spirituality and Medicine

Since the beginning of recorded time, religion, spirituality, and medicine have shared a close, even unified, relationship. In fact, only in our highly developed Westernized culture have they become separate. The earliest records reveal that there were individuals in villages or tribes who served not only as spiritual leaders, but also as medicine men and women. Referred to as "shamans," there are many cultures today, such as in South America, where they still serve both of these roles for their community. Five thousand years ago, *Ayurveda* emerged from the *Vedic* literature—a spiritual text. The ultimate purpose of *Ayurveda* is said to be "enlightenment." In other words, the intent of *Ayurveda* is to teach you how to achieve an extraordinary state of balance and health in the mind and body, so that you can achieve union with the Creative Source or God.

Major religious figures throughout time, such as Jesus, as well as numerous saints, including St. Teresa of Avila, were known for their remarkable healing abilities, as much as for their spiritual leadership. For long periods of history from before the Middle Ages to the time of the American colonies, physicians were often also priests and ministers. Even today, many hospitals are run by religious organizations. However, it is now rare to find a physician in Western cultures who will even mention spirituality to their patients. In fact, many patients will even find it off-putting if they do. I remember my mother, a very devout Christian and church organist, saying that when her surgeon asked to pray with her before he operated on her, it made her nervous, because she worried that he wasn't confident enough of his abilities!

Research into Spirituality and Health

Although scientist can't accurately measure or quantify the impact of your relationship with a higher power and your health and longevity, they have made attempts to by analyzing some rough indicators, such as the influence of religious service attendance. For example, a study published in 1999 found that women who frequently (at least once a week) attended religious services were, over the duration of the study, 49 percent less likely to die and men were 37 percent less likely compared to those who don't attend. Another study published the following year looked at the influence of engaging only in private spiritual activities, such as prayer and meditation, on longevity. The researchers found that those who had private spiritual practices also had a survival advantage.

According to a landmark study published in 2012 in the journal *ISRN Psychiatry*, research shows that spiritual practices are associated with many health benefits. This study reviewed thousands of studies published between 1872 and 2010 that explored the relationship between religion/ spirituality and mental and physical health. The researchers noted that approximately 80 percent of the research involved studies on mental health. These studies found that those who are spiritual tend to have a more positive outlook, a better sense of well-being, and happiness. They also are more hopeful and optimistic, and have a better sense of purpose and self-esteem. In addition, those who are spiritual also show a greater ability to enjoy life, even in the midst of physical symptoms from health issues, including pain. They suffer less from mood disorders, such as depression and anxiety, as well as from substance abuse. According to numerous other studies, spirituality also appears to enhance recovery from illness and surgery, and to improve the ability to cope with disease, bereavement, and death.

Many of the world's religions emphasize the importance of taking care of your body. For instance, the Bible (Corinthians 6:19–20) describes the body as the "Temple of the Holy Spirit." Therefore, it would be expected that those who appreciate this belief would tend to have healthier habits. Research does indeed show that religion and spirituality are associated with better health habits. For instance, those who are spiritual tend to not smoke cigarettes or engage in risky sexual behavior. They are also more likely to exercise and eat a healthy diet. These healthier behaviors, as well as the psychological and emotional benefits from spiritual practices, have been shown to reduce the risk of numerous diseases, including:

- Cardiovascular disease, including high blood pressure, heart attacks, and strokes
- Alzheimer's disease and other forms of dementia
- Immune system dysfunction
- Endocrine dysfunction
- Cancer

Meditation

Meditation can be considered a spiritual practice, because it is a part of certain religions—for instance, Buddhism. A number of studies have shown that Buddhist mindfulness and compassion meditations are associated with stress reduction, as well as many other health benefits. As you may recall from chapter 3, the most researched form of meditation is Transcendental Meditation (TM). Although it is not a religious practice, the state of consciousness that is experienced when transcending—called the "fourth state of consciousness"—is thought to be one that merges with Spirit. Those who practice just twenty minutes of TM, twice a day, are found to have significant reductions in worry, stress, anxiety, hostility, and depression. According to a Canadian study, practitioners of TM have 56 percent fewer hospital admissions for all diagnoses, including cancer and accidents. For cardiovascular disease, including strokes and heart attacks, the reductions in admissions were even greater: 87 percent. A study published in the journal *Stroke* found that the simple practice of TM could actually reverse coronary artery disease.

Spiritual Healings

There are endless accounts of "miraculous" healings that have occurred from spiritual healings. The healings have come from major religious figures such as Jesus and saints, as well as faith healers, psychic surgeons, and shamans. Simple prayer and spontaneous healings following spiritual insights have also resulted in what we think of as miracle healings. We think of all of these healings, which don't fit into our Western paradigm and understanding of physical laws, as miracles. But, as Jesus said, he was simply showing us what is within all of us. That means each of us has the power to heal ourselves, as well as others, by connecting with the Creative Source. The hard and fast rules we think that exist according to the Newtonian physics turn out to be bendable. Quantum physics explains more of the truth of how the universe operates. However, the Spirit realm has the ultimate control, and your relationship to that Source is capable of manifesting anything.

Around 2000, I read an article in one of my medical journals about a psychic surgeon/ healer in Brazil named João de Deus or "John of God." Immediately skeptical, I read in amazement about a group of American physicians and scientist who traveled to Abadiânia, Brazil, where John of God sees thousands of people every week from all over the world at his spiritual healing center, the Casa Dom Inácio de Loyola. The physicians described various case studies of patients who came to be healed. One case was of a man with a large inoperable cancerous tumor in his lung. He had an MRI scan documenting his tumor. He was then treated by John of God using "psychic surgery." Following the treatment, he had another MRI, which showed the tumor was gone. That really piqued my interest.

For years after reading this article, I sent friends to see John of God, but could never seem to work it out with my schedule to go myself. Then one day in 2011, a friend sent me a video of an interview with Anita Moorjani. Anita was diagnosed with terminal cancer. She had gone into a coma and had been given just hours to live. But she didn't die. Instead, she says that she experienced "crossing over and coming back." She shares her vivid near-death experience in her book, *Dying to Be Me: My Journey from Cancer, to Near Death, to True Healing,* as well as in many interviews on YouTube (www.youtube.com/watch?v=Oz4NUe_hv2M). Anita said that while on the "other side" she was told that she had been living her life to make others happy. Instead, she was instructed to live her life for herself—to be the authentic expression of her unique self and to love herself for exactly who she is. Anita was sent back to her body, and within three days, there were no traces of cancer in her body.

Anita is a living example that each of us has the potential to heal, even from life-threatening illnesses. The key for her was her extraordinary spiritual experience in which she realized the emotional shift she needed to make in her life. As a physician, I believe that all illnesses symbolically give us clues about emotional and spiritual issues that must be addressed for healing to occur. When we fully confront those issues and ask for help and guidance from Spirit, the possibility of healing is profound.

After watching Anita's video, my eyes glanced to the related videos on the right, where I noticed a video of an interview with Wayne Dyer, best-selling self-health author and motivational speaker, about his diagnosis of leukemia. I didn't know that Wayne had leukemia. Alarmed, I clicked on the video to get the details. In his interview, he spoke about his experience of being cured of leukemia by John of God (www.youtube.com/watch?v=VzCy5B_1QpM). Even more amazing was that Wayne didn't go to Brazil. He didn't believe in John of God's ability to heal. Instead, a woman physician friend of Wayne's went to Brazil and had "psychic surgery" performed on her—intended for him—while he was in Maui, Hawaii. His story is amazing, and I highly recommend you watch his interview. Wayne Dyer recently died (2015) at the age of seventy-five, reportedly from a heart attack—not leukemia. In that moment, I decided I could wait no longer to see the remarkable healer, John of God. I flew to Brazil a few months later and what I experienced there was completely life altering.

John of God—the man—is a simple individual with only a second-grade education, but who has a powerful gift. He is a medium who has the ability to allow spirits, called "entities," to use his body to help heal others. He says that he does not heal, God does. If you don't know about him, I recommend that you watch the videos of the interviews by Oprah, which can be found on YouTube at the following links: www.youtube.com/watch?v=5sSJ2wqVJz0 and www.youtube.com/watch?v=wMQHzOB9RrY&list=PLF755B576B6F91F11.The main reason I wanted to see him was to witness an alternative reality filled with "miracles." My desire was completely fulfilled.

Emma, my guide for the trip, said that only about 10 percent of people receive instantaneous healings. A larger percentage of people make many trips and experience gradual healing, because their illness is an important part of their spiritual journey. Some conditions don't improve because their illness is their spiritual path. The most important key to receive healing, Emma said, is to surrender to God and receive.

Rather than coming to see John of God only as an observer, I wanted to personally experience how God works through him to heal. There were a few minor conditions I requested to be healed, including a small hernia on my abdomen. After asking for the healing, I realized I didn't know how to completely surrender to God and receive. So, I cried and prayed for hours asking to be shown. I was. When I met with John of God, he told me I needed "surgery." The surgery he recommended was no ordinary surgery—it was invisible. In other words, no surgeon, no scalpels, and no physical person who touches you. Instead, I sat on what looks like a church pew with many others who are also there for invisible surgery. Prayers and invocations were given at the beginning of the session. Mediums sat in front of the room to hold the meditative state of consciousness that facilitates invisible spirits or entities to enter the room. We were instructed to close our eyes, place our hands on the affected area of our body or on our hearts, and then receive. Trust, surrender to God, allow and receive.

I felt hands touching me, although no physical hands actually were. The invisible entities worked on closing my hernia above my belly button, and it hurt so much I felt nauseated. Waves of joy passed over me. And there was so much more . . . but the point of this story is this: beyond a shadow of a doubt, I know that each of us has angels and beneficent guides that love us and watch over us. Talk to your angels and guides, God, or Spirit. Ask for guidance and to be shown the path to your healing. Then, surrender, trust, and open yourself to receive. Even if you have an advanced stage of cancer and would like to live many more years, do not give up. Plenty of people, such as Anita Moorjani, who was in a coma and given just hours to live, go on to live long, productive lives.

(Pages 264–266 adapted from *Waking the Warrior Goddess* by Christine Horner, M.D., used with permission of Basic Health Publications.)

Modern Medical System
Combines with Spiritual Approaches

Brazil has developed a medical system that combines Western medicine with spiritual approaches. Their approach to mental healthcare, for instance, provides a great example. Most mental health issues are thought to originate from a spiritual crisis. Mental health personnel work closely together with spiritual counselors, who include mediums somewhat like John of God. These mediums work with the "unseen entities" to remove negative energy from the patients and provide them with other types of spiritual healings. The outcomes have been extraordinary. Emma Bragdon, Ph.D., a psychologist from the U.S. who served as my guide when I saw John of God, organizes tours every year of the psychiatric facilities in Brazil for Western mental healthcare. She has even written a medical text book about the mental health system used in Brazil and conducts frequent workshops. To learn more about Emma Bragdon, visit her website at www.emmabragdon.com.

Angels in the OR

When I worked as a surgeon, the presence of the unseen help was profound. I had so many experiences in the operating room of such powerful and direct Divine guidance, I'd often say out loud to the nurses, "Wow, the whirl of the guardian angel wings in here is deafening." I'll share a couple of stories with you, so that you have a clear idea of what I mean.

As a plastic surgeon, I worked with patients who were paralyzed and in wheelchairs and had developed pressure sores that required surgery to heal. The operations to close these wounds involve removing the dead tissue, shaving down the underlying boney prominence that is the source of the pressure, and then rotating a "flap" of healthy tissue composed of skin and muscle from an adjacent area to close the wound. These muscle flaps are kept alive by blood vessels, so knowing exactly where they are is crucial.

Muscle flap surgery for pressure sores is not a common operation for most plastic surgeons. For example, a typical plastic surgeon might only perform one of these operations every year or two. In addition, there are dozens of possibilities of where pressure sores may form and each requires a different muscle flap to repair them properly. So, when a patient presents with a pressure sore, most plastic surgeons have to review the multivolume text book to either remind themselves, or learn for the first time, what operations are the best options, as well as all the steps required for that surgery.

One day, I took a paraplegic patient to the operating room to close a pressure sore that had developed on his buttocks. The night before, I reviewed the muscle flap options in the text book, selected the one I thought was best, and reviewed how to do it. The anesthesiologist put the patient to sleep, and we turned him over in preparation for the operation. The bright operating room lights revealed scars from a previous operation that wasn't listed in his medical records and which hadn't been previously visible in the dim lights of his hospital room. The scars appeared to cut right across the area of the blood supply for the muscle flap I had planned to perform.

Any surgeon in their right mind would have turned the patient over, woke him up, and rescheduled the operation for another day—after studying the steps for an alternative muscle flap. But I heard clear voices in my head that said, "We want you to do a different operation using a muscle flap from the leg."

I told them silently, "But I didn't read about how to do it last night—I glanced at it, but didn't study it. So I have no idea how to do it and don't know where the blood supply is."

They said, "Don't worry, we'll guide you every step of the way."

Looking back on this now, it still amazes me that I decided to go ahead with the operation I hadn't studied, and therefore didn't know how to do, yet I never felt any fear or lack of confidence. As I performed the operation, I heard instructions such as, "Cut here," and "stop now." The operation went smoothly and the muscle flap fit into the wound perfectly. After completing it, I looked up the procedure in the textbook and discovered I had done it exactly how it was described!

The next story is of a spiritual phenomenon that happened frequently—in fact, 100 percent of the time when I saw patients with facial skin cancers. When a patient presents a skin cancer on their face, they are often sent to a specialized dermatologist called a "Mohs surgeon" to have it removed. The Mohs technique has far superior outcomes than traditional surgical excisions performed by a surgeon working with an independent pathologist, so I preferred to use this method. After a patient had their cancer removed by the Mohs surgeon, he or she would come to my office that same day to have his or her wound repaired. I never knew what the shape or size of their wound would be prior to removing the bandage.

To close wounds on the face, just like the muscle flaps for pressure sores, there are numerous options that use various geometrical designs based on the natural tension lines in the face. The goal is to close the wounds so that they appear as natural as possible without pulling on or distorting the facial features. With each of these patients, I would remove their bandage and stare at their wound and within minutes the incision lines for the operation would "magically" appear on the patient's face. I'd mark the lines with a surgical marker and then perform the surgery. The lines I "saw" for the incisions worked out perfectly every time.

I tell you these stories as another example of how Spirit is intimately connected to your health and healing. There is no separation. Asking for help from God or Spirit, and then trusting and receiving that help, is something that is available for you at every moment. There is so much more to this world than what you can see. And the power of the "unseen" has the ability to defy any natural laws. I believe it is best to receive the guidance from Spirit every day to help you to make the best choices for your health and your life. This way of living is the ultimate path of good health and serenity. If you have been off this path, know that Spirit is infinitely compassionate and is always there to help you when you are ready to get back on.

Living from Your Heart

Spiritual teachings tell us we need to live from our hearts. Your heart holds your truths and is all about love—giving *and* receiving love. Many of us, especially women, naturally tend to give more than we receive, so learning how to receive may be one of the more difficult and important tasks to master. It's tough for most of us, because we are taught by parents and religions that it is better to give than receive. Giving is thought of as noble and the highest form of altruism. We give awards and recognition to those who are the biggest givers. Receiving is thought of as selfish. But it is not; it is necessary and life-sustaining. Giving without an equal balance of receiving is life-draining.

Receiving from the Divine is an extraordinarily important ability for you to learn how to allow. There is no greater source of power, healing, and love from which to draw. Being rooted in Spirit supplies you with an infinite source of love, healing, and strength. All stress melts away when you know that every step you take is one that you take with walking hand in hand with God or Source. Yes, there are lots of challenges in life. But the more closely connected you are to Spirit, the more quickly you will be able to see your circumstances from a more expanded perspective and find the lessons and the blessings. In *Ayurveda*, the state of always being in Divine consciousness is called "enlightenment." For me, it is also the definition of living life with grace—and who wouldn't want to do that?

> *"The reality of all life is interdependence. We need to compose our lives in such a way that we both give and receive, learning to do both with grace, seeing both as parts of a single pattern rather than as antithetical alternatives."*
>
> ~MARY CATHERINE BATESON

Embracing Your Femininity

Another realization I had after returning from Brazil was that all the qualities that are important for receiving love and healing from Spirit/God are feminine in nature. However, our culture in general reveres masculine qualities and views feminine qualities as weak. As a direct result, women usually find it easy to express outer attributes of femininity, but simultaneously suppress inner feminine qualities such as trusting in a higher power. Asking and receiving, and working in cooperation holds much more power than the masculine approach of forcing things to happen on your own.

Finding Your Path

I find that reminding myself that I am on a spiritual journey helps with all sorts of challenges and traumas that life throws at me. Through the years, I have developed several spiritual practices that work for me. They include prayer, meditation, shamanic journeying, sweat lodges, and consulting with healers, to name a few. Your spiritual journey is your journey—no one else's. Only you can decide what is right for you. Explore and find what makes you feel closer to God. Pray often. Ask for help. Your prayers will be heard.

Sometimes we don't get everything exactly how we ask for it, but trust that what is delivered to you is in your best interest. You are loved. You are being guided. Listen to the guidance with your heart, and you will intuitively know exactly what you need to do in the next step of your journey to extraordinary health and longevity. There is no greater source for your health and happiness than the infinite power available through the Divine.

CHAPTER 12

Youthful Glowing Skin

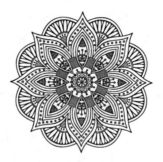

The Reward of Inner Radiant Health and Outer Care

Beauty is not in the face;
Beauty is a light in the heart.

~KAHLIL GIBRAN

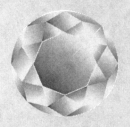

THE TWELFTH GEM—DIAMOND

The final gemstone in your breastplate is a diamond and is considered the "king of the crystals." In ancient times, it was recognized as a "stone that enhances invulnerability." With everything you have learned in this book, represented by the completion of collecting every stone in your breastplate, you now have all the elements that will help to protect you from being vulnerable to disease and accelerated aging.

When you incorporate everything into your life that helps to bring you into balance, enhance your health, and support a profound spiritual connection, your face takes on a radiant glow. Your skin appears luminous, because it reflects the extraordinary state of your inner health. The radiant light emanating from your face is the end result of the combination of all the elements necessary for extraordinary health—just as a diamond reveals that the brilliant light it reflects is actually composed of prisms of different colors.

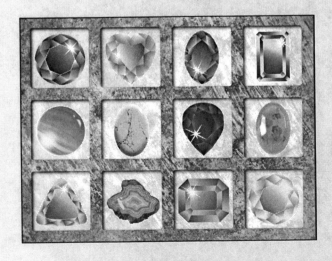

You might think the key to achieving radiant glowing skin centers on expensive time-consuming topical skin care, including facials, moisturizers, and sunscreens. When I began my plastic surgery practice, I thought this was true, too—along with the help of lasers, chemical peels, and surgery. But when I began to learn about natural health, I soon realized that while important, these "outside" treatments aren't the real secrets to radiant skin. Rather, it's how you take care of your "inside" that counts the most.

Your Skin Reveals Your Health

Your skin is a window to your internal health. If you eat mostly nutrient-depleted, inflammation-producing junk foods with lots of highly refined sugars; are under a lot of stress; stay up too late at night; drink a lot of alcohol and colas; and drink very little water—there's no doubt that your skin doesn't look that great. The reflection staring back at you in the mirror is more than likely on the sallow side. The texture of your skin is probably dry. The lines on your face may be increasing in number and depth at an alarming rate, and you may be wondering why you are still getting break-outs at your age.

If you've ever had a time when you've done the opposite—for example, taken a week off your hectic schedule and gone on a relaxing vacation that included plenty of outdoor exercise balanced with rest; consumed lots of pure water, and nutritious fruits and vegetables; and enjoyed time laughing with people you love—no doubt when you got back home, your friends exclaimed how much younger and more relaxed you looked.

Nothing Is More Beautiful Than *Ojas*

According to *Ayurveda,* all of the health-promoting techniques presented throughout this book bring balance to your body, enliven your inner healing intelligence, and produce something called *ojas. Ojas* is a Sanskrit term that describes the most refined subtle physical essence of perfect health. It is the substance created as the end result of perfectly digested foods, which occurs when your diet is filled with highly nutritious foods and your body is finely balanced. You can think of *ojas* as your body's most powerful internally created health- and longevity-promoting elixir. When your *ojas* is high, your health, energy, stamina, and immune system are all at their peak. And it shows on your face. Your eyes will be clear and bright, and your complexion will look supple, luxurious, and glowing.

The Structure and Function of Your Skin

Your skin is composed of three basic layers. The epidermis is the outer layer. The dermis lies beneath the epidermis and makes up 90 percent of the thickness of the skin. Under the dermis is a fat layer, called the "hypodermis."

The epidermis is composed of five layers. Starting with the outermost layer and moving inward, they include:

1. **Stratum corneum**—the exposed surface layer, which is made up of dead skin cells, called "corneocytes." This layer provides protection and helps to keep the skin hydrated.

2. **Stratum lucidum**—a thin layer of clear-appearing dead cells that is only present in the palms of your hands and soles of your feet

3. **Stratum granulosum**—contains granular cells that help to bind keratin fibrils together. It also takes part in creating a barrier that prevents water absorption.

4. **Stratum spinosum**—the formation of keratin begins in this layer.

5. **Stratum germinativum** (also called "stratum basale," or basal layer)— this is the deepest layer of the epidermis and contains the stem cells that create the skin cells, called "keratinocytes." It also holds melanocytes, which are the pigment-producing cells; Langerhans cells, which are involved in the immune system; and touch receptors, called "Merkel cells."

The dermis lies beneath the epidermis and contains nerve endings for touch and temperature; hair follicles; sweat glands; sebaceous glands that secrete sebum, an oily substance that lubricates and waterproofs the skin and hair; apocrine glands that produce the substance responsible for the odor in the armpits and groin; and lymphatic channels and blood vessels.

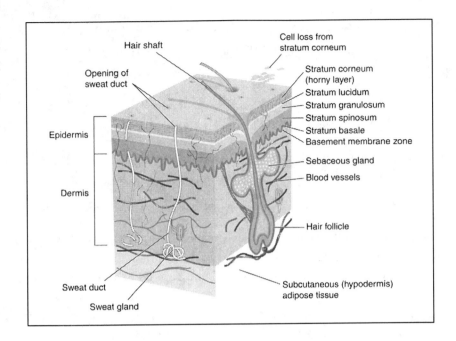

More Than Just Protection

Your skin is the largest organ in your body and has many different functions. Not only does your skin provide protection for the internal structures of your body, but it also:

- Regulates your body's temperature
- Controls evaporation of fluids
- Contains sensory nerves that allow you to feel touch, pressure, vibration, heat, cold, and tissue injury
- Contributes to your immune system and fighting off pathogens
- Manufactures vitamin D
- Helps your body detoxify by eliminating waste products and toxins
- Prevents water-based substances from entering into your body
- Allows absorption of selective substances into your body
- Provides communication to others by showing mood, physical state, and attractiveness

"Nature gives you the face you have at twenty;
it is up to you to merit the face you have at fifty."

~COCO CHANEL

Three Major Contributors to Aging

Researchers have identified three factors that accelerate aging of the skin: UV light, oxygen free radicals, and inflammation.

UV Light

UV light damages the DNA in skin cells. This damage can lead to wrinkles, thick leathery skin, pigmented "age spots," and skin cancers. In fact, nothing ages the skin more rapidly than UV light from the sun or tanning beds. To minimize the damage from UV light, avoid excessive sun exposure, especially during the peak hours from 10 a.m. to 2 p.m., wear protective clothing and nontoxic sun screens, and never use a tanning bed.

Sunscreens, especially those that use chemicals, have become a source of controversy for several reasons. First, research shows that if you use sunblock every time you go out, you prevent your skin from manufacturing vitamin D. Low vitamin D levels are associated with dozens of cancers and chronic diseases. Furthermore, those who regularly expose their skin to "safe" amounts of UV light have actually been found to have less skin cancers, including melanoma—the deadly type. Secondly, many brands of popular sunscreens use toxic chemicals that can increase your risk of cancer and damage your health in other ways.

The Environmental Working Group (EWG) tests sunscreens every year and releases a guide on their website, www.ewg.org. In their last report, two-thirds of the sunscreens analyzed by EWG did not work well or contained potentially hazardous ingredients. Some of the top-selling brands, including Neutrogena, Rite Aid, Walgreens' "Well" brand, "Up and Up" brand from Target, and Coppertone were among those that made the most toxic list. The common chemicals in sunscreens that should be avoided are:

- Oxybenzone: a hormone disrupter and can increase the risk of cancer

- Retinyl Palmitate: may increase the risk of skin cancer

- Parabens and phthalates: hormone disrupters that mimic estrogen and increase the risk of hormone-driven cancer in women, such as breast cancer

I recommend only using sunscreens that use nontoxic substances that provide a physical barrier to UV light, such as zinc and titanium. A sunscreen that has an SPF of 15 will block out 98 percent of the harmful UV rays. You don't need an SPF higher than this. In fact, products with a higher SPF have chemicals that are so concentrated, they can cause skin reactions, in addition to the more serious toxic effects mentioned above. Also, you should avoid spray-on sunscreen products. Most of them contain toxins that you can inhale and that are flammable. There are safe herbs that can help give additional protection against the damaging effects of UV radiation, which I will discuss later.

Oxygen Free Radicals

As you may recall from previous chapters, oxygen free radicals are tiny, unstable molecules of oxygen that are created in your body as normal byproducts of metabolism. When they are found in excess—when there are too many of them—they can be highly destructive, even deadly. Oxygen free radicals attack cell membranes and DNA, creating damage that researchers have estimated contributes to 80 to 90 percent of all chronic degenerative disorders, including Alzheimer's disease, arthritis, and cancer, as well as accelerated aging and wrinkles. Excessive oxygen free radicals are formed by UV radiation, smoking, drinking alcohol, eating red meat (especially grilled meats), eating junk food, staying up too late at night, and exposure to environmental pollutants, to name a few.

The best protection from excessive oxygen free radicals is to avoid these free radical promoters and consume plenty of antioxidants. Excellent sources of antioxidants are fresh, organically grown fruits, vegetables, and whole grains and certain supplements like vitamin C, vitamin E, alpha-lipoic acid, selenium, and CoQ10. There are also a variety of powerful herbal antioxidants that are discussed in the next section.

Inflammation

Inflammation has also been identified as a key factor in the initiation and progression of most chronic degenerative disorders. Oxygen free radicals and inflammation engage in a symbiotic circular dance of destruction: inflammation is promoted by the damage caused by oxygen free radicals, and oxygen free radical formation is promoted by inflammation.

Recent studies have shown that taking anti-inflammatories can dramatically lower the risk of many chronic disorders, including arthritis, dementia, heart disease, and cancers of the prostate, colon, and breast. Anti-inflammatories have also been shown to help protect the skin and reduce signs of aging. These studies reveal pharmaceutical anti-inflammatories are effective, but have potentially serious side effects. As you may recall from chapter 5, there are herbal anti-inflammatories that research shows may be just as effective. And instead of dangerous side effects, they have many side benefits.

All of these processes damage the connective tissue in your skin, which is composed of elastin and collagen fibrils. Elastin and collagen are what give your skin elasticity and firmness. When they are damaged, your skin loses tone and develops wrinkles. With age, the dermis become thinner and loses water content, which also contributes to wrinkles.

Herbal Protection

One of the reasons I became so excited about natural medicine is because of the remarkable medicines contained in plants. Nature has masterfully crafted thousands of plants with a multitude of powerful medicinal qualities *without* the severe side effects of pharmaceutical medication. For example, there are a variety of foods and nutrients that act as "natural sunscreens," because they can protect your skin from the damaging effects of ultraviolet light.

Just like human beings, plants also need to protect themselves from the damage that too much sunlight can cause. They developed numerous natural chemicals that work in a variety of ways to reduce the damaging effects of ultraviolet radiation. Some of these plant chemicals, or "phytochemicals," include carotenoids, polyphenols, and isoflavones. In chapter 4, you learned that all of these phytochemicals have potent antioxidants and anti-inflammatory properties. They can protect your skin from excess oxygen free radicals caused by UV radiation and decrease the inflammation associated with sunburn. Other types of phytochemicals reduce your risk of sunburn by absorbing some of the UV radiation.

Carotenoids are naturally occurring pigments in plants that provide UV protection. For example, lycopene is the red color in tomatoes and watermelons, beta-carotene in the orange color in carrots and sweet potatoes, and lutein is the yellow color in egg yolks and zucchini squash. According to a 2007 study published in the journal *Molecular Biotechnology*, carotenoids protect your skin by decreasing its sensitivity to UV radiation. So, if you eat a diet high in carotenoids, your skin will be more resistant to burning.

The amount of protection carotenoids provide isn't small. A study published in 2001 in the *Journal of Nutrition* found that test subjects who ate 40 grams of tomato paste (high in lycopene) for ten weeks had a 40 percent reduction in sunburn. The superfoods, spirulina and chlorella, also discussed in chapter 4, contain the carotenoid astaxanthin, which has an antioxidant power 550 times greater than vitamin E! Research shows astaxanthin strongly protects your eyes and skin from UV radiation. The carotenoid beta-carotene has also been shown to defend against free radicals and lower the risk of skin cancer.

Polyphenols are found in high amounts in many foods, including teas (catechins), cacao beans (cocoa/chocolate), grape seeds (proanthocyanidins), grape skins (resveratrol), pomegranates (ellagitannins), apples (epicatechin and quercetin), and onions (quercetin). In a 2010 study published in the *Archives of Dermatology*, polyphenols were found to have a variety of anticancer effects that protect against the development of skin cancer. Several studies show that tea drinkers have a significantly lower incidence of skin cancer. One study found that two or more cups of either black or green tea a day reduced the risk of squamous cell skin cancer by 30 percent. Dark chocolate contains four times more polyphenols than tea, so it, too, protects your skin from UV radiation and can significantly reduce your risk of skin cancer. A study of the polyphenols in grape seeds, proanthocyanidins, found that they not only reduce the risk of skin cancer, but also maintain the elastin in your skin, which helps to keep it toned. Proanthocyanidins also work synergistically with both vitamins C and E (see below). Resveratrol from grape skins provides strong antioxidants that protects against ultraviolet radiation and damage, including skin cancer.

There are many other plants and nutrients with research-proven skin benefits. Here are some of the best:

- Cruciferous vegetables, such as broccoli, cauliflower, and kale contain a chemical called "sulforaphane," which is an antioxidant that reduces oxygen free radical damage.

- Omega-3 fatty acids found in flaxseeds and wild-caught salmon contain powerful anti-inflammatory and antioxidant properties. They protect your skin from sunburns and lower the risk of melanoma—the deadly form of skin cancer.

- Vitamins C and E are antioxidants naturally found in the skin that can protect against sunburn. Vitamin C and E also prevent premature aging and malignant changes of the skin by reducing oxygen free radicals. One way that vitamin E protects against sunburn is by reducing the absorption and penetration of UV radiation. A study published in 2010 in the journal *Nutrients* found that the protective effects of vitamins C and E against sunburns are synergistic. In other words, if you take them at the same time, they have greater effects together than if you take them at separate times. Vitamin C is water soluble and doesn't absorb into the skin. However, it can be chemically combined with oil, creating a vitamin C ester, which will absorb easily into the skin. When applied topically, vitamin C esters can greatly improve skin tone by repairing damaged elastin and collagen fibrils.

- Vitamin A, also known as retinoids, helps skin cells to function normally, reduces sebum production and acne, and reverses and treats sun damage, stretchmarks, and cellulite.

- Vitamin D is manufactured in your skin by a chemical reaction caused by sunlight. It acts like a hormone and is involved in hundreds of different processes in the body, including supporting the immune system. Vitamin D has strong anticancer effects and lowers the risk of dozens of cancers, including skin cancer.

- Alpha-lipoic acid is called "the universal antioxidant," because it is both fat and water soluble. Its antioxidant power is 400 times greater than vitamin E and C. Alpha-lipoic acid also has strong anti-inflammatory effects and can prevent tissue damage caused by sugar. Because it is fat soluble, it absorbs especially well into the skin cells and can be used topically.

- CoQ10, as discussed in chapter 5, is a vitamin-like substance naturally created by your body and is used for energy production. It also has strong antioxidant capabilities and has been shown to protect against damage from UV radiation. It also reduces inflammation, protects against oxygen free radical damage to the mitochondria, and regulates genes, which slow aging. CoQ10 can absorb through the skin and, therefore, can be used topically too.

The following minerals are particularly important for skin health:

- Zinc assists in the structure of proteins, collagen, and cell membranes; improves wound healing; has anti-inflammatory and antioxidant effects; supports the immune system; and protects against UV radiation.

- Sulfur is involved in collagen synthesis, which gives the skin its structure and strength.

- Silica helps form collagen.

- Selenium is a part of the structure of glutathione peroxidase, an enzyme necessary for the antioxidant function of glutathione—one of the major antioxidants in the body that protects against cellular damage from oxygen free radicals that cause inflammation, aging, and skin cancer.

Topical Protection Too

Research shows that many types of polyphenols can also protect against UV radiation and skin cancer when applied topically. For example, grape seed extract, resveratrol, silymarin from milk thistle, as well as the Indian spice, turmeric, all have excellent research documenting their skin protecting benefits. Aloe vera has been used for centuries for sunburns and has been proven by research to be beneficial before, during, and after excessive sun exposure to reduce the severity of the burn.

There are a number of plant oils that can be used topically as sunscreens, too. For example, sesame oil blocks out 30 percent of UV rays, while coconut, peanut, hemp seed, and olive oils block out about 20 percent. According to a 2011 study published in *Pharmacognosy Reviews*, the following oils have research-proven skin health benefits.

Borage Oil

Borage (*Borago officinalis*) oil stimulates skin cell activity and encourages skin regeneration. It contains high levels of gamma-linoleic acid (GLA), making it useful in treating all skin disorders, particularly allergies, dermatitis, inflammation, and irritation. Borage penetrates the skin easily and benefits all types of skin, particularly dry, dehydrated, mature, or prematurely aging skin.

Evening Primrose Oil

Evening primrose (*Oenothera biennis*) oil has a high GLA content that promotes healthy skin and skin repair. It is usually yellow in color and soothes skin problems and inflammation, which makes it a good choice for people with eczema, psoriasis, or any type of dermatitis. Evening primrose skin oil discourages dry skin and premature aging of the skin.

Avocado Oil

Avocado (*Persea americana*) oil is rich in vitamin E, beta-carotene, vitamin D, protein, lecithin, and fatty acids. These ingredients are rich in antioxidants and soothe and protect the skin from UV damage.

Tea Tree Oil

Tea tree (*Melaleuca alternifolia*) oil is an ancient aboriginal remedy known for being antiseptic, fungicide, and germicide. It is a popular component of many sunscreen formulations that relieve sunburn by increasing blood flow in capillaries and bringing nutrients to damaged skin.

Pomegranate Oil

The fruit of the tree *Punica granatum,* grown mainly in the Mediterranean region, has been shown to possess many medicinal properties, including antioxidant and anti-inflammatory. It has also been shown to be effective at diminishing the damage of UVA and UVB rays, as well as reducing the risk of skin cancer.

Porphyra

Porphyra (*Bangiales, Rhodophyta*), a delicious red algae widely consumed in eastern Asia, contains high levels of free amino acids. When it is exposed to intense radiation, it synthesizes UV-absorbing secondary metabolites, such as mycosporine-like amino acids. Porphyra is 334 times more potent at absorbing UV rays than aloe vera gel.

Sea Buckthorn Oil

Sea buckthorn is a thorny shrub with long linear leaves and bright yellow/orange fruits (false berries). It is indigenous to Eastern Europe and northern Asia. The first documented use of sea buckthorn was over one thousand years ago in Tibet and Mongolia. It was also used by the ancient Chinese (600 AD), Romans, and Greeks. According to ancient Greek history, sea buckthorn was a key part of the diet for race horses. In fact, it was sea buckthorn's ability to do wonders for the horses' outer appearance that led to its botanical name *Hippophae rhamnoide*. *Hippophae* means "shiny horse." According to mythological legends, sea buckthorn leaves were one of the preferred foods of the flying horse, Pegasus.

Pegasus may have loved the leaves, but the most medicinal part of sea buckthorn is its berries and the seeds. Ancient cultures used sea buckthorn berries most frequently to treat diseases of the skin and digestive tract. Modern research confirms that this remarkable plant is indeed a powerful medicine for the skin and all mucous membranes, especially those that line the digestive and urogenital tract.

Sea buckthorn berries have a rich supply of nutrients important to skin health, including antioxidants (vitamin C, vitamin E, beta-carotene, and lycopene) and several micronutrients (sulfur, selenium, zinc, and copper). They also contain a very high percentage (30 to 50 percent) of a fatty acid rarely found in significant quantities in plants called "palmitoleic acid," an omega-7 fatty acid fundamental to healthy human skin fat. Linolenic acid, an omega-3 fatty acid with important healing and anti-inflammatory qualities, is found in equally large amounts (30 percent).

Studies show that sea buckthorn retards skin aging, smoothes skin wrinkling, and cures or alleviates acne, impetigo, atopic dermatitis, and dry skin. It also enhances wound healing. A 1990 study found that sea buckthorn significantly decreased damage to DNA caused by highly toxic agents, indicating that it may also protect the DNA in your skin from environmental toxins. Because of its ability to repair and rejuvenate skin, for the past thirty years, sea buckthorn has been used in many hair and skin formulas in Scandinavia, Eastern Europe, and China.

Two other beneficial plant compounds include almond oil, which decreases the aging effect caused by UV light, and a tropical fern, called "golden polypody" or "golden serpent fern," which decreases damage from UV radiation and the risk of skin cancer.

Buggy Beauty Secrets

Another "inside" secret to beautiful skin might surprise you. It has to do with bugs—specifically, the ones that live in your intestinal tract. Believe it or not, you have more bugs—bacteria—in your body than the human cells. Your body depends on these "healthy" microbes to help it function properly. These friendly critters do a lot of important tasks, including helping digestion by breaking down and processing your food, and improving its absorption and assimilation.

Reduces Inflammation

These health-promoting bacteria also prevent inflammatory toxins from leaking into your bloodstream. Inflammation not only promotes virtually every chronic disease, it is also an enemy to a beautiful complexion by causing acne, redness, rashes, wrinkles, and other signs of accelerated aging.

Probiotics

You might be wondering how you get more of these desirable bugs in. Do you actually have to eat bugs? Well—yes, but it's not as bad as it sounds. The bugs come in food that can be delicious or simply taken in a pill called "probiotics." Probiotics are defined as live microorganisms—the good guys—which are found naturally in certain foods, including yogurt and kefir. Fermented foods such as sauerkraut, miso soup, tempeh, and the beverage kombucha are also brimming with beneficial bugs.

Not a fan of fermented foods? No worries. You can also get your probiotics by taking a supplement. The most common and well-studied bacteria that are found in most probiotic supplements are *Lactobacillus* and *Bifidobacterium*. Some probiotic supplements contain many other additional bacterial strains—called "mega probiotics." Mega probiotics are thought to be even more beneficial; however, research hasn't confirmed any statistical advantage. For the best results, look for a probiotic supplement with at least 20 billion live organisms per dose.

PROBIOTICS IMPROVE ACNE AND ECZEMA

Research shows that probiotic supplements improve skin conditions, including acne and eczema. Two specific ways that probiotics improve acne is by strengthening your immune system and directly killing off harmful bacteria, viruses, and fungi—including ones that cause acne. Clinical studies of acne patients confirm the benefits of probiotics. For example, a prospective, randomized study published in 2013 evaluated acne patients given pharmaceutical medication, with, and without probiotics. The researchers found that those patients taking probiotics showed the most improvement.

Probiotics may also help prevent eczema in infants. Researchers from the Norwegian University of Science and Technology found that mothers who drank milk with probiotics during pregnancy, and while breastfeeding for an additional six months, cut their children's odds of developing eczema by nearly 50 percent.

Protects Against Sun Damage

As you are well aware, ultraviolet radiation from sunlight is known to be a top contributor to premature aging of the skin and skin cancer. Probiotics may protect against its damaging effects, too. A 2013 study published in the *British Journal of Nutrition* found that probiotics boosted the immune system and protected against the tumor-inducing effects of ultraviolet radiation.

The Ayurvedic Approach to Skin Care

Thousands of years ago, the ancient texts from *Ayurveda* described advanced techniques of topical skin care designed not only to enhance the attractiveness of one's external appearance, but also to contribute to achieving extraordinary health and longevity. Daily, as well as seasonal, skin care routines using herbalized oils, pastes, and waters were recommended to slow the aging of the skin, smooth its imperfections, increase its tone and hydration, and cause it to look radiantly healthy.

I'm always fascinated to learn Sanskrit words from 5,000 years ago that describe incredibly evolved concepts in health, beauty, and consciousness. These words give insights to the ancient *Vedic* culture—the thoughts that occupied their minds and their perceptions of the world, which were startlingly sophisticated and deep compared to our culture today. For example, according to a study published in 2010 in the *Journal of Ayurveda and Integrative Medicine,* there are eight different qualities recognized by *Ayurveda* that various plants may possess, which enhance the beauty and radiance of skin and slow its aging:

1. *Vayasthapana* literally means "maintaining youthfulness or arresting age." It refers to ingredients that have an overall anti-aging effect by nourishing the skin and improving all of its physiological functions. *Vayasthapana* herbs support the skin by keeping all three *doshas—vata, pitta,* and *kapha*—in balance. Gotu kola (*Centella asiatica*) is the most notable *vayasthapana* herb. It has many different anti-aging effects, including enhancing collagen synthesis.

2. *Varnya* means "youthful radiance." The principal herbs that enhance the radiance or give a healthy glow to the complexion include:

   • Sandalwood—an aromatic wood from a sacred tree in India, it is antibacterial, antiseptic, anti-acne, emollient (reducing skin drying and itchiness), anti-inflammatory, anti-aging, and evens skin tone and helps wound healing.

   • Vetiver—a fragrant grass similar to lemon grass, vetiver helps to clear acne, promote skin regeneration, strengthen the connective tissue, assist wound healing, and benefit aging skin.

   • Indian madder—a species of flowering plant, it is anti-inflammatory; reduces acne, freckles, and skin discoloration; and supports wound healing.

   • Indian sarsaparilla—a member of the milkweed family, this herb tastes somewhat like root beer, is anti-inflammatory and antibacterial, and improves acne and psoriasis.

3. *Sandhaniya* means "protection from normal wear and tear." Herbs that are in this category are healing and regenerative. For instance, "sensitive plant" enhances healing and regeneration of the nerves by 30 to 40 percent.

4. *Vranaropana* means "deep healing." Gotu kola and sensitive plant are two examples of herbs that enhance the deeper healing abilities of the skin.

5. *Tvachya* means "enhancing and nurturing." Herbs of this type support moisture balance and provide overall nourishments to the skin. The best examples are:

   • Gotu kola (*Centella asiatica*)—used in India for thousands of years to heal wounds, improve mental clarity, and treat skin conditions such as leprosy and psoriasis. Extracts have been found to calm inflammation, speed wound healing, stimulate new cell growth, build collagen, and improve circulation.

   • Silk cotton tree—is anti-inflammatory and used topically on burns and blistering to prevent scarring. The flowers are also said to be good for the skin and complexion.

   • Costus root—also known as Indian aloe, reduces skin discoloration and blemishes.

   • Rose petal—is anti-inflammatory, antibacterial, toning, moisturizing, and high in antioxidants.

6. *Shothahara* means "anti-inflammatory." As you are aware, inflammation is one of the major causes of aging, so all anti-inflammatory substances have an anti-aging effect. Rose petal, silk cotton tree, *Boswellia serrata*, and aloe vera are *shothahara* herbs with excellent anti-inflammatory properties.

7. *Tvachagnivardhani* literally means "to enhance the luster of the skin by enhancing the skin's metabolism." With age, the metabolism of the skin slows down and can cause an accumulation of toxins called *ama*. *Ama* clogs the channels in the skin, creates dullness, and can lead to wrinkles, dryness, and other signs of aging. Application of gotu kola enhances

enzymes and improves your body's ability to remove *ama*. *Ayurveda* says that by assisting the removal of *ama* and deep impurities, gotu kola also helps to prevent varicose veins, cellulite, aging skin, and weakened immunity to allergens and skin diseases.

8. *Tvagrasayana* literally means "skin *rasayana*" or that which prevents aging of the skin. (In *Ayurveda,* the term *rasayana* means "that which negates old age.") The plant amalaki (*Phyllanthus emblica*) is considered a *rasayana* and one of the best rejuvenating herbs for a beautiful complexion.

Topical Skin Care: West Meets East

Early in my plastic surgery career, my specialty was just beginning to recognize that the results from any facial rejuvenating surgery were greatly enhanced and sustained with a good topical skin-care regimen. Most plastic surgeons, including myself, hired aestheticians to provide facials and other types of noninvasive skin-care treatments. At the time, only light chemical peels, such as glycolic acid peels, and a couple of professional skin-care lines were available. Over time, a variety of other effective noninvasive treatments became available.

My approach includes the best of both Western and Eastern techniques. In general, daily topical skin-care routines for all skin types involve a nondrying cleanser, a toner, and a day and night moisturizer. All of these products should be nontoxic and, ideally, made from mostly organic natural plants. I also recommend a facial, approximately once a month, to exfoliate, deeply cleanse, and tone the skin.

The following are some of the topical products with which I have had personal experience and recommend. Some of them are only available through a physician's office or medical spa, or by prescription only. Others are widely available over-the-counter products that can be purchased on the Internet. There are also several noninvasive technologies that have impressive rejuvenating effects.

Retin-A

Generically called "retinoic acid" or "tretinoin," it is derived from vitamin A and available only by prescription. Retin-A first became popular more than twenty years ago as an acne treatment. But after its users also reported significant improvements in skin texture, including diminished wrinkles and brown spots, Retin-A became popular for its anti-aging effects. The first double-blind study of Retin-A was published in 1988 and showed a significant improvement in the photo-damage of the skin after four months of daily application. Retin-A helps to normalize the function of cells, prevents the breakdown of and repairs collagen, improves skin texture, and fades dark spots and freckles. Studies also show that it also helps to prevent skin cancers.

Apply Retin-A once a day as a thin layer before you go to bed. Don't apply other moisturizers or creams for at least one hour. Retin-A can initially cause skin drying, redness, and flakiness. You may be tempted to stop using it at this stage, but if you continue, these mild reactions will go away within a few weeks and your skin will look noticeable better. To minimize this reaction, I recommend gradually introducing your skin to Retin-A. Begin by using it only one day a week, then two, then three, and so on until you are using it every night. Renova is a brand of Retin-A that is more emollient and causes less drying. It's the one I personally use and recommend.

Glycolic Acids

Glycolic acids are naturally occurring compounds found in foods, such as fruits and milk that help to exfoliate the skin. When topically applied, they may help to reduce the appearance of fine lines, wrinkles, and hyper-pigmentations (or brown spots). Higher, more effective concentrations of glycolic acids are only available through physicians or aestheticians. Less concentrated, weaker solutions are available over the counter for home use.

Vitamin C

Not only is vitamin C beneficial for your skin when you ingest it, but it also has wonderful anti-aging effects when applied topically. Research shows it counteracts skin aging by increasing blood flow, decreasing inflammation, protecting against UVA and UVB damage, promoting collagen production, supporting structures in the dermal layer of your skin—which help to keep your skin looking plumper and more youthful, and by improving wrinkling and age-related hyper-pigmentations, such as brown spots. Vitamin C is added to many moisturizers. I recommend using a high-quality vitamin C serum once a day in the morning. Then apply a good moisturizer of your choice, such as one of those I mention below.

Galvanic Skin Devices

These handheld devices produce a low-voltage DC current that changes the electrical charge of the skin causing the moisture content to increase. They are also thought to diminish the appearance of fine lines and improve skin tone by working with the electrical endplates between nerves and muscles. I personally use a galvanic device made by Nu Skin Enterprises. For more information, email info@drchristinehorner.com.

Microcurrent Therapy

This device provides an electrical current that stimulates nerves and muscles. When applied to the skin and muscles on the face and neck, it has been shown to:

- Increase collagen (12 percent) and elastin (45 percent) production
- Smooth and firm the skin
- Improve blood circulation (39 percent) and hydration
- Diminish appearance of fine lines and wrinkles
- Increase muscle tone in the facial muscles
- Lift sagging jowls and eyebrows

Microdermabrasion

This process uses a handheld device to physically remove the dead surface layers of the skin and to stimulate an increase in collagen production. Many patients see dramatic improvements in the tone, texture, and color of treated areas after just one treatment.

Topical Skin-Care Products

There are several companies I recommend that make excellent topical skin-care products depending on your desired results and budget. Here are a few of them:

makana Skin Cream

makana uses organic oils from plants that grow in Hawaii. It contains no chemicals, preservatives, or other potentially harmful chemicals. The main ingredients include:

- **Tamanu oil**, which promotes wound healing and speeds the formation of new healthy skin

- **Kukui oil**, which is high in antioxidants and diminishes fine lines by improving elasticity

- **Macadamia nut oil**, which is naturally rich in vitamin E, and helps soften fine lines and wrinkles

- **Jojoba seed oil**, which enhances the suppleness of the skin

- **Unrefined shea butter**, which is rich in vitamins A, E and F, and helps promote new collagen

- **Cocoa seed butter**, which is dense with polyphenols antioxidants

You can read more about it and order the product at www.drchristine-horner.com/shop-oils.cfm

Youthful Skin Cream

Youthful Skin Cream, an *Ayurvedic* formulation, contains gotu kola, sensitive plant, silk cotton tree (*Bombax*), Indian madder, and *Woodfordia fruticosa*, which helps enhance the skin's resistance to photosensitivity. It also contains other herbs that help the skin resist environmental irritants, while providing deep nourishment to the skin and decreasing the effects of oxygen free radicals and aging. It can be purchased on www.mapi.com (use the code: "radianthealth" for 10% discount).

Sarada Ayurvedic Remedies

Sarada Ayurvedic Remedies (www.saradausa.com) are made by a mother and daughter partnership in Ojai, California. The daughter has been an *Ayurvedic* practitioner for the past twenty-three years and studies with *vaidyas* in India. The products are all natural *Ayurvedic* ingredients that have been traditionally prepared and are free of chemical, artificial, or preservative additives. Their herbal oils are made using traditional methods combined with the understanding of modern science. The herbs and oils are ethically sourced, sustainable, and organic, and include herbs such as amla, ashwagandha, turmeric, licorice, neem, and tulsi.

Beautiful Skin Requires a Holistic Approach

If you want your skin to look more beautiful and radiant, remember it begins from the inside. Yes, how you treat your skin topically matters, too. But, because your skin reflects your inner health, you can never achieve a youthful glowing complexion with topical skin care alone. The payoff of following all of the advice in this book is not just extraordinary health and longevity, but also radiantly beautiful skin—no matter your age.

The following are my top-10 tips for healthy skin from the inside:

1. **Eat a healthy diet filled with organically grown plants.** Fruits, vegetables, whole grains, nuts, and seeds provide the best nourishment for your body and skin. These nutrient-dense plants are packed with essential vitamins and minerals required by your body to stay healthy. They are also alkaline, anti-inflammatory, and high in antioxidants, which help your body ward off disease and slow aging.

2. **Avoid junk foods.** Processed foods, sugar, colas, excessive red meat, caffeine, and alcohol create oxygen free radicals and promote inflammation. They accelerate aging and can cause your complexion to look dull and sallow. Oxygen free radicals and inflammation also contribute to the development of every chronic disorder, including heart disease, dementia, diabetes, and certain cancers, especially cancers of the breast, prostate, and colon. So staying away from these "bad" foods is also important for your overall health.

3. **Drink plenty of pure water every day.** Staying hydrated is essential for your body to function properly. The adult body is composed of more than 70 percent water and, therefore, drinking an adequate amount of purified water every day is critical for your organs to function properly. Most experts recommend that you drink a minimum of 8 cups of water each day. If you are active—especially if you enjoy rigorous activities that

make you sweat—you will need to consume much more. Drinking adequate amounts of water improves circulation and, therefore, the delivery of nutrients to your cells and the removal of waste products. It also helps to keep your skin moist, smooth, pumped, toned, and elastic.

4. **Consume good fats.** Fat is another macronutrient that is essential for your body to function properly. Your cell membranes, hormones, and the protective layer of your nervous system and body are all composed of fat. The type of fat you predominately consume is very important because it becomes the construction material for your body. Saturated animal fats and man-manipulated hydrogenated fats and trans-fats increase inflammation and cause your cell membranes to become stiff and not function properly. Whereas healthy fats, especially essential omega-3, omega-9, omega-7, and evening primrose oil have the opposite effect. They make your cell membranes flexible, decrease inflammation, and improve the function of your cells. These nourishing fats also keep your skin cells plumper and help to make your complexion look moist and luxurious.

5. **Add superfoods to your diet.** The term "superfoods" refers to foods that contain an unusual concentration of nutrients. Some of the superfoods that are especially good for your skin include:

- Green tea (contains powerful antioxidants, anti-inflammatories, and protects against ultraviolet radiation)
- Tomatoes (high in the antioxidant lycopene)
- Berries (packed full of antioxidants and low on the glycemic index)
- Avocados (great source of healthy oils and biotin—a B vitamin essential for skin health)
- Salmon (rich in the antioxidant astaxanthin and omega-3 fatty acids)
- Eggs (high in protein and biotin)
- Pomegranate (teeming with powerful antioxidants)
- Legumes (good source of protein needed for cell repair)

6. **Take key supplements.** Taking certain vitamins, minerals, and other beneficial compounds is one of the most effective ways to treat skin

conditions and improve the health of your skin. There are several nutrients that are known to play a key role in your skin health. They include:

- Vitamin A—or retinol, a powerful antioxidant that is one of the most important nutrients for healthy skin. It supports optimal growth and function.

- Vitamin B complex—works in a variety of ways to support skin health, including decreasing oxygen free radicals, improving circulation, protecting against stress, enhancing sleep, and helping many enzymes.

- Vitamin C—an antioxidant involved in collagen synthesis, it protects against UV damage, and improves skin appearance by increasing hydration and decreasing skin wrinkling.

- Vitamin E—the most abundant fat-soluble antioxidant found in the skin, a potent anti-inflammatory that protects against UV radiation damage.

- Selenium—a mineral component of glutathione peroxidase, an enzyme necessary for the antioxidant function of glutathione, one of the major antioxidants in the body that protects against cellular damage from the oxygen free radicals that cause inflammation, aging, and promote skin cancer.

- Alpha-lipoic acid—called "the universal antioxidant" because it is both fat and water soluble; it is 400 times more powerful than vitamin E and C.

- Resveratrol—from grape skins, provides strong antioxidants that protect against ultraviolet radiation and damage, including skin cancer.

- Zinc—assists in the proper structure of proteins and cell membranes, improves wound healing, has anti-inflammatory effects, and protects against ultraviolet radiation.

- Sulfur—involved in collagen synthesis, which gives the skin its structure and strength.

- Silica—a mineral that helps form collagen.

7. **Exercise regularly.** Moving your body is fundamentally important for good health, including the health of your skin. Aerobic activities every day improve the circulation of your blood and, therefore, the delivery of nutrients to your skin and the removal of cellular waste material. Be careful not to overexercise because it can cause an increase in oxygen free radicals, which accelerates aging.

8. **Minimize stress.** Nothing is more damaging to your health than severe stress. Chronically high levels of stress hormones wreak havoc on your body and skin by increasing inflammation and oxygen free radicals, decreasing circulation and causing your body to become acidotic. Take an inventory of your life and write down everything that is stressful for you. For those items over which you have some control, make changes that will reduce your stress. Because there are many stressful events in everyone's life over which you have no control, it is important to practice an effective stress-reducing technique daily such as meditation, yoga, tai chi, or breathing exercises. These techniques tone down the response of your nervous system and minimize the release of stress hormones. Certain herbs called "adaptogens," such as holy basil and ashwagandha, protect against the damaging effects of stress and are a great idea to take during times that are especially stressful.

9. **Make the most of your sleep.** The quality of your sleep has a profound effect on your health. When you sleep, your body not only rests but also detoxifies and rejuvenates. The exact times you sleep are just as important as the total number of hours. Research shows that going to bed before 10 p.m. and getting up by 6 a.m. are the optimal hours for sleep. Most people do best with seven to eight hours of sleep. Sleeping less or more than this is associated with an increased incidence of many diseases, including heart disease, diabetes, obesity and cancer. You can improve your sleep by engaging in only light, calming activities in evening, and avoiding stimulating exercise, computer work, or emotionally disturbing movies and television programs. Be sure to turn off all your lights in your bedroom and pull down the shades. Melatonin, your sleep hormone, is very sensitive to light. If you are a night owl, go to bed 15 minutes earlier every week to gradually train your body to go to sleep before 10 p.m.

10. **Get the toxins out.** Toxins are released as a natural process of metabolism from all of your cells. In addition, you are exposed every day to an assortment of chemical toxins found in your food, cleaning products, personal-care products, and the environment. Toxins clog up your system and prevent your body from functioning well. Too many toxins will make your skin break out and/or look dull. They are also known to contribute to numerous diseases. That's why it is important to detoxify on a regular basis. The major organs of detoxification are your liver, colon, kidneys, and skin. You can promote healthy elimination by consuming plenty of fiber, fresh fruits, vegetables, and purified water every day. Because the bacteria in your colon play a vital role in your digestive and immune health, probiotics can make a big difference in your health and skin. You can boost the elimination of toxins with yoga, aerobic exercise, massages, and sweating. Research shows infrared saunas are the most effective for helping your body eliminate toxins through sweat.

The more of these tips you follow, the better your health and the quality of your skin will be. The good news is that for most people, the skin's response is rapid. In other words, just a few days of a healthy diet and lifestyle can really show on your face. If you make all of these tips your daily habits, you'll enjoy the pleasure of consistently feeling and looking great—no matter what your age.

CHAPTER 13

Putting It All Together

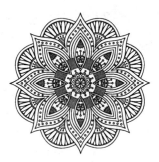

Dr. Horner's 30-Day Program for Radiant Health and Ageless Beauty

Yesterday is a dream, tomorrow but a vision.
But today well-lived makes every yesterday
a dream of happiness, and every tomorrow
a vision of hope. Look well, therefore, to this day.

~Sanskrit Proverb

CONGRATULATIONS!

You have now finished gathering all the elements for your breastplate of protection and are ready to begin putting them all together in your 30-day program.

> *"The secret of getting ahead is getting started."*
>
> ~MARK TWAIN

It's time to begin your 30-day program. I promise it will be fun, adventurous, inspiring, and you will be amazed by how much better you will look and feel. This program is designed to help you successfully adopt all the important aspects to extraordinary health and longevity presented in this book. It's structured to be easy and stress-free. There's no *right* way to do the program, nor is there an advantage of doing the program in the order that it's presented—except I recommend completing the first three days in the order presented. After the first three days, if you want to mix up the order of the days, that's perfectly fine. You may want to choose the suggestions for the days that come most easily and naturally to you first, and later, choose the more personally challenging ones—or vice versa.

People are usually better at sticking with programs that are time-sensitive. So, I challenge you to make a commitment to complete the program in thirty days. You can do it over a longer time if you need to, but the chances of your completing it will not be as a good. It's just a matter of human psychology. The fact is that most people are more successful at adopting new habits if they have a structure and a timeframe in place for achieving their goals.

Another tip for success is to have an accountability partner or buddy—a friend, family member, or your significant other—to do the program with you. For example, research shows having a partner for weight-loss programs and/or exercise programs is associated with a much higher rate of success. You can easily talk yourself out of going for a walk or to the gym. But, if you have a buddy that's doing these activities with you, chances are very good that you'll show up—even when you don't want to.

"Every human being is the author
of his own health or disease."

~Swami Sivananda Saraswati

DAY 1   Love and honor yourself.

Today is the day that you've decided to begin a new relationship with yourself. It is a sacred moment. As Antoine de Saint-Exupéry said, "A single event can awaken within us a stranger totally unknown to us. To live is to be slowly born." This day is the moment of conception for the birth of a new you, an even more extraordinary person than you already are; a person with deep understanding and reverence for your body, mind, and soul.

Each of us is a unique expression of the Divine. It is time to love and honor yourself as much as you do your child or dearest friend. The natural tendency of the mind is to wander into negative chatter. If you have let your inner critics run wild, it will take some rigorous discipline to tame them. But you can! If you have been your worst critic, now is the time for you to become your best friend.

Your success on this program to radiant health and ageless beauty will be easy if you base it on a foundation of self-love. The truth is—this entire program is an act of self-love. Honoring yourself by taking the best care of yourself that you can, in every way, is the highest expression of self-love.

Activity

Start paying close attention to your "self-talk." Are you talking to yourself as a supportive friend or as a judgmental critic? Each time you catch yourself saying something negative or critical—stop! Immediately say something positive and supportive instead. Make this a practice from this day forward. Become rigorous about paying attention to your self-talk.

Whenever you notice that your inner critics have taken over—put a gag on them immediately. Counteract whatever they just said to you with something loving and supportive. For instance, if your inner critics are telling you that your body isn't attractive—tell them to zip it and counteract their negativity by telling your body how much you appreciate all the wonderful ways it serves you. With time, you will notice that your inner critics will become much quieter. Eventually, you'll rarely hear a peep out of them. Inner peace and serenity are the gifts of living every day in gratitude and appreciation—especially for yourself.

DAY 2   Discover your constitutional *dosha*.

In chapter 1, you learned about the *doshas* or governing principles called *vata, pitta,* and *kapha*. If you need to review this information, do so now. Almost everyone has certain *doshas* that occur in higher amounts than others. Knowing your dominant or "constitutional" *dosha* type will help direct you to more specific guidelines that can more effectively help you to keep your body in balance.

Activity

Go to www.banyanbotanicals.com/info/prakriti-quiz/ or www.mapi.com/doshas/vpk-explanation.html#gsc.tab=0 and take the simple quiz. Answer the questions for your lifetime tendencies to determine your *dosha* constitution, also known as your *prikriti*. You can also take the same test to determine your current *dosha* balance, called your *vikriti*, by answering the questions based on how you are now. For example, if your hands and feet have tended to be cold most of your life, but recently have been warm, answer the question about your natural tendency for the temperature of your hands and feet as "cold" if you want to determine your *prikriti*, and "warm" if you would are determining your *vikriti*.

DAY 3   Balance your *doshas* with food.

Now that you have determined your *dosha* constitution (*prikriti*), you can look up what foods you should favor and which you should avoid that will help bring your body into balance. For instance, if your *pitta dosha* is predominant you will want to favor foods that are cool and liquid, and minimize hot spicy foods. Cook with olive oil and coconut oil. Choose grapes, cherries, melons, coconuts, pomegranates, and sweet plums; avoid citrus, olives, papayas, and sour plums. Favor vegetables that are sweet—for example, carrots, beets, parsnips, artichokes, and asparagus. Also enjoy vegetables that are bitter, such as dandelion greens, arugula and other leafy greens. Avoid pungent vegetables, including green chilies, horseradish, leeks, green onions, hot peppers, and radishes.

Activity

Go to www.mapi.com to read more about your predominant *dosha* and the foods you should favor and avoid.

- If you are *vata*, the direct link is www.mapi.com/ayurvedic-recipes/dietary-guidelines/vata.html#gsc.tab=0

- If you are *pitta*, the direct link is www.mapi.com/ayurvedic-recipes/dietary-guidelines/pitta.html#gsc.tab=0

- If you are *kapha*, the direct link is www.mapi.com/ayurvedic-recipes/dietary-guidelines/kapha.html#gsc.tab=0

For the next week, eat only those foods that are balancing for your predominant *dosha*. Notice if your digestion and energy improve. If not, you might want to try a different *dosha* diet that would correspond to your current balance or *vikriti*, which you determined from the quiz you took yesterday. In other words, if your predominant *dosha* is *pitta*, but your current balance or *vikriti* is *vata*—try a *vata*-pacifying diet for a week.

DAY 4   Enhance your social network.

Having a strong support system and social network has consistently been shown to be one of the most important attributes of those who enjoy extraordinary longevity. For many, time with friends falls to the wayside as work and other responsibilities take over. If this has happened to you, today is the day you are going to begin correcting that imbalance.

Activity

Make a list of friends you enjoy who you haven't connected with for a long time. Now chose one or two of those friends and call them today. Emailing, texting, or communicating by Facebook messaging doesn't count. You must talk with your friend in real time. Better yet, schedule a time to physically get together if you can. If you have friends or family who live at a distance, I highly recommend using Skype. I have family members who live in other countries, and communicating with them via Skype—which is free—has allowed us to stay in close contact. When you connect with this friend, schedule the next time you will speak or get together, so that you don't let your relationship fall between the cracks again.

Next, spend some time thinking about ways that you can increase your social network—especially if you don't have much of one currently. For example, I started playing tennis and taking ballroom dancing lessons to expand my social network. I also started going to the gym and hiking with my sister-in-law. Prior to this, I generally did all of my regular physical activity alone. You could also join a group, such as a church group or a book club, or participate regularly in a meet-up group. If you haven't participated in groups before, you will be amazed by how enjoyable and satisfying they can be.

> *"One word frees us of all the weight and pain of life:*
> *That word is love."*
>
> ~SOPHOCLES (496–406 BC)

DAY 5   Practice random acts of kindness.

When you do something kind for someone else, research shows the person who gets the most benefits—is you! Today is the day you will begin the practice of purposefully doing something kind for someone every day. For instance, you could let someone in the grocery line go ahead of you, open the door for someone, or simply smile at a person you pass in the street. You have no idea how much that act will affect that person or how much it will impact you. Wayne Dyer told a story once about his daughter letting a woman go ahead of her in the line at the grocery store. The woman said that she and her family were just about to move back to the town they had recently left, because no one in this town seemed to be kind. She asked for a sign that morning. She told Wayne's daughter that her act of kindness was her sign, and now her family would stay. This simple act of kindness had a huge impact on an entire family. Your simple act of kindness could end up affecting people all over the world!

*"Constant kindness can accomplish much.
As the sun makes ice melt, kindness causes
misunderstanding, mistrust, and
hostility to evaporate."*

~ALBERT SCHWEITZER

Activity

Make a list of random acts of kindness that you can do. Write down the act you will do for each day of the week for the next week. With each act of kindness you give, notice the reaction of the person who received it, as well as how you felt. Share your miracles with others to inspire them to do the same. Continue giving acts of kindness as often as you can.

DAY 6   Create joy in your life.

To-do lists usually aren't filled with tasks that are centered on joy. If you find that your life is filled with activities that don't bring you joy, then this activity is especially important for you.

Activity

Take some time thinking about what brings you joy. Perhaps it is watching the sunset, walking in nature, and or getting a massage. Make a list. Now, add at least one activity that brings you joy to your to-do list every day. I started doing this a few years ago, and then realized after several months that I have the opportunity to bring joy into everything I do. This practice helped me to see my world differently and taught me how to experience joy consistently throughout the day.

*"If you wouldst live long, live well;
for folly and wickedness shorten life."*

~BENJAMIN FRANKLIN

DAY 7   Minimize your stress.

There's no question that life in the Western world is filled with stress—from commuting in heavy traffic to work, dealing with a difficult boss, and having unexpected expenses to dealing with a health issue, losing your job, or grieving the death of a loved one. Some of the chronic stress you experience may be from factors over which you have some control. For example, you have taken on too many responsibilities, or have allowed certain people to stay in your life who treat you badly.

Activity

Make a list of everything you currently find stressful in your life. Mark those over which you have some control. Now think of a few creative ways that could help reduce the stress you experience with each of these situations. For instance, your work demands that you have to frequently stay late. By the time you get home, you are exhausted and have no time or energy to cook—not to mention running errands or cleaning. You could lower your stress by hiring someone for just a couple hours a week to help you out, such as a retired older woman or a college student. For instance, she could cook all your meals for the week and stock them in your freezer or refrigerator and/or run some errands for you, such as grocery shopping or picking up the dry cleaning. Perhaps you have taken on too many volunteer positions. Review everything you are doing and determine which activities you can let someone else do.

"Tension is who you think you should be.
Relaxation is who you are."

~CHINESE PROVERB

DAY 8   Learn and practice an effective stress-reducing technique.

In chapter 3, you learned about several techniques that can help to minimize the stress response. For instance, yoga, tai chi, qigong, and meditations have all been documented by research to lower stress hormones. The key is that these practices must be done daily to keep your nervous system in a more relaxed state.

Activity

Review the "Summary of Techniques to Reduce Stress" at the end of chapter 3. Select one or two of the techniques that you think you can commit to every day. For instance, if you choose breathing exercises, practice the *pranayama* technique described on page 67 for ten minutes a day. Choose a time, such as soon as you get up in the morning, during a work break, or right after you get home, to always practice your technique. Having a scheduled time is extremely important, because it is easy to forget or let other things in your life interfere. When you have mastered ten minutes, expand the time to twenty minutes.

"The time to relax is when you don't have time for it."

~SYDNEY J. HARRIS

DAY 9 Learn to tap.

An extremely easy and effective technique for releasing emotional stress is called the "Emotional Freedom Technique" (EFT), or tapping. It can be done anywhere and is free. The technique can be easily learned from a short instructional YouTube video.

Activity

Go to https://www.youtube.com/watch?v=IWu3rSEddZI and learn how to do the EFT technique. Choose a topic that causes you to feel mild stress—not a major issue—and test out the technique to see how it works. Then practice the technique with several other minor issues until you feel comfortable with the process. For the next week, choose one issue every day to practice the technique. Whenever you feel triggered in the future, use the tapping technique to help release the charge of your emotional reaction.

DAY 10   Expand your choice of vegetables.

Researchers at the Washington Center for Obesity Research have found that most Americans routinely eat no more than thirty different foods. And they generally cycle through all of them in about four days. To put this in perspective, the Maya ate 1,200 different types of plants. You were designed to eat a diversified diet. Each plant has hundreds of phytochemicals that act as natural medicines. By eating a diversity of plants, you will be supplying your body with a much larger number of disease-fighting chemicals. Remember that you should always choose organically grown, fresh plants as much as possible.

Activity

Go to your local grocery that carries organic produce. If your community has a farmer's market, that's an even better place to get your organic produce, because it is generally fresher. Go through all the vegetables they carry and then select a few that you normally don't eat. Look up recipes on the Internet to discover various ways that the vegetable can be prepared. Be adventurous! You may discover vegetables you have never tried that become your favorites. Try to prepare different types of vegetables every day. Think of a friend or two who might want to participate on this adventure with you. You can share your recipes and experience with new vegetables with each other.

DAY 11   Discover new fruits.

Just like vegetables, fruits are also loaded with antioxidants and other nutrients that are extremely beneficial for your health, but most people consume only a limited variety.

Activity

Go to your grocery store or farmer's market and look for organic fruits you have never tried before. Make a list and try a new fruit every week. As you did on Day 9 with vegetables, do the same with fruits—chose a different type of fruit to consume each day for one week. Try to find a dozen fruits you like. Make a schedule that rotates all of these fruits over the course of a couple of weeks.

DAY 12   Supercharge your diet with superfoods.

There are a variety of foods that are so nutrient dense they are called "superfoods." I highly recommend adding superfoods to your diet every day to supercharge your nutrition. Review the superfood section in chapter 4. Choose a few superfoods you would like to try.

Activity

An easy way to consume some of the more exotic superfoods is in a smoothie. Many of them can be purchased as powders that are available at certain grocery stores or the Internet. I buy many of mine from discount retailers, for example Amazon.com and Vitacost.com. To make a smoothie, add a cup of water to a blender, then add a tablespoon of a few powdered superfoods, such as pomegranate, acai, maqui, camu camu, or maca. Next, add a cup or so of fresh or frozen organic berries—strawberries, blueberries, raspberries, and/or blackberries. Push the button on your blender and let it do its magic until it is the consistency you desire, usually about a minute or two. I like to also add a scoop of organic whey protein powder, but you can use a plant-protein powder if you prefer.

DAY 13   Take an *Ayurvedic rasayana.*

As you may recall from chapter 5, a *rasayana* means "that which negates old age." The purpose of a *rasayana* is to improve your strength, immunity, and vitality and help you resist disease and enjoy a long healthy life. The most powerful *rasayana* is a 5,000-year-old formula called *Amrit Kalash*. *Amrit Kalash* is also very helpful for those who are currently undergoing cancer treatments, by enhancing the effectiveness of the Western treatments while, at the same time, taking away many of their side effects.

Activity

Go to www.mapi.com and order one bottle each of Amrit Kalash Nectar and Ambrosia tablets. You can also try the paste, but the taste can be challenging for some people. Use the code "radianthealth" at checkout for a 10% discount. Take one tablet each of the ambrosia and nectar every day, twice a day, for one month. Notice how you feel at the end of the month. Many people report a significant improvement in energy levels and overall well-being.

DAY 14   Boost your immune system with medicinal mushrooms.

Medicinal mushrooms are extraordinarily powerful at supporting your immune system. You can eat them, but in all practicality, you are not going to eat them every day in the dose that is needed to be effective. This is an example of why taking a supplement can be important. Taking a medicinal mushroom supplement every day is a simple and easy way to help keep your immune system strong. My favorite formula is AHCC, which stands for active hexose correlated compound. AHCC has been the subject of hundreds of studies and has been shown to be extremely effective at fighting bacterial and viral infections, as well as cancer. In fact, AHCC is prescribed in hospitals in Japan for cancer patients, because it significant improves their chances of survival. I take it every day because I believe it is one of the best supplements to help keep my immune system in top form.

Activity

Try an AHCC supplement. I personally use the one made by Quality of Life Labs and, for your convenience, have it available on my website: www.drchristinehorner.com. If you'd like to try one from another company, that's fine. AHCC is made by a single source in Japan, so its quality doesn't vary. Check to see how much AHCC is contained in the supplement. A daily dose of at least 1,000 mg is recommended. If you are ill, you should take more, such as 2,000–4,000 mg per day.

DAY 15   Start your morning with omega-3s.

Omega-3 fatty acids are critical for your health and nearly impossible to get enough of without taking a supplement. I recommend that everyone take an omega-3 fatty acid supplement every day. There are a variety of different sources for omega-3 fatty acids. I like the Omega Swirl products made by Barlean's Organic Oils because they are organic and processed with techniques that are of the freshest and highest quality. Because I'm a vegetarian, I take flax oil, but there are also fish oils available.

Activity

Go to your local grocery store that contains organic produce. Look in the refrigerated section for Barlean's Omega Swirl products. You can also ask about an omega-3 supplement that comes as capsules if you prefer. If you don't have a store that carries Barlean's products near you, you can order them on the Internet and have them shipped to your doorstep.

DAY 16   Find an invigorating body movement you love.

Moving your body every day—especially in ways that causes your heart rate to go up—is one of the most important aspects to good health. Conversely, being sedentary is one of the most destructive choices for your health. Sitting more than five hours at a time is associated with a higher risk of disease and early death—even if you exercise daily. So be sure to get up every hour and stretch your legs. Even as little as two minutes of moving every hour can make a big difference.

Activity

If you must sit for work, set a timer on your phone or computer to remind you to get up every thirty to sixty minutes and walk and stretch for three to five minutes.

> *"There is no substitute for exercise as part of your plan to stay healthy. Just accept it, work it into your routine, and enjoy it."*
>
> ~J. J. GOLDWAG

DAY 17   Maximize your sleep.

Research shows that the absolute hours you sleep are just as important as the number of hours you sleep. Going to bed by 10 p.m. and getting up by 6 a.m. are the optimal hours for sleep.

Activity

If you have been a night owl, now is the time to start backing your bedtime up. Go to bed fifteen minutes earlier every week, until you are going to bed before 10 p.m. This helps your body to naturally adjust to the earlier bedtime. Make sure to turn off all your lights and make your bedroom as dark as possible. Also do not have any electronic equipment near you, including an electric alarm clock to avoid the EMFs they produce.

DAY 18   Create a bedtime ritual.

Ensuring a night of luxurious restful sleep requires conscious preparation. You can't eat a large meal, engage in strenuous activity, or watch a disturbing movie and expect to fall asleep immediately and have a wonderful night's rest. Instead, you must work with the natural rhythms of your body and gradually slow down your activities in the evening.

Activity

Commit to trying a bedtime ritual for seven days straight to observe the effects it has on your sleep and how your energy and mood are during the day. Eat a light dinner at least three hours before you go to bed. Go for a walk after dinner. If you need to check your emails or do some computer work, finish the work at least two hours before you go to bed. Engage only in activities in the evening that are quieting, such as taking a bath, reading uplifting material, listening to soothing music, doing a needle craft or other relaxing activity, having a pleasant conversation with a friend, or whatever you find most relaxing. Go to bed at the same time every night before 10 p.m. and get up at the same time every morning before 6 a.m. After you experience how much better you sleep and feel with this ritual, it will be easy for you to continue doing it.

DAY 19 Change a daytime habit to enhance your sleep.

What you do during the day also affects the quality of your sleep. For instance, exercising in the morning, eating three meals a day that are easily digestible, taking naps that are no longer than twenty minutes before 4 p.m., avoiding caffeine after midday, breathing fresh air and getting some direct sunlight, avoiding heavy and/or spicy foods for dinner, and practicing a stress-reducing habit in the morning or late afternoon, such as meditation, are all associated with helping you get a better night's sleep.

Activity

Take a look at all the daytime habits above that can help you get a better night's sleep. Do any of them that stand out as one that might make a big difference for you? If so, make the change. For instance, if you work indoors during the day and never go outside, go outside for ten to twenty minutes during your lunch hour. If you normally exercise in the late afternoon or evening, try getting up earlier and exercising in the morning instead. If you usually reach for some caffeine in the late afternoon or evening, drink purified water instead. Try this new habit for at least a week to see what difference it may make in your quality of sleep.

DAY 20 Detoxify for three days.

If you have never tried a detoxification program, you might be amazed at how quickly you will feel and look better if you do. Everyone in the world today is exposed to toxins. Toxins can clog your channels, obstruct your inner healing intelligence, slow down your digestion, dull your skin and eyes, and zap you of your energy. Even a short, three-day detoxification can be effective enough to make you feel remarkably better.

Activity

For the next three days, stop eating meat, processed foods, sugar, refined carbohydrates, dairy, and alcohol. Instead, consume only fresh, lightly cooked, organically grown vegetables and other easily digestible plants, fresh vegetable soups and juices, purified water, and herbal teas. Do not engage in any strenuous activities. Instead go for brisk walks and enjoy some light yoga. If you would like, take some detoxifying herbs such as milk thistle, dandelion root, and turmeric. Try a sauna for twenty minutes if available and/or get a massage using organic sesame oil to help facilitate the release of more toxins.

At the end of three days, evaluate if you would like to continue this detoxification for a few more days. If this is your first time, I recommend only trying this type of detoxification for a week. If you are experienced at detoxification, you could follow this program for two or three weeks. For the future, plan at least one week, three times a year to detoxify. Review chapter 8 for other types of detoxification programs you can do.

DAY 21   Take a sauna.

Saunas, especially infrared saunas, enhance the release of toxins and heavy metals from your cells and facilitate their removal from your body through your sweat. Many facilities are now offering infrared sauna sessions. You will have to investigate if your community has one.

Activity

If you have access to an infrared sauna, do twenty-minute sessions at a temperature of at least 130 degrees Fahrenheit several times a week. Don't overdo it. If you feel too hot or lightheaded, please shorten your session until you can build up to the longer time. You will need to make sure you drink plenty of purified water and add minerals, such as magnesium, which are lost in your sweat. If you don't have access to an infrared sauna, you can use moist or dry sauna instead. Many fitness centers have saunas. Again, you will have to check to see what is available in your community. Many companies make infrared saunas for home use. I recommend saunas made by Sunlighten (www.sunlighten.com).

To help your body eliminate even more heavy metals, take chlorella— a type of algae discussed in chapter 5. You can purchase it from your local health food store or online. Start with 10 small tablets of chlorella every day for thirty days. Over time, you can increase the dose if you would like.

DAY 22   Discover your ideal body weight.

Standardized charts are not always accurate for determining what your ideal body weight should be. There are so many variables based on your body constitution, bone structure, and muscle mass that need to be considered.

Activity

Schedule an appointment with a personal trainer or a facility where they have a more sophisticated technology to determine your percent body fat and metabolic rate. You'll have to research where these facilities are in your community. A noninvasive scanner is one of the most accurate ways to measure your body fat. A bioelectric impedance test is also fairly accurate. Avoid skin-fold measurements and calipers, because their accuracy is much less.

DAY 23   Reach your ideal weight.

It's no secret that the vast majority of Americans are overweight. In fact, more than 66 percent of us are. If you are overweight, losing the excess pounds is extremely important for your health and longevity. There are many chronic diseases associated with obesity, including diabetes, hypertension, heart disease, Alzheimer's disease and certain cancers, to name a few. The most successful weight-loss programs are ones where you work with a coach, as well as having the support of others. Trying to lose weight completely on your own is tough, especially if you have a significant amount of weight to lose.

Activity

If you have only ten to twenty pounds to lose, you might find that by simply avoiding sugar, processed foods, and fast foods, and instead favoring a plant-based, nutrient-dense, lower-calorie diet along with some moderate exercise, such as brisk walking, will easily get you to your ideal weight. These habits are also the ones that will help you achieve and maintain your best health. If you have more than twenty pounds to lose, I recommend working with a weight-loss program, such as Weight Watchers. Be sure to see you doctor first.

DAY 24   Go for a brisk walk for at least thirty minutes every day.

Brisk walking is one of the best exercises you can do every day. Research shows that just thirty minutes a day can have profound effects on your overall health, risk of chronic disease, and longevity. The good news is you can achieve similar benefits whether you do the thirty minutes at one time, or if you break the thirty minutes up to several chunks—for instance, walking briskly for ten minutes, three times a day.

Activity

Determine the best way that you can get 30 minutes of brisk walking in a day. Make the schedule and then stick to it. One of the best times to walk is in early morning. Try to find someone to walk with you, so that you keep each other committed to your walks. If you need to break up your scheduled walks, choose three times during the day that you can walk for ten minutes. Perhaps you can walk for ten minutes in the morning, again at lunchtime, and in the early evening. Find what works best for you.

"I had to wait 110 years to become famous.
I wanted to enjoy it as long as possible."

~JEANNE LOUISE CALMENT (1875–1997)

DAY 25   Find an activity you enjoy that gets your heart rate up.

If you don't like going to the gym—don't go! If you are bored with whatever activity you normally have been doing and find it difficult to do it—stop trying to do it!

Activity

Find a new form of exercise that is fun for you. For example, take dancing lessons, learn how to play tennis, or join a hiking group or a baseball team. Keep trying different activities until you find one you really enjoy. Then make it a regular habit. Find a friend or family member to participate with you if you can, because having an exercise buddy helps you to stick with it.

DAY 26   Experience energy healing.

Because we are made of energy, working with subtle energy can cause profound healing. If you have never experienced energy healing, this is the day to arrange an appointment.

Activity

Energy healers fall under the category of many different subspecialties, including acupuncture, Healing Touch, Therapeutic Touch, Reiki, and cranial sacral therapy. There are many other forms of energy healing as well. To find a good therapist in your area, check Internet sites such as Yelp or ask your friends and family for a referral.

DAY 27   Take an EMFs tour of your house.

Electromagnetic frequencies emit from all wired and wireless devices, including household appliances, computers, cell phones, cordless phones, and clock radios. These frequencies interact with the electrical charges in your body and can contribute to serious health problems. So, minimizing your exposure to EMFs is very important.

Activities

Take a tour of your home and identify all the wired and wireless devices in your home. Also check for transformers outside your home. There are meters you can purchase to measure the amount of EMFs in the various areas of your home. When you find places with high EMFs, see what you can do to minimize them. I recommend EMFs protection devices made by GIA Wellness (www.drchristinehorner.com/shop-emfprotection.cfm). Change electric clocks to battery operated, use a bluetooth for your cell phone, and when you use appliances, keep a safe distance from them if you can. Make sure there are no electrical devices in your bedroom, especially near your head, because the EMFs can interfere with your ability to sleep.

DAY 28   Start a gratitude journal.

Keeping a gratitude journal has been shown to be one of the most effective ways to create happiness. It's a simple practice that can help to keep you focused on all your blessings, rather than on all of your complaints. Happiness is not a result of your external circumstances, but rather from your internal perspective, which can be cultivated through gratitude.

Activity

Go to your local bookstore, look through their journals, and find one that calls to you for your gratitude journal. Every day take a few minutes to write down in your journal what you're grateful for that day. Do not use this journal for any other purpose. If you'd like to write down your daily events and thoughts, do that in another journal. This journal is to be purely about gratitude.

Even if your life is very difficult right now, you can find at least three things for which you are grateful. Viktor Frankl wrote in his classic book, *Man's Search for Meaning,* how he was able to stay positive while in a Nazi concentration camp. So no matter your circumstances, you too can find many blessings for which you can be grateful. For example, the blue sky, a flower, the warm sun on your face, your pet, someone in your life, or a roof over your head. Be inspired by people who have a much more challenging life than you do, but are able to be in gratitude. I had a very ill quadriplegic patient who said something profound to me one day that has stayed with me ever since. He said, "I woke up breathing, so today is a good day."

You can write as many items for which you are grateful as you would like each day. Try to list a minimum of three. Tony Robbins, for example, said that he only writes down three things he is grateful for every day, but then spends time really feeling the emotion of gratitude for each one. He always chooses one that is very simple and ordinary, such as the look in his child's eyes. When you focus on your blessings every day and notice the beauty in the mundane, as well as in the more significant, you'll soon notice that you generally feel more peaceful, calm, and uplifted.

DAY 29   Take ten.

Take just ten minutes out of your day for prayer or for some quiet reflective time. This practice can be amazingly effective at helping you to stay connected to Spirit and in a more relaxed and serene state.

Activity

Choose a consistent time every day to spend at least ten minutes in prayer or quiet reflection. I like to do this every morning as I begin my day. It helps me to center myself in the bigger picture and in a place of compassion, serenity, and conscious intention for the day. But if you find it works better for you to take ten minutes at another time of the day—do it then. What's most important is that you do it every day.

Depending on your spiritual beliefs, you can address the higher power or simply say to yourself the prayers or desires you have for yourself and for the other people in your life. Ask for guidance; pray for peace and happiness for those you feel have wronged you in some way, pray for those who are sick or struggling, and for your own well-being and ability to trust in the higher power. Whatever else you would like to pray for and contemplate, do so. Commit to doing this for 30 days and observe what happens in your life. I'm sure you'll be amazed by the miracles.

DAY 30   Upgrade the care of your skin.

Beautiful, radiant skin is one of the incredible gifts of this 30-day program. Good skin care begins by working from the inside, but also includes taking good care from the outside. The first outer care step is to cleanse your skin with a nontoxic, nondrying cleanser at least twice a day, depending on your activity. Apply a nontoxic, moisturizer made with mostly organic natural ingredients. Two examples of these types of moisturizers include, makana (www.drchristinehorner.com/shop-oils.cfm) and Youthful Skin Cream made by the company, Maharishi Ayurveda Products International (www.mapi.com). Use the code "radianthealth" at checkout for a 10% discount.

Activity

If you have been using chemically based products on your face—throw them out! Order nontoxic natural skincare products from one of the companies listed above. Both are reasonably priced. After applying the moisturizer in the morning, gently spread a nontoxic sunscreen that uses a physical barrier, such as zinc, over your face and neck. If you wear makeup, you can apply it now. As with the skincare products, you should use also use nontoxic products. Most health food stores and groceries have a section with nontoxic makeup lines.

Congratulations! You have finished the 30-day program and established a foundation of habits that will bring you radiant health, and ageless beauty. You now have all the skills you need to create extraordinary health and longevity. The key is to stay on the path! Invite your friends and family to join you in this lifelong program. Having the support of others is the easiest way to continue with all of the healthy changes you have made. In addition, you will be gifting those whom you love with a much better state of health; there is nothing more sacred or valuable. I wish for you the blessings of extraordinary health and happiness and hope that you share it with the world. Namaste.

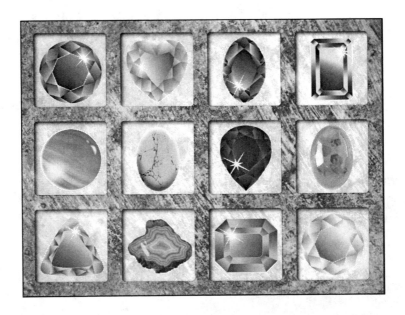

Appendices

According to *Ayurveda* all chronic diseases begin as imbalances that stem from "mistakes of the intellect" or *pragyaparadh*. These mistakes generally refer to poor choices in diet and lifestyle. If you follow the diet and lifestyle advice presented in this book, your likelihood of developing any chronic disease will be extremely low. If you have a chronic disease, making healthy changes will help to bring balance back to your body and gradually reverse your condition. There are also a variety of herbs and nutritional supplements that can also help to restore balance and improve your symptoms. But keep in mind that herbs and supplements don't work well without a foundation of a healthy diet and lifestyle. As one of my favorite sayings goes, "You can never mop the floor dry, unless you turn off the faucet first."

This book focuses on health rather than disease. However, I thought it might be helpful to include an appendix that addresses some of the most common chronic conditions and the specific nutritional supplements that research shows can be of help. They are not meant to be a replacement for your medications. If you have one of these conditions, it is extremely important that you do not go off your medications without your doctor's consent. Work with your doctor. As your health improves, your doctor will advise you on the adjustments you may be able to make in your medications. Ideally, you should also work with an integrative or holistic physician who can help monitor your progress and dietary supplements.

APPENDIX A

Natural Help
for Menopausal Symptoms

Menopause is a natural process that, for some women, brings on a myriad of uncomfortable symptoms. These symptoms generally come from imbalances in your physiology that usually stem from poor choices in diet and lifestyle. Common perimenopausal complaints include:

- Weight gain
- Fatigue
- Hot flashes
- Headaches
- Loss of libido

- Dry skin
- Vaginal dryness
- Mood swings
- Anxiety
- Depression

- Memory problems
- Insomnia or sleep difficulties
- Joint and muscle aches and pains

After menopause, the risk of osteoporosis and heart disease also increases dramatically.

The Western Approach

To combat perimenopausal symptoms, Western medicine developed synthetic feminine hormones. Hormone replacement therapy (HRT) was promoted as the fountain of youth. It was said to lower the risk of heart disease, strokes, Alzheimer's disease, and osteoporosis. But several studies in the early 2000s, including the Women's Health Initiative, found that mostly the opposite is true: Women who take HRT have an increased risk of heart disease, strokes, blood clots, gall bladder disease, and invasive breast (30 to 100 percent higher) and ovarian cancer (80 percent higher). HRT does help osteoporosis, but not any more than a little weight-bearing exercise and a diet rich with nutritious plants can.

The Eastern Approach

Traditional systems of medicine, including *Ayurveda*, tell us that menopause should be a time of gentle and easy transition. The hormonal changes at menopause are part of the natural progression of life. Symptoms appear only if you are out of balance—usually arising from poor diet and lifestyle choices.

Therefore, the best way to improve and control menopausal symptoms is to restore balance to the physiology through healthy diet and lifestyle choices—in essence, everything presented in this book. Then, if any symptoms are still present after you have made these changes, herbs and supplements may be added. If you don't correct your habits that are creating the imbalances first, then herbs and supplements usually don't work very well.

Herbal Help

Here are some of the top research-proven herbs that can help to balance your hormones and alleviate uncomfortable menopausal symptoms.

Black Cohosh

This root was discovered centuries ago by Native Americans to help improve menstrual cramps and menopausal symptoms. A member of the buttercup family, the German Commission E has approved it for menstrual discomfort, as well as the physical and psychological symptoms of menopause including hot flashes, irritability, mood swings, anxiety, vaginal dryness and sleep disturbances.

Maca

Grown in the high plateaus of the Andes, maca comes from the root of a cruciferous vegetable. For centuries it has been used by the people of Peru for hormonal imbalances, menstrual irregularities, fertility, and menopausal symptoms including hot flashes, vaginal dryness, depression and loss of energy and libido. Maca contains no plant hormones, but works by helping the endocrine system maintain hormonal balance.

Chaste Tree Berry

Also known as vitex, the German Commission E has approved its use for irregularities of the menstrual cycle, premenstrual disturbances, and breast tenderness (mastodynia). Research shows it may also help with anxiety, hot flashes, and night sweats and improve sleep quality.

Dong Quai

Used in Asia for thousands of years as a tonic for the female reproductive system, modern research shows that this member of the celery family promotes uterine health and regulates the menstrual cycle. Best used in combinations with other herbs, dong quai has been shown to help with depression, hot flashes, night sweats, and vaginal dryness.

Flax Lignans

Lignans are plant compounds found abundantly in a variety of fruits and vegetables. Flax seeds contain 100 times more lignans than any other known edible plant. A subject of hundreds of studies, lignans have been found to have many health benefits including balancing feminine hormones. In a clinical trial, 100 women given flax lignans reported improvement in PMS and perimenopausal symptoms including breast tenderness, bloating, hot flashes, mood swings, and "brain fog."

Red Clover

This wild plant belongs to the legume family and has been found to contain isoflavones, which help to regulate estrogen. Research shows red clover may help to alleviate hot flashes. It also supports cardiovascular and bone health.

Schisandra Berry

Produced on a woody vine, this red berry has been revered in China for thousands of years because of its many health benefits. Widely known as a longevity herb and aphrodisiac, research shows it may also be beneficial for menopausal symptoms by reducing hot flashes and night sweats, as well as depression, fatigue and insomnia.

Shatavari

Considered one of the most powerful rejuvenating herbs in *Ayurveda*, this member of the asparagus family is commonly used in India for conditions affecting the female reproductive system. Shatavari may also help mood swings and irritations associated with PMS and menopausal hot flashes, insomnia and osteoporosis.

Ashwagandha

Also called "Indian ginseng," this important *Ayurvedic* herb has been prescribed for more than 3,000 years. Ashwagandha grows as a small woody shrub and is considered an "adaptogen," because it helps to protect against stress. Research shows it may also be of benefit for anxiety, insomnia, and fatigue; and may stimulate libido and cognitive function.

Shilajit

Prized by both traditional Indian and Chinese medicines, the Chinese consider shilajit a "Jing" tonic, which aids physical energy and sexual drive. The high-potency extract is packed with nutrients, amino acids, and antioxidants. One of its antioxidants is fulvic acid. It is known to promote vitality by stimulating cellular ATP production—the molecule your cells use for energy. Shilajit is also known to alleviate anxiety, lift mood, and stimulate overall health.

Cynanchum wilfordii

This herb is a key component of a famous Chinese herbal tonic that has been used for more than a thousand years to enhance vitality. It is also used in traditional Korean medicine to promote healthy aging.

Phlomis umbrosa Root

This plant has also been used in China for thousands of years to support liver health and detoxification. Because of its strong anti-inflammatory properties, Phlomis is useful for a variety of other health conditions, including pain relief.

Angelica gigas Root

Also called "Dang Gui," Angelica is an herb traditionally used in Korea to improve gynecological, cardiovascular, and immune system health.

Pollen Extracts

In addition to all the herbs described above, there is also a very interesting, relatively new plant-based product available in the U.S. made from flower pollen that appears to be very beneficial for menopausal symptoms, too.

It was discovered by accident when a Swedish beekeeper noticed that his bees seemed more energetic when they consumed the pollen from a particular flower. He then wondered if it would have the same effect on people. So he gave it to men and women, and although he was unimpressed by the pollen's ability to improve energy, he was quite impressed and surprised to find that it appeared to provide great relief for menopausal women.

The first pollen extract product was released in Europe in 1999. Made from the extracts of several Swedish flowers—specifically from the grass (*Poaceae*) family, including rye (*Secale cereale*)—this product was recently introduced in the U.S. with the trade name Relizen. To date, more than 1 million women worldwide have used this type of product with great satisfaction, and it is currently the number-one non-hormonal menopausal product used in France. In the U.S., more than 2,000 gynecologists have recommended it to their patients. Just to note, the manufacturer says they use a highly effective process to remove the allergenic husk so there is no need to worry if you have pollen allergies.

Numerous clinical studies have been published—some in peer-reviewed medical journals—including a randomized, double-blind, placebo-controlled study in 2005 and a large controlled clinical trial in 2015 that was conducted by ninety gynecologists. These studies have found that Relizen works through non-estrogenic pathways to help alleviate menopausal symptoms, including hot flashes, night sweats, sleep disturbances, mood swings, and fatigue. Exactly how the pollen extract works is not fully understood, but it has been found to be high in antioxidants and anti-inflammatories. In addition, according to a study published in 2016, it also increases serotonin, a neurotransmitter that stabilizes mood and improves symptoms of depression. Because it is non-hormonal, it is considered safe for women who have had breast cancer.

No Need to Suffer

There's no need to suffer with menopausal symptoms. This natural transition of life is meant to go smoothly. For most women, making a few healthy diet and lifestyle changes can dramatically improve or resolve symptoms. If you find that you still need some help, consider taking an effective herbal formula, or flower pollen product, such as Relizen (www.relizen.com).

APPENDIX B

Natural Help for Healthy Bones

*A*s you age, it is normal for your bones to lose density. When you are young, your bones continue to grow and add mass until you are about thirty years old. Sometime between thirty and forty-five, more bone starts to absorb than is replaced, causing your bone mineral density to decrease. However, too much bone loss, a condition called "osteoporosis," can cause your bones to become porous and fragile, which increases your risk of fractures. The National Osteoporosis Foundation estimates that 54 million Americans currently have osteoporosis or low bone density. Every year, approximately 1.5 million suffer osteoporosis-related bone fractures. Studies suggest that approximately one in two women and up to one in four men age fifty and older will break a bone due to osteoporosis.

What Causes Excessive Bone Loss?

There are many factors that have been found to increase your risk of osteoporosis, including:

- Low body weight
- Advanced age
- Estrogen, progesterone, and testosterone imbalances
- Amenorrhea
- Anorexia nervosa
- Autoimmune diseases, including rheumatoid arthritis, lupus, multiple sclerosis, and ankylosing spondylitis

- Gastrointestinal issues, including celiac disease, weight-loss surgery, and inflammatory bowel disease
- Certain medications, such as corticosteroids and anticonvulsants
- Cigarette smoking
- Endocrine disorders, including diabetes, hyperthyroidisms, hyperparathyroidism, and Cushing's disease
- Inactivity
- Yo-yo dieting
- Excessive consumption of alcohol
- Drinking colas
- Consuming excessive animal protein—particularly red meat

Western Approaches

There is a lot of controversy when it comes to the Western approach to bone loss and its prevention and treatments. John Abramson, M.D., explains in his book, *Overdosed America: The Broken Promise of American Medicine,* how the pharmaceutical companies have done an excellent job creating the illusion that normal bone loss with age is a disease that needs pharmaceutical treatment. However, studies show that in general these drugs do not significantly lower your risk of fractures. The full explanations are beyond the scope of this book, but in short, these medications add strength to the outer layer of your bone (cortical bone), whereas the strength of your bone actually comes from the inner layer (trabecular bone). In fact, studies show that women who take bisphosphonate drugs, such as Fosamax, Actonel, Boniva, and Reclast, for more than five years have almost a three times higher incidence of hip fractures! In addition, these medications are associated with a number of serious side effects, including eye problems, osteonecrosis (destruction) of the jaw, liver and kidney damage, cardiac arrhythmias, and low calcium, to name a few. The good news is there are many natural approaches without dangerous side effects that can help to keep your bones strong.

Natural Approaches

Good bone health begins with good nutrition. Research shows that eating a wide variety of fresh, organically grown plants—fruits, vegetables, nuts, and seeds help to supply your bones with the nutrients they need to stay strong. There are also a number of dietary supplements that research shows can help preserve your bone density and lower your risk of osteoporosis. In the past, it was thought that supplemental calcium was all that was needed. However, as our knowledge of bone physiology has advanced, we now understand that magnesium, vitamin D, and vitamin K2 are also critically important. In fact, these four nutrients interact together and support each other. Taking excess amounts of one, while being deficient in another, can have serious consequences, including increasing your risk of heart attacks and strokes.

Magnesium

Magnesium is a mineral that is vital for your overall health. It is involved in more than 300 different enzymes in your body and is essential for the most basic processes of your body—from protein synthesis, energy production, metabolism, and digestion to the function of your bones, muscles, and nerves. Taking extra calcium without also taking adequate amounts of magnesium can cause muscle spasms and even lead to heart attacks and sudden death. Magnesium not only helps to maintain your bone density, but also lowers the risk of numerous other diseases and conditions, including diabetes, hypertension, heart disease, migraine headaches, depression, fatigue, and possibly colorectal tumors. The daily recommended amount is 310–320 mg per day for women and 400–420 mg for men. Good food sources include seaweed and green leafy vegetables, such as spinach and Swiss chard, as well as avocados, beans, nuts, and seeds especially pumpkin, sunflower, and sesame seeds. You can't take pure magnesium supplements, because magnesium has to be combined with another substance, such as glycinate, chloride, carbonate, or citrate. Each substance affects how well the magnesium is absorbed and used by your body. For example, magnesium glycinate is a chelated form that is highly absorbable and bioavailable. Magnesium chloride contains only 12 percent magnesium, but has better absorption than many other forms. Magnesium citrate is also well absorbed and has a laxative effect. Magnesium can be bitter, so I recommend either tablets or a delicious powdered form mixed with water such as Natural Calm made by Natural Vitality.

Vitamin D

Vitamin D, like magnesium, has profound effects on your entire body. As discussed in chapter 5, it acts more like a hormone and has been shown to interact with thousands of genes. Vitamin D helps your bone density by increasing the absorption and retention of calcium. A study from Iceland published in the *Journal of the American Medical Association* in 2005 found that if you don't get enough vitamin D, it doesn't seem to matter to your bones how much calcium you get. In other words, even high doses of calcium won't do much good in preserving your bone density if you don't get enough vitamin D. When your vitamin D levels are sufficient, the amount of calcium you require to maintain ideal bone health may be far less.

A subject of thousands of recent studies, vitamin D is essential not only for good bone health, but also for your overall health. It has been shown to lower your risk of most chronic diseases, including Parkinson's disease, Alzheimer's disease, and certain cancers. Vitamin D is unique because your body can manufacture it when your skin is exposed to sunlight. But the vast majority of Americans are found to be deficient, so taking supplemental amounts is recommended. Vitamin D is found naturally in only a few foods such as fatty fish and mushrooms. There are several foods—for example, milk, orange juice, and cereal—that are fortified with vitamin D. To get enough daily vitamin D from these foods, large volumes of them would have to be consumed, so taking supplemental vitamin D is also important. Experts now believe that healthy individuals need at least 2,000 IU of vitamin D3 (the active form) per day, and if you are sick, you may need much more.

Vitamin K2

Vitamin K comes in two forms: K1 and K2. Vitamin K1 is found in green vegetables and helps your blood to clot. Vitamin K2 is manufactured by bacteria and helps to keep calcium in its appropriate place. Specifically, it helps your bone hang on to calcium by supporting your osteoblasts (cells that build bone) and quieting your osteoclasts (cells that absorb bone).

Vitamin K2 also prevents calcium from being deposited on the walls of your arteries, and therefore, lowers your risk of cardiovascular disease. If you take calcium without vitamin K2, it may deposit in the wrong places and increase your risk of heart disease and other problems. Taking mega doses of vitamin D3 without taking vitamin K2 can cause you to become vitamin D toxic. Experts recommend you take 100–150 mcg of vitamin K2 for every 1,000 IU of vitamin D3 you take. Natural sources of vitamin K2 include fermented foods, especially natto. Because the taste of natto can be disagreeable for many, I recommend a vitamin K2 supplement.

Other substances that research shows may help keep your bones fit include omega-3 fatty acids, tea, soy, and flaxseeds.

Omega-3 Fatty Acids

Many studies have found that omega-3 fatty acids improve bone health, including a study published in the *British Journal of Nutrition,* which found that docosahexaenoic acid (DHA) is important for healthy bone marrow and bone density.

Tea

A study published in the *American Journal of Clinical Nutrition* in 2000 found that older women (ages sixty-five to seventy-six) who drank tea had significantly greater bone density than those who did not drink tea.

Soy

A double-blind, placebo-controlled, randomized study published in the journal *Menopause* in 2004 found that soy isoflavones maintained hip bone mineral content in postmenopausal women.

Last but not least, exercise, especially weight-bearing exercises that put stress on your bones, such as jogging and weight lifting, is extremely important for maintaining bone density. It's also a good idea to include balance and coordination exercises, too, because they can help to prevent falls.

Remember that your bone density naturally decreases with age and doesn't mean you have a disease. If you are at risk for too much bone loss, the best approach is to prevent it naturally. Avoid pharmaceutical medications because of their significant side effects and questionable benefits. Instead, eat plenty of fresh, organic green vegetables; go for brisk walks every day—in the sunshine if possible; and make sure to take adequate amounts of calcium, magnesium, and vitamins D3 and K2.

Natural Help for a Healthy Heart

*H*eart disease is the leading cause of death for both men and women in the United States. Every year about 610,000 people die of heart disease—that's one in every four deaths. Coronary heart disease (CHD) is the most common type of heart disease and is responsible for 370,000 deaths annually.

Risk factors include high blood pressure, high cholesterol, inflammation, and smoking. About half of Americans (47 percent) have at least one of these three risk factors. Several other medical conditions and lifestyle choices can also increase the risk for heart disease, including:

- Diabetes
- Overweight and obesity
- Poor diet
- Physical inactivity
- Excessive alcohol use

The Western Approach

Because there have been so many studies showing that diet and lifestyle significantly influence the risk of heart disease, most Western physicians recommend healthier habits to their patients. In addition, Western doctors may prescribe various pharmaceutical medications to lower blood pressure or cholesterol, and/or improve other cardiovascular factors. Surgery may also be recommended to treat different disease conditions, such as blockages of the coronary arteries or malfunctions of the heart valves.

Natural Approaches

Cardiologist, Dean Ornish, M.D., was the first to document that cardio-vascular disease could be reversed through diet and lifestyle changes alone. In the 1980s, Dr. Ornish conducted a randomized-controlled trial, which studied the effects of a comprehensive lifestyle change on coronary artery disease (CAD). The changes included a 10 percent-fat, whole-foods, vege-tarian diet; aerobic exercise; stress-management training; smoking cessa-tion; and group psychosocial support.

By following all the diet and lifestyle approaches presented in this book, you can minimize your risk of heart disease. In addition, there are a variety of nutritional supplements that may be of help.

Omega-3 Fatty Acids

Omega-3 fatty acids, which were presented in detail in chapter 4, are par-ticularly beneficial for heart disease. Several hundred studies have shown that consuming foods high in omega-3s, especially fatty fish and flaxseeds, not only reduces risk factors for heart disease, but also decreases the risk of death from coronary artery disease. Omega-3 fatty acids promote heart health in several different ways. They:

- Improve heart rhythm
- Prevent clot formation and plaque buildup in arteries
- Lower blood pressure
- Reduce blood triglyceride levels by 25 to 30 percent
- Increase plasma levels of "good" HDL cholesterol
- Possess profound anti-inflammatory properties

A review of randomized, controlled trials published in August 2005 revealed that omega-3 fatty acids consistently lower elevated plasma triglyc-eride levels in a dose-dependent fashion. Improvements were seen with just 300 mg per day, while even better results were observed with 2,000–3,000 mg per day.

Plant Sterols

Plant sterols (phytosterols) are substances that are structurally similar to cholesterol. Because they compete with the absorption of dietary cholesterol, they can decrease its intestinal absorption and enhance its elimination. Studies show that consuming plant sterols can cause reductions in serum cholesterol levels and lower the risk of cardiovascular disease. A comprehensive review of forty-one trials comparing plant sterols to placebo concluded that consuming only 2 grams of sterols per day can reduce "bad" LDL cholesterol by 10 percent. The researchers of this study stated that the ability of plant sterols to lower cholesterol is greater than that of either diet or medications. The evidence that plant sterols reduce cholesterol is so strong that the National Cholesterol Education Program and the American Heart Association recommended plant sterols for reducing cholesterol. Examples of foods naturally high in sterols include wheat germ, flaxseeds, coconut, nuts, legumes, and certain oils (flax oil, olive oil, and coconut oil). You can also take a plant sterol nutritional supplement.

Coenzyme Q10 (CoQ10)

In chapter 5 you learned that CoQ10 is an antioxidant and vitamin-like substance involved in energy production in the mitochondria, or "powerhouses," of your cells. Specifically, CoQ10 assists in making energy (called "adenosine triphosphate" or ATP) from carbohydrates and fats. CoQ10 has many other important functions—from stabilizing membranes to decreasing the amount of oxidized "bad" LDL cholesterol that is implicated in atherosclerosis. It is also useful for preventing damage to your heart during periods of stress. CoQ10 is depleted in patients with a variety of heart conditions, as well as in those taking cholesterol-lowering statin drugs. Supplemental CoQ10 can be very valuable for these patients for not only preventing, but also treating cardiovascular disease. Preventive doses usually range from 30–100 mg per day, depending on the form that is taken. Natural fermented forms are far more bioavailable than the dry synthetic forms, and therefore, much lower doses are needed. The recommended therapeutic dose of CoQ10 is 100 mg or greater per day.

Red Yeast Rice

The cardiac benefits of red yeast rice—a delicacy in Japan—have been known for more than 1,000 years. This bright, reddish-purple rice acquires its color from a fermentation process with a mold called *Monascus purpureus*. Red yeast rice can also be consumed in supplemental form and has been shown to reduce several risk factors for cardiovascular disease. For example, it lowers total cholesterol, "bad" LDL cholesterol, and fasting triglycerides, and diminishes the triglyceride response to meals. One study showed that red yeast rice (1,200 mg per day) reduced the triglyceride response to a fat-rich meal by 45 to 50 percent. Unlike cholesterol-lowering statin drugs, which can increase the risk of and/or worsen diabetes, red yeast rice extracts seem to have the opposite effect. A Chinese study found that red yeast rice extract may improve type 2 diabetes by lowering insulin and blood glucose.

Lycopene

Lycopene is a powerful antioxidant found in many fruits and vegetables. It is responsible for the red color in tomatoes and has been shown to have many health benefits. They include lowering the risk of certain cancers such as those of the breast and prostate, and protecting against cardiovascular disease. Studies show that those with high lycopene levels have lower incidences of cardiovascular disease, while those with the lowest levels of lycopene have more than a three-fold greater risk of having an acute coronary event or stroke.

L-Carnitine

L-carnitine is an amino acid made in your body from lysine and methionine. Similar to CoQ10, carnitine is depleted in patients with various heart conditions and taking supplemental amounts can be very beneficial. L-carnitine assists in transporting fat into the mitochondria to be burned as fuel for the muscles in your body, including your heart. It is very helpful for hypoxic conditions—severe reductions in the amount of oxygen in tissues—that can lead to damage. Studies show that for people with moderate to severe heart failure, supplemental l-carnitine improves both exercise tolerance and oxygen consumption. Recommended doses are approximately 2 grams per day.

Magnesium

This mineral is essential for every cell in your body to function properly. It is involved with hundreds of enzymes (proteins that speeds up biochemical reactions) and is also important for your muscles, including your heart. If your magnesium levels drop too low, you can develop many serious health problems, including congestive heart failure, atherosclerosis, angina, high blood pressure, cardiac arrhythmias, heart muscle disease (cardiomyopathy), heart attacks, and even sudden cardiac death. Magnesium supplements can help to prevent and reverse all of these conditions. If you have a cardiac condition, magnesium is very important for you to take. Recommended doses are 400 mg per day.

Nattokinase

Nattokinase is an enzyme that is produced during a fermentation process involving soy and a bacterium called *Bacillus natto*. For more than 1,000 years, it has been consumed in a popular Japanese fermented cheese-like food, called "natto," and used as a folk remedy for cardiovascular diseases. Studies show that nattokinase can not only help to prevent unhealthy coagulation of the blood, but can also decrease blood pressure. It can be very beneficial for cardiovascular diseases, including heart disease, high blood pressure, stroke, chest pain (angina), deep vein thrombosis (DVT), hardening of the arteries (atherosclerosis), hemorrhoids, varicose veins, poor circulation, and peripheral artery disease (PAD).

Vitamin D

Vitamin D deficiency is associated with several cardiovascular risk factors, including high blood pressure, atherosclerosis, diabetes mellitus, and inflammation. It also contributes to heart attacks, strokes, and congestive heart failure. Therefore, raising your vitamin D levels by taking supplemental vitamin D3 can help to protect against all of these conditions.

Vitamin K2

Vitamin K comes in two forms: K1 and K2. Vitamin K1 is found in green vegetables and helps your blood clot. Vitamin K2 is manufactured by bacteria and helps to keep calcium in its appropriate place. Not only is it good for healthy bone density as discussed in appendix B, but it is also good for your heart heath. Vitamin K2 works through the matrix GLA protein (MGP), which is responsible for protecting your blood vessels from calcification. If the soft lining of your blood vessels become damaged, an inflammatory process is initiated that can cause calcium to deposit into the damaged tissue. If calcium builds into a plaque, it can eventually cause a heart attack or stroke. Vitamin K2 helps to prevent calcium from depositing on your artery walls. Remember that vitamins K2 and D3, as well as calcium and magnesium all work together.

If you take vitamin D3 without taking vitamin K2, it may actually increase your risk of heart disease. Experts recommend you take 100–150 mcg of vitamin K2 for every 1,000 IU of vitamin D3 that you take. Natural sources of vitamin K2 include fermented foods, especially natto. Because the taste of natto can be disagreeable for many, I recommend a vitamin K2 supplement.

Guggul

Guggul is a gum resin from a tree (*Commiphora mukul*), which has been used by *Ayurveda* for thousands of years. The ancient *Ayurvedic* text, the *Sushruta Samhita*, describes the use of guggul for a wide variety of conditions, including rheumatism, obesity, and atherosclerosis. Studies show that guggul does have many medicinal effects. It has been shown to reduce total cholesterol up to 30 percent and LDL by 35 percent, and increase HDL by 20 percent within twelve weeks. Guggul also has strong anti-inflammatory properties and can improve the redness and swelling that occurs in certain types of acne.

Garlic

Many studies have suggested that garlic and garlic extracts lower blood cholesterol and triglycerides, and slightly elevate "good" HDL cholesterol. Garlic extract (1.2 grams three times per day for two weeks) significantly reduces the oxidation of "bad" LDL cholesterol. In addition, garlic contains strong antioxidants, particularly in the form of aged extracts.

Green Tea

Numerous studies show that green tea may reduce your risk of heart attacks and strokes. It has been shown to decrease several cardiac risk factors, including cholesterol, blood pressure, and atherosclerosis (hardening of the arteries). A study of 40,530 Japanese adults found that those who drank more than five cups of green tea a day had a 26 percent lower risk of death from heart attack or stroke and a 16 percent lower risk of death from all causes, when compared to those who drank less than one cup of green tea a day. A 2011 meta-analysis found that people who drank the most green tea had a 28 percent lower risk of coronary artery disease, compared to those who drank the least green tea. Black tea had no effect on heart risk. Another 2011 meta-analysis of fourteen randomized, placebo-controlled clinical trials found that green tea significantly lowers LDL cholesterol and triglyceride levels. Many of the studies included in this meta-analysis used capsules containing catechins, the active polyphenols in green tea, rather than with the beverage itself.

Niacin

Niacin, also known as vitamin B3, is naturally involved in carbohydrate and fat (lipid) metabolism. In supplemental doses, niacin is a potent vasodilator that causes blood vessels to increase in diameter and lowers blood pressure. Niacin also significantly lowers blood levels of "bad" LDL cholesterol and triglycerides and increases "good" HDL cholesterol. Effective doses range from 50–200 mg per day.

Arginine

Arginine is a natural amino acid that is needed to synthesize a very potent substance called "nitric oxide," which relaxes and dilates blood vessels and lowers blood pressure. It also has antioxidant properties and inhibits platelet aggregation that can cause blood clots leading to heart attacks and strokes. This amino acid also improves endothelial function (the lining of arteries) in patients with coronary artery disease and dilates blocked coronary arteries. Studies have found that 6 grams per day (2 grams consumed three times per day) for ten days can prevent the vascular dysfunction associated with consumption of a high-fat meal. A recent review concluded that the main benefit of arginine supplementation is to restore optimal function to your blood vessels, reduce high blood pressure, and prevent atherosclerosis.

Hawthorn Extract

The flowers and berries of the hawthorn plant have been used to treat a variety of cardiovascular conditions for thousands of years. Hawthorn is best known for its ability to relax and dilate your blood vessels, which reduces blood pressure and increases blood flow. A recent randomized study found that 1,200 mg per day of hawthorn extract for sixteen weeks significantly reduced blood pressure in patients with diabetes, when compared to those who took a placebo.

As with all chronic diseases, improving your diet and lifestyle is the foundation for minimizing your risk of heart disease or helping to reverse it. In addition, there are many dietary supplements, particularly those presented in this appendix that can help to significantly reduce your risk. If you are taking medications for your heart, do not go off of them without your doctor's approval. Work with your doctor as you improve your health, so that he or she can make the proper adjustments in your medications. Remember, cardiovascular disease is reversible, so even if you have it, making healthy diet and lifestyle changes along with the help of nutrition supplements may not only improve your symptoms, but may also cure your disease.

Natural Health for Diabetes

*D*iabetes is a chronic disease that occurs either when your pancreas does not produce enough insulin (type 1) or when your body cannot effectively use the insulin it produces (type 2). Ninety percent of diabetics have type 2, and the incidence in the U.S. has doubled in the last two decades. Currently 11 percent of adults over the age of twenty are diabetic. Type 2 diabetes is primarily caused by being overweight as the result of consuming too many calories and not exercising enough. Almost 90 percent of diabetics are overweight or obese, and approximately one-third of those who are overweight have the disease. A study from the Harvard School of Public Health found that being even slightly overweight increased diabetes risk five times, and being seriously obese increased it sixty times.

If left untreated, the high blood sugars associated with diabetes can have serious health consequences, including comas and death. Even when the disease is treated, poor sugar control can damage organs and cause serious complications. Diabetes is the seventh-leading cause of death and a major cause of kidney failure, blindness, limb amputations, heart disease, and strokes. It also increases the risk of numerous other chronic disorders, including dementia, arthritis, and cancers of liver, colon, pancreas, endometrium, breast, and kidney.

The Western Approach

Because type 2 diabetes mainly develops from excess weight caused by a poor diet and lifestyle, it can be significantly improved or cured by improving these factors. Depending on the severity of the disease, either insulin or antihyperglycemic drugs such as sulfonylureas, biguanides, alpha-glucosidase inhibitors, thiazolidinediones, and meglitinide are also prescribed.

The Natural Approach

Along with all of the diet and lifestyle advice presented in this book, there are a number of nutritional supplements and herbs that have also been found to be of benefit. They include:

Chromium Picolinate

Chromium is required for normal carbohydrate metabolism and is a critical cofactor for insulin. It is also a component of the glucose tolerance factor (GTF), which plays a role in glucose metabolism. Studies show this trace mineral tends to be low in diabetics. Diabetics given chromium supplementation (200–1,000 mcg/day) show significant improvements in insulin resistance, blood sugar levels, vascular inflammation, and blood lipids. A double-blind, placebo-controlled study published in the journal *Diabetes Technology and Therapeutics* found that chromium supplementation significantly reduces hunger and food cravings in overweight adult women with carbohydrate cravings, and may help with weight loss.

Vanadium

Named after the Norse goddess of beauty, Vanadis, because of its beautiful natural colors, this trace element is involved in various aspects of carbohydrate metabolism, including glucose transport, glycolysis, glucose oxidation, and glycogen synthesis. Vanadium has been shown to facilitate glucose uptake and metabolism, as well as lipid and amino acid metabolism. It also improves thyroid function and enhances insulin sensitivity. Recommended doses range from 100–200 mg per day.

L-Carnitine

Made in the body from the amino acids lysine and methionine, l-carnitine has been shown to enhance glucose uptake with doses of 1,000–3,000 mg per day. It also helps to transport fatty acids into mitochondria to be used for fuel. In a study published in *Diabetes Care* in 2005, l-carnitine was found to improve pain, nerve regeneration, and vibratory perception in patients with chronic diabetic neuropathy.

Alpha-lipoic Acid

A powerful antioxidant discussed in detail in chapter 5, alpha-lipoic acid has been shown to improve glucose metabolism, insulin sensitivity, and diabetic neuropathy. Double-blind trials have found that diabetics who take 600–1,200 mg of lipoic acid per day have improved insulin sensitivity and the symptoms of neuropathy. In a preliminary study of patients with type 2 diabetes, those who took 600 mg of alpha-lipoic acid per day for eighteen months had a much slower progression of kidney damage when compared to those who did not.

Magnesium

Known for being essential for all of the tissues in your body (see appendix B), this trace mineral also improves blood sugar in diabetics by enhancing glucose transport across cell membranes. Approximately 400 mg per day are recommended.

Ginseng

In a small pilot study, patients with type 2 diabetes were given a high-glucose drink, with either 3 grams of American ginseng or a placebo. Those who took the ginseng had significantly lower blood sugar levels. A double-blind trial found that 200 mg of Asian ginseng per day improved blood sugar levels in people with type 2 diabetes.

Fenugreek

A traditional *Ayurvedic* herb, fenugreek has been shown to help lower cholesterol and blood sugar levels in people with moderate cardiovascular disease and type 2 diabetes. Double-blind trials have found that fenugreek helps improve blood sugar control in patients with both type 1 and type 2 diabetes.

Bitter Melon

Studies show that bitter melon contains many different substances that can help lower blood sugar and benefit those with type 2 diabetes.

Aloe Vera

Two small controlled human trials found that aloe, either alone or in combination with the oral hypoglycemic drug, glibenclamide, effectively lowers blood sugar in people with type 2 diabetes.

Ginkgo biloba

Preliminary research shows that *Ginkgo biloba* extract may be useful for the prevention and treatment of early-stage diabetic neuropathy.

Gymnema

The hypoglycemic (blood-sugar-lowering) action of gymnema leaves was first documented in the late 1920s. Animal studies show that it helps to enhance the regeneration of the cells in your pancreas that secrete insulin and increases the flow of insulin from these cells. It has also been found to reduce glucose absorption from the intestine, improve uptake of glucose into cells, and prevent adrenal hormones from stimulating the liver to produce glucose, thereby reducing blood sugar levels.

Prickly Pear Cactus

Also called "nopal," the young cactus leaves are used in traditional Mexican dishes. Research shows it may be helpful for diabetes, high cholesterol, obesity, and hangovers. A study published in *Diabetes Care* found that prickly pear cactus can decrease blood sugar levels in people with type 2 diabetes by 17 to 48 percent. Because it contains fiber and pectin, it can decrease the absorption of sugar in the stomach and intestine. A study from the University of Vienna in Austria found that prickly pear decreased total cholesterol by 12 percent, LDL by 15 percent, triglycerides by 12 percent, blood glucose by 11 percent, and insulin by 11 percent.

Garlic

In a 2013 study, garlic was found to lower blood sugar and lipids (total cholesterol, triglyceride, and low-density lipoprotein) in type 2 diabetics. In addition, it lowers C-reactive protein (an indicator of inflammation), which suggests that garlic is valuable not only for controlling blood sugar levels, but also for the prevention of long-term complications of diabetes.

Green Tea

A 2013 study published in the *Diabetes and Metabolism Journal* found that people who drank six or more cups of green tea a day were 33 percent less likely to develop type 2 diabetes compared to those who drank less than one cup a week. A 2012 study conducted at Pennsylvania State University reported that animals that were given EGCG, a polyphenol found in green tea, before they were fed a high-carbohydrate meal had a 50 percent lower spike in their blood glucose compared to the control animals.

Cinnamon

In a study in the journal *Diabetes Care,* diabetic patients were given a quarter teaspoon of cinnamon every day. After forty days, they experienced a significant drop in their blood sugars, and a 30 percent reduction in their blood cholesterol and triglycerides. One study found that cinnamon increased glucose metabolism by twentyfold! Cinnamon prevents blood glucose spikes by slowing the emptying of your stomach and the rate of absorption of glucose from the food you eat, and also improves insulin sensitivity.

Because type 2 diabetes is generally caused by being overweight as the result of consuming too many calories and not exercising enough, you can significantly improve or cure this chronic disease through diet and lifestyle changes. Diabetes can be extremely dangerous, so do not go off your medications without your doctor's approval. It is very important that you work with your doctor as you gradually restore your health. With the help of some of the nutritional supplements discussed above, you may be able to lower your dose of your prescription medications. But, again, be sure to work closely with your doctor. Keep in mind that by simply taking better care of yourself, there's an excellent chance that you will be able to reverse this dangerous disease and enjoy a long healthy life.

APPENDIX E

Natural Help for Healthy Breasts

*B*reast cancer is a hormonally driven tumor this is closely linked to diet and lifestyle. In fact, research shows that about 95 percent of the cancers of breast cancer could be prevented by diet and lifestyle alone. What increases the risk of breast cancer or protects against it has a similar influence on the risk of prostate and colon cancers. To learn about all the approaches to lower your risk, please refer to my book, *Waking the Warrior Goddess: Dr. Christine Horner's Program to Protect Against and Fight Breast Cancer.* Here are just a few dietary supplements that have been shown to help:

Vitamin D3

Most famous for making bones and teeth strong by helping the body to effectively use calcium and phosphorus, vitamin D also supports breast health. Numerous studies have found that low vitamin D levels are associated with a higher risk of breast cancer. In fact, the impact of having deficient amounts of vitamin D can be quite significant. In a study published in 2013, Australian women with the lowest levels of vitamin D compared to women whose levels were optimal had up to a 2.5 times higher risk of breast cancer. A study presented by the American Society of Oncology found that women low in vitamin D were twice as likely to have their cancers spread and 73 percent more likely to die compared to women who had healthy levels of this vitamin. Prospective studies show that supplemental vitamin D3 may drop the risk of breast, prostate, and colon cancers by over 50 percent. Recommended doses are 2,000–8,000 IU per day.

Research shows that vitamin D supports breast health in the following ways:

- Helps to make breast cells more resistant to damage by toxins

- Decreases the ability of breast cells to divide

- Stops tumor cells from growing (anti-proliferative)

- Decreases the ability of tumor cells to invade into surrounding tissues and spread to other areas of the body (anti-metastatic)

- Causes the death of tumor cells through apoptosis

- Prevents new blood vessels from growing into a tumor (anti-angiogenic)

- Boosts the immune system, especially the activity of natural killer (NK) cells

- Decreases the activity of the COX-2 inflammatory enzyme

- Lowers tumor-growth factor IGF-1

- Inhibits the aromatase enzyme

- Modulates the estrogen receptor

- Supports the immune system

Iodine

Iodine is a trace element that is normally only taken up by the thyroid gland to make thyroid hormones. Breast cells have a temporary ability to uptake and concentrate iodine during pregnancy and lactation—the purpose being to supply the baby with this important substance through the breast milk. Researchers have found that iodine is also significantly taken up by breast cancer cells, but *not* normal breast cells or any other cells in the body. Iodine has been shown to be toxic to breast cancer cells and can cause cell death. A Korean case-controlled study in 2010 showed an inverse association between iodine-rich seaweed intake and the risk of breast cancer. Recommended doses are 180–220 mcg per day.

Research shows that iodine supports breast health in the following ways:

- Toxic to breast cancer cells. Japanese researchers in a study published in the *International Journal of Clinical Oncology* in 2005 reported that the iodine in seaweed killed breast cancer cells more effectively than common chemotherapeutic drugs.

- Involved in the production of antioxidants that protect cells from oxidative damage that can lead to cancer.

- Suppresses the development and growth of both benign and cancerous breast tumors.

Turmeric

More than 8,000 studies published in medical journals confirm that turmeric (member of the same botanical family as ginger: *Zingiberaceae*) possesses numerous anticancer qualities and healing benefits. Research shows that turmeric inhibits the growth of dozens of different cancers, including cancers of the breast, prostate, colon, uterus, ovary, lung, mouth, esophagus, liver, kidney, skin (melanoma), head and neck (squamous cell cancers), nervous system, connective tissue (sarcoma), lymph (lymphoma and multiple myeloma), and blood (leukemia). An article published in the *American Association of Pharmaceutical Scientists* journal listed every known way that turmeric has been shown to selectively kill tumor cells. They described over thirty different ways. The recommended dose is 1,000–2,000 mg per day.

Research shows that turmeric supports breast health in the following ways:

- Blocks the COX-2-enzyme, which is involved in inflammation and strongly promotes tumor growth

- Potent antioxidant qualities (300 times the power of vitamin E)

- Stimulates the immune system

- Blocks the activity of phase 1 enzymes in the liver and breast tissue, reducing the number of carcinogens formed or activated, and enhances the action of phase 2 enzymes, which eliminate more carcinogens

- Helps the body to detoxify mutagens

- Blocks the estrogenic effects of pesticides and other chemicals

- Downregulates the estrogen receptor, reducing its response

- Inhibits the growth of breast tumors that are estrogen/progesterone positive or negative, HER2/neu positive, and triple negative

- Induces apoptosis of tumor cells

- Inhibits cell proliferation

- Prevents tumor cell invasion

- Anti-angiogenic

- Dissuades tumor migration and metastasis

- Blocks the production of the tumor-proliferating cytokine: interleukin-6 (IL-6)

- Increases the effectiveness of both chemotherapy and radiation by making cells more sensitive to their killing effects, while at the same time protecting normal healthy cells against their damaging effects

- Helps to promote weight loss through thermogenesis. Obesity raises the risk of many cancers, including breast cancer, so keeping a normal weight lowers the risk.

Green Tea Extract

Research has shown that green tea is very effective in hampering the growth of at least eleven different types of cancer, including cancers of the esophagus, stomach, colon, bladder, prostate, skin, ovaries, uterus, and breast. Green tea also reduces the risk of lung cancer in smokers, non-Hodgkin's lymphoma, and leukemia. Cancers of the digestive tract are as much as 68 percent lower in tea drinkers. Researchers believe that most of the health benefits of green tea come from substances within it called "polyphenols." The three polyphenols considered most important are gallocatechin (GC), epigallocatechin (EGC), and epigallocatechin gallate (EGCG). Of the three, EGCG is the most potent. Recommended doses are 500–1,000 mg per day.

Research shows that green tea supports breast health in the following ways:

- COX-2 anti-inflammatory

- Antioxidant

- Blocks phase 1 liver enzymes and enhances phase 2 enzymes

- Improves function of liver enzymes that detoxify toxins

- Enhances the immune system to make it more effective at identifying and destroying cancer cells

- Improves DNA repair

- Increases the number of sex-hormone binding globulin (SHBG) proteins in the blood. SHBG binds estrogen and prevents it from attaching to estrogen receptors in the breast.

- Downregulates the alpha-estrogen receptor

- Lowers estradiol levels

- Decreases several tumor-promoting growth factors, including IGF-1

- Influences the expression of twelve different genes in breast cancer cells that help to reduce their growth

- Enhances the effectiveness of chemotherapy

Flax Lignans

Lignans are natural plant compounds that have over dozen anticancer qualities. They are found abundantly in certain fruits, vegetables, beans, seeds, and legumes. Flaxseeds contain at least 100 times more lignans than any other known edible plant. Research shows that women with the highest amounts of lignans in their urine—a reflection of how much they consume in their diet—have the lowest risk of breast cancer. If a woman who consumes high amounts of lignans develops breast cancer, she is far less likely to be diagnosed with invasive, aggressive, and/or triple negative tumors and her survival is better. The recommended dose is 250–1,000 mg per day.

Research shows that flax lignans support breast health in the following ways. They:

- Decrease production of estrogen
- Act as a "selective estrogen receptor modulator" blocking estradiol and environmental estrogens from attaching to estrogen receptors
- Have an anti-inflammatory effect
- Impart antioxidant benefits
- Improve 2-OH estrone to 16-OH estrone ratio
- Cause breast cells to be more resistant to environmental toxins
- Decrease three different growth factors that speed up the growth of breast cancer: VEGF, epithelial growth factor, and IGF-1
- Kill tumor cells through apoptosis
- Serve as an anti-proliferative
- Act as an anti-metastatic
- Increase amount of sex-hormone binding globulin in the blood
- Lengthen the time between menstrual cycles
- Block the aromatase enzyme
- Decrease tumor growth and invasion
- Decrease breast density
- Reduce the risk of other cancers, including cancers of the prostate and colon

Diindolylmethane (DIM)

Indole-3-carbinol (I3C) is a substance found in high quantities in cruciferous family of vegetables and has been shown to have strong anticancer qualities. When I3C is ingested, it is converted by stomach enzymes to a substance called "diindolylmethane" (DIM). DIM is two molecules of indole-3-carbinol joined together, and has a stronger effect on the body than I3C. For example, DIM appears to be much more powerful at blocking the estrogen receptors compared to I3C. According to a study published in the *Journal of Nutritional Biochemistry* in 2006, DIM was twenty times stronger. Recommended amounts are 120 mg per day.

Research shows that I3C and DIM support breast health in the following ways. They:

- Stop breast cancer cells from growing by shutting off a key enzyme (cyclin-dependent kinase) necessary for the cells to grow.

- Downregulate the estrogen receptor: decreasing the cell division rate in response to activation.

- Increase production of 2-OH estrone compared to 16-OH estrone in the liver. Researchers have found that 16-OH estrone—a breakdown product of estrogen—is a significant contributor of breast cancer. In one study, the amounts of 2-OH estrone and 16-OH estrone were measured in healthy women and women with breast cancer. Those with breast cancer had almost twice as much 16-OH estrone as the healthy women.

- Turn on a "tumor-suppression gene," which sends messages that prevent tumor cells from invading bodily tissues, spreading to other areas of the body, and from adhering together. A 2011 Canadian study found two other genes involved in cancer growth that diindolylmethane (DIM) quiets transcription factor Sp1 and fatty acid synthase.

- Block the estrogen receptor, preventing strong natural or chemical estrogens from attaching to it and turning it on.

- Encourage the production of p21, which stops cell growth in both estrogen- and progesterone-positive and negative tumors.

- Prevent the initiation of tumor growth by stimulating immune function in many different ways, including increasing interferon, amplifying production of immune cells in the spleen, and improving macrophage function.

- Dissuade the growth of new blood vessels into tumors by as much as 76 percent.

- Inhibit the COX-2 enzyme and therefore, all of its cancer-promoting effects.

Resveratrol

Resveratrol, discussed in chapter 4, is an antioxidant found in abundance in the skins of grapes, peanuts, raspberries, and mulberries. There were more than 400 studies in the medical literature detailing the anticancer effects of resveratrol. Only a few human clinical trials have been done using resveratrol supplements, and the results of all of them are encouraging. Resveratrol has been shown to reduce the growth of several types of cancer, including cancers of the colon and breast. The recommended amount is 100 mg per day.

Research shows that resveratrol supports breast health in the following ways:

- Antioxidant: A clinical trial found that 40 mg of resveratrol significantly reduced the markers of oxidative (free radicals) and inflammatory stress when given to healthy people for six weeks.

- Anti-inflammatory and blocks the COX-2 enzyme

- Anti-proliferative: Resveratrol has been shown to promote normal cell replication. Studies document that it inhibits colon, breast, liver, lung, lymphocyte, and prostate cancer cell replication by halting the cell replication cycle.

- Decreases the production of the tumor-growth factor IGF-1

- Kills tumor cells by apoptosis

- Anti-angiogenic

- Inhibits the aromatase enzyme

- Prevents tumor cell adhesion

- Anti-invasive

- Anti-metastatic

- Improves cytotoxic effects of radiation and chemotherapy

- Improves cytotoxic effects of vitamin D3

- Prevents the transformation of breast cancer stem cells and normal breast cells into cancer cells

- Suppresses lymphoid and myeloid cancers; multiple myeloma; cancers of the breast, prostate, colon, liver, stomach, pancreas, thyroid, cervix, and ovary; head and neck squamous cell carcinomas; and melanoma

Shiitake Mushroom Extract

More than 100 studies have been published documenting the antitumor and immunomodulatory actions of the mycelia of shiitake mushrooms (*Lentinus edodes*). Clinical studies show that those who regularly consume the extract of shiitake mushrooms have a lower incidence of numerous types of cancer, including breast cancer. Shiitake mushroom extracts have also been shown to improve survival statistics and quality of life when given in combination with postoperative adjuvant chemotherapy. In Japan, shiitake mushroom extracts (administered as an injection or orally) have been approved as an adjuvant treatment for cancer patients. An alpha-glucan-rich compound isolated from the mycelium of several subspecies of shiitake called "active hexose correlated compound" (AHCC) is the second most popular complementary and alternative medicine used by cancer patients in Japan.

Research shows that shiitake mushroom extract supports breast health in the following ways:

- Anti-proliferative
- Apoptotic cells death
- Immunomodulation

Maitake Mushrooms

Maitake mushrooms (*Grifola frondosa*) grow in clusters on hardwood trees and are indigenous to the Northern Hemisphere. In Japanese, "maitake mushrooms" means "dancing mushrooms." As legend has it, the name comes from how the ancients danced for joy when they found these extremely valuable mushrooms. Most of the medicinal effects of this mushroom are thought to come from a special polysaccharide (a type of sugar). Found in what scientists call the "D fraction" in the maitake mushroom, the polysaccharide contains a substance called "beta-glucans," which research shows stimulates the immune system and has direct tumor killing effects.

In a human study, patients diagnosed as having stage-2, stage-3, or stage-4 breast cancer were given a combination of whole maitake powder and the "D fraction" of maitake mushrooms. Tumors shrank and symptoms improved in 68.8 percent of the patients.

Researchers have found that the maitake mushrooms also helps to shrink cancers of the prostate, liver, and lung. In addition, maitake mushroom extract has been shown to reduce the side effects of chemotherapy. In a study of 165 cancer patients, 90 percent reported an improvement in nausea, vomiting, and hair loss associated with cancer treatments and 83 percent reported pain reduction.

Research shows maitake mushrooms support breast health in the following ways. They:

- Kill tumor cells by apoptosis

- Act as an anti-metastatic

- Serve as an anti-invasive

- Boost the immune system by increasing the number and function of natural killer (NK) cells, macrophages, and T cells

- Reduce side effects of cancer treatments

I recommend maitake-D fraction supplements made by the company Mushroom Wisdom. The recommended daily dose is 20–40 mg of the extract and 600 mg of dried maitake powder.

For the best protection, I recommend a combination formula such as two that I helped to formulate. Protective Breast Formula made by Integrative Therapeutics contains turmeric, green tea, maitake mushrooms, vitamin D3, DIM, calcium D-glucarate, and grape seed extract. ProShield is made by the Institute for Vibrant Living (www.IVLproducts.com) and contains turmeric, green tea, iodine, flax lignans, resveratrol, DIM, vitamin D3, and shiitake mushrooms.

Acknowledgments

irthing a book is one of the most difficult journeys I have ever undertaken. Having made it through a general surgery residency—that's saying a lot! I swore I would never do it again, but I did. This book seemed even more difficult than the first. It is a journey that cannot be taken alone, and there are so many people who helped me along the way.

The process began with the book proposal, and I am in awe and gratitude of all the people who generously donated their time and expertise giving me feedback and editing. It is a reminder of how truly blessed I am. There were several of my book proposal editors who also generously volunteered to review my book.

Jay P. White—novelist, poet, copywriter, general expert in the English language, entrepreneur, fellow natural health enthusiast, undying optimist, humorist, and profound friend. I am so grateful for your tremendous writing and editing talents, which you graciously offered for not only the proposal, but also the book. I can't imagine making it through this process without all of your support—both professionally and personally. It's a sign of a true friend who can stick with me through all the difficult times—and there were lots of them on this journey! I will forever be grateful.

Bette Craig—former English teacher and counselor, wise woman, inspirer, and one of my dearest friends. You have contributed so much to my life in so many ways. Thanks for your brilliant input and editing on the proposal and book; and for your incredibly supportive friendship through the years.

Deborah Horner—teacher, musician, devoted and loving wife to my dear brother, extraordinary mother, business partner, exercise buddy, best sister-in-law ever, and one of my all-time closest friends. Can't thank you enough for everything you do for me and for all the ways you make my life more rich and joyful. I'm so glad you married my brother!

Dotti Posillico—world's best supporter and my dearest friend. Thanks for not only editing my book proposal, but for all of your unconditional love and support. I am so grateful to have such a kind and loving soul walking together with me on this journey. Your friendship means everything. Love you dearly, sister.

Shoshana and David Olsen—kind and generous friends, kindred spirits, health enthusiasts, and beacons of light. Thank you both for all your time and hard work editing my proposal and for your wonderful friendship.

Irene Bauer—amazing woman, Rotarian, and dancer with a gleam in her eyes. Thanks so much for helping to edit my proposal. I so appreciate your skills and intellect. You are a gem!

Kelly Rudy—former pilot, race car driver and motorcycle adventurer (aka adrenaline junky), exotic traveler, premier pet-sitter, father, grandfather, and loving friend. Thanks so much for your help with my proposal. I'm especially grateful for you being a wonderful "Uncle Kelly" to Sita and for your deep friendship throughout the years. Have fun on your adventure and come back safely from South America!

Karen Overton—former executive secretary to a military general and a super meticulous editor. Can't believe everything you found! I so appreciate your kindness and generosity for offering to edit my book proposal and book. You are fabulous!

Keri Goldsmid—dear friend, gifted artist, spiritual seeker, soul sister, beach-walk companion. Thanks so much for the extraordinary job you did along with your super-talented brother, Scott Ressler, creating all the drawings of the gemstones and bejeweled breastplates. You rock! And thanks even more for your sweet spirit and the richness you add to my life. Every time I'm with you I feel lighter and more peaceful. You are a unique and rare gem in my life.

Much appreciation goes out to all my amazing colleagues who provided endorsements for my book: Dr. Memhet Oz, Dr. Joseph Mercola, Dr. Christiane Northrup, Dr. Nancy Lonsdorf, Dr. John Doulliard, and Dr. Hyla Cass.

Thanks to my extraordinary agent Jeanne Fredericks for supporting my book and me during the process of pitching publishers. Can't thank you enough for all of your hard work and excellent advice. You are truly one of the best!

I have an immense amount of gratitude for Carol Killman Rosenberg and her exceptional talent as a copyeditor, along with her equally talented husband, Gary Rosenberg, for the cover design and typesetting. Thanks for helping me take the "Independent" leap! My heartfelt thanks also goes to my former publisher, Norman Goldfind, for his mentorship and dear friendship.

Finally, my gratitude goes to two of the most generous and kind human beings I have ever known, Rita Starr and Ivor Rose. Without their extraordinary support, this book would not have been possible. As I have said to you many times—I counted my lucky stars the day I met you, Rita Starr. Thank you for your amazing friendship, extraordinary support and generosity that are beyond words. I love you both dearly. Thank you so much for believing in me.

Recommended Reading

Anti-aging and Longevity

Buettner, Dan. *The Blue Zones*. Washington D.C.: National Geographic, 2008.

De Grey, Aubrey, Ph.D. *Ending Aging*. New York, NY: St. Martin's Press, 2007.

Fossel, Michael M.D., Blackburn, Greta. Woynarowski, Dave, M.D. *The Immortality Edge*. Hoboken, New Jersey: John Wiley & Sons, Inc., 2011.

Ayurveda

Bhishagratna, Kaviraj Kunjalal. *The Sushruta Samhita: An English Translation Based on Original Texts*. New Delhi: Cosmo Publications, 2006.

Chopra, Deepak, M.D. *Perfect Health*. New York, NY: Harmony Books, 1991.

Dreyer, Ronnie. *Vedic Astrology*. York Beach, ME: Samuel Weiser, 1997.

Emoto, Masaru. *The Message from Water: The Message from Water is Telling Us to Take a Look at Ourselves 1*. Tokyo: Hado, 2000.

Hagelin, John, Ph.D. *Manual for a Perfect Government*. Fairfield, IA: Maharishi University Management Press, 1998.

Lad, Vasant. *Secrets of the Pulse: The Ancient Art of Ayurvedic Pulse Diagnosis*. Albuquerque, NM: The Ayurvedic Press, 1996.

Lad, Vasant. *Ayurveda: The Science of Self-Healing*, Santa Fe, NM: Lotus Press,1984.

Levacy, William. *Beneath the Vedic Sky*. Carlsbad, CA: Hay House, 1999.

Lonsdorf, Nancy, M.D. *A Women's Best Medicine for Menopause*. New York, NY: Contemporary Books, 2002.

Lonsdorf, Nancy, M.D., Veronica Butler, M.D., and Melanie Brown, Ph.D. *A Woman's Best Medicine*. New York, NY: Putnam, 1995.

O'Connell, David, Ph.D., and Charles Alexander, Ph.D. *Self Recovery: Treating Addictions Using Transcendental Meditation and Maharishi Ayur-Veda*. Binghamton, NY: Harrington Park Press, 1994.

Roth, Robert. *Transcendental Meditation*. New York, NY: Donald Fine, 1994.

Sharma, Hari, M.D. *Freedom from Disease*. Toronto, Canada: Veda Publishing, 1993.

Sharma, Hari, M.D., and Christopher Clark, M.D. *Contemporary Ayurveda*. New York, NY: Churchill Livingstone, 1998.

Sharma, Ram Karan and Dash, Bhagwan. *Caraka Samhita: Text with English Translation & Critical Exposition Based on Cakrapani Datta's Ayurveda Dipika* (7 Volume Set). Vapanasi: Chowkhamba Sanskrit Series, 2009.

Tirtha, Swami Sada Shiva. *The Ayurvedic Encyclopedia.* Bayville, NY: Ayurveda Holistic Center Press, 1998.

Wallace, Robert, Ph.D. *The Neurophysiology of Enlightenment.* Fairfield, IA: Maharishi International University Press, 1991.

Wallace, Robert, Ph.D. *The Physiology of Consciousness.* Fairfield, IA: Maharishi International University Press, 1993.

Emotional and Spiritual Health

Arylo, Christine. *Madly in Love with ME: The Daring Adventure of Becoming Your Own Best Friend.* Novato, CA: New World Library, 2012.

Bragdon, Emma, Ph.D. *Spiritual Alliances: Discovering the Roots of Health at the Casa de Dom Inacio.* Woodstock, VT: Lightening Up Press, 2002.

Bragdon, Emma, Ph.D. *Spiritism and Mental Health: Practices from Spiritist Centers and Spiritist Psychiatric Hospital in Brazil.* Philadelphia, PA: Singing Dragon, 2012.

Hunt, Valerie. *Infinite Mind: Science of the Human Vibrations of Consciousness.* Malibu, CA: Malibu Pub, 1996.

McTaggart, Lynne. *The Intention Experiment.* New York, NY: Free Press, 2007.

Motz, Julie. *Hands of Life: Use Your Body's Own Energy Medicine for Healing, Recovery, and Transformation.* New York, NY: Bantam, 2000.

Moorjani, Anita. *Dying to Be Me: My Journey from Cancer, to Near Death, to True Healing.* New York: Hay House, 2012.

Myss, Carolyn, Ph.D. *Anatomy of the Spirit: The Seven States of Power and Healing.* New York, NY: Harmony Books, 1996.

Myss, Carolyn, Ph.D. *Sacred Contracts.* New York, NY: Three Rivers Press, 2002.

Myss, Carolyn, Ph.D. *Why People Don't Heal and How They Can.* New York, NY: Three Rivers Press, 1997.

Ornish, Dean, M.D. *Love and Survival.* New York, NY: Harper Collins, 1995.

Pert, Candace, Ph.D. *Molecules of Emotion.* New York, NY: Touchstone. 1997.

Tipping, Colin. *Radical Forgiveness.* Marietta, GA: Global 13, 2002.

Tolle, Eckhart. *The Power of Now.* Novato, CA: New World Library, 1999.

Tripodi, Jonathan. *Freedom from Body Memory.* 3rd ed. Virginia Beach, VA: Three Feet Publications, 2012.

Yogananda, Paramhansa. *Autobiography of a Yogi.* Kolkata: Yogoda Satsanga Society of India, 2001.

Food and Nutrition

Boyens, Ingeborg. *Unnatural Harvest.* Toronto, Canada: Doubleday Canada, 1999.

Cummins, Ronnie, and Ben Lilliston. *Genetically Engineered Food*. New York, NY: Marlowe and Company, 2000.

Garrett, Howard. *J. Howard Garrett's Organic Manual*. Fort Worth, TX: The Summit Group, 1993.

Gastelu, Daniel, and Fred Hatfield, Ph.D. *Dynamic Nutrition for Maximum Performance*. Garden City Park, NY: Avery Publishing Group, 1997.

Gittleman, Louise. *The Fast Track Detox Diet: Boost Metabolism, Get Rid of Fattening Toxins, Jump-Start Weight Loss and Keep the Pounds Off for Good*. New York, NY: Morgan Road Books, 2006.

Hospodar, Miriam. *Heaven's Banquet: Vegetarian Cooking for Life Long Health the Ayurveda Way*. New York, NY: Dutton, 1999.

Johari, Harish. *The Healing Cuisine: India's Art of Ayurvedic Cooking*. Rochester, VT: Healing Arts Press, 1994.

Richard, David, and Dorie Byers. *Taste Of Life! The Organic Choice*. Bloomington, IL: Vital Health Publishing, 1998.

Robbins, John. *The Food Revolution*. Berkeley, CA: Conari Press, 2001.

Schlosser, Eric. *Fast Food Nation*. New York, NY: Houghton Mifflin, 2001.

Smith, Jeffrey. *Genetic Roulette: The Documented Health Risks of Genetically Engineered Foods*, (4th edition). White River Junction, VT: Chelsea Green, 2007.

Smith, Jeffrey. *Genetic Roulette: The Gambles of Our Lives*. DVD. Fairfield, IA: Institute for Responsible Technology, 2012.

Steinman, David. *Diet for a Poisoned Planet*. New York, NY: Harmony, 1990.

General Health

Abramson, John, M.D. *Overdosed America: The Broken Promise of American Medicine*. New York, NY: HarperCollins, 2005.

Quantum Physics and Energy

Greene, Brian. *The Elegant Universe*. New York, NY: Vintage Books, 1999.

Gittleman, Louise. *Zapped: Why Your Cell Phone Shouldn't Be Your Alarm Clock and 1,268 Ways to Outsmart the Hazards of Electronic Pollution*. New York. NY: Harper One, 2010.

Women's Health

Gottfried, Sara. *The Hormone Cure: Reclaim Balance, Sleep, Sex Drive and Vitality Naturally with the Gottfried Protocol*. New York, NY: Scribner, 2013.

Love, Susan, M.D. *Dr. Susan Love's Hormone Book*. New York, NY: Times Books, 1998.

Northrup, Christiane, M.D. *Women's Bodies, Women's Wisdom*. Revised edition. New York, NY: Bantam Books, 1998.

Northrup, Christiane, M.D. *The Wisdom of Menopause*. New York, NY: Bantam Books, 2001.

Resources

AHCC SUPPLEMENT

Quality of Life Labs, Inc.
2975 Westchester Avenue, Suite G-01
Purchase, NY 10577
Phone: 877-937-2422
Websites: www.qualityoflife.net or
  www.drchristinehorner.com

ALPHA-LIPOIC ACID

Integrative Therapeutics
825 Challenger Drive
Green Bay, WI 54311
Phone: 800-931-1709
Fax: 920-469-4444
Websites: www.integrativepro.com or
  www.drchristinehorner.com

AMRIT KALASH

Maharishi Ayurveda Products Int'l
1680 Highway 1 North, Suite 2200
Fairfield, IA 52556
Phone: 800-255-8332
Fax: 719-260-7400
E-mail: info@mapi.com
Website: www.mapi.com
**Use the code "radianthealth" for
a 10% discount**

ANTIOXIDANT SUPPLEMENTS

**Maharishi Ayurveda Products
  International**
1680 Highway 1 North, Suite 2200
Fairfield, IA 52556
Phone: 800-255-8332
Fax: 719-260-7400
E-mail: info@mapi.com
Websites: www.mapi.com or
  www.drchristinehorner.com

New Chapter
90 Technology Drive
Brattleboro, VT 05301
Phone: 800-543-7279
Fax: 800-470-0247
E-mail: info@new-chapter.com
Websites: www.new-chapter.com or
  www.drchristinehorner.com

AYURVEDIC HEALTH EDUCATION

California College of Ayurveda
700 Zion Street
Nevada City, CA 95959
Phone: 530-478-9100
Fax: 530-478-9105
E-mail: info@ayurvedacollege.com
Website: www.ayurvedacollege.com/

Maharishi University of Management
1000 N 4th St.
Fairfield, IA 52557
Phone: 641-472-7000
Website:
  https://www.mum.edu/academic-
  departments/physiology-and-
  health/ms-in-maharishi-ayurveda-
  and-integrative-medicine/overview/

**National Ayurvedic Medical
  Association**
8605 Santa Monica Blvd. #46789
Los Angeles, CA 90069-4109
Phone: 800-669-8914
E-mail: nama@ayurvedaNAMA.org
Website: www.ayurvedanama.org/

The *Ayurvedic* Institute
11311 Menaul Blvd. N.E.
Albuquerque, NM 87112
Phone: 505-291-9698
Website: www.ayurveda.com

AYURVEDIC HEALTH SPAS

AuroMesa, LLC
101 Coyote Loop
P.O. Box 567
Arroyo-Hondo, NM 87571
Phone: 575-776-2212
E-mail: Tizia@auromesa.com
Website: www.auromesa.com

The Ayurvedic Institutes
11311 Menaul Blvd., N.E.
Albuquerque, NM 87112
Phone: 505-291-9698
Website: www.ayurveda.com

Ayurvedic Natural Health Center
1342 North Fairfield Road, Suite B
Beavercreek (Dayton), OH 45432
Phone: 937-429-WELL (9355)
E-mail: ayurveda429WELL@
   sbcglobal.net
Website: www.midwestayurveda.com

Dr. John Douillard's LifeSpa
6662 Gunpark Drive East, Suite 102
Boulder, CO 80301
Phone: 303516-4848 or 866-227-9843
E-mail: info@lifespa.com
Website: lifespa.com

The Raj
1734 Jasmine Avenue
Fairfield, IA 52556
Phone: 800-248-9050 or
   641-472-9580 (in IA)
E-mail: theraj@lisco.com
Websites: www.theraj.com

For European health spas that offer
   ***panchakarma*, visit:**
www.ayurveda.de/mag_forsch.htm
www.ayurveda-badems.de/english/
   haus/index.php
www.maharishi-european-
   sidhaland.org.uk

AYURVEDIC SUPPLEMENTS

Banyan Botanicals
6705 Eagle Rock Ave NE
Albuquerque, NM 87113
Phone: 800-953-6424
E-mail: info@banyanbotanicals.com
Website: www.banyanbotanicals.com

Maharishi Ayurveda Products Int'l
1680 Highway 1 North, Suite 2200
Fairfield, IA 52556
Phone: 800-255-8332
Fax: 719-260-7400
E-mail: info@mapi.com
Website: www.mapi.com

BREVAIL SUPPLEMENT

Barlean's Organic Oils
3660 Slater Road
Ferndale, WA 98248
Phone: 800-445-3529 or
   360-384-0485
Fax: 360-384-1746
Websites: www.barleans.com or
   www.drchristinehorner.com

CALCIUM D-GLUCARATE SUPPLEMENTS

Enzymatic Therapy
825 Challenger Drive
Green Bay, WI 54311
Phone: 800-783-2286
Fax: 920-469-4444
Websites: www.eticonsumer.com or
   www.drchristinehorner.com
Available in Protective Breast Formula.

CARNOSINE SUPPLEMENTS

NOW Foods
Corporate Offices
244 Knollwood Drive, Suite 300
Bloomingdale, IL 60108

Phone: 888-669-3663
Website: www.nowfoods.com

Source Naturals
Customer Service Department
23 Janis Way
Scotts Valley, CA 95066
Phone: 800-815-2333
Website: www.sourcenaturals.com

COENZYME Q10/UBIQUINOL SUPPLEMENTS

Enzymatic Therapy
825 Challenger Drive
Green Bay, WI 54311
Phone: 800-783-2286
Fax: 920-469-4444
Website: www.eticonsumer.com

New Chapter
90 Technology Drive
Brattleboro, VT 05301
Phone: 800-543-7279
E-mail: info@new-chapter.com
Website: www.new-chapter.com

CONJUGATED LINOLEIC ACID (CLA)

NOW Foods
Corporate Offices
244 Knollwood Drive, Suite 300
Bloomingdale, IL 60108
Phone: 888-669-3663
Website: www.nowfoods.com

DETOXIFYING SUPPLEMENTS

Enzymatic Therapy
825 Challenger Drive
Green Bay, WI 54311
Phone: 800-783-2286
Fax: 920-469-4444
Website: www.eticonsumer.com
Whole Body Cleanse

Maharishi Ayurveda Products International
1680 Highway 1 North, Suite 2200
Fairfield, IA 52556
Phone: 800-255-8332
Fax: 719-260-7400
E-mail: info@mapi.com
Websites: www.mapi.com or
  www.drchristinehorner.com
Digest Tone, Herbal Cleanse, Elim-Tox, Elim-Tox-O, Genitrac

DIGESTIVE FORMULAS

Enzymatic Therapy
825 Challenger Drive
Green Bay, WI 54311
Phone: 800-783-2286
Fax: 920-469-4444
Website: www.eticonsumer.com

New Chapter
90 Technology Drive
Brattleboro, VT 05301
Phone: 800-543-7279
Fax: 800-470-0247
E-mail: info@new-chapter.com
Website: www.new-chapter.com

Maharishi Ayurveda Products Int'l
1680 Highway 1 North, Suite 2200
Fairfield, IA 52556
Phone: 800-255-8332
Fax: 719-260-7400
E-mail: info@mapi.com
Website: www.mapi.com
Use the code "radianthealth" for a 10% discount

EMF PROTECTION DEVICES

GIA Wellness
5939 Darwin Court, Suite #103
Carlsbad, CA 92008
Websites: www.drchristinehorner
  .com/shop-emfprotection.cfm
www.drchristinehorner.com/
  dangersofemf.cfm
www.giawellness.com

EMOTIONAL AND RELATIONSHIP EDUCATION AND PRACTITIONERS

An Adventure in Intimacy
Hedy and Yumi Schleifer
Website: www.hedyyumi.com/
  workshops

Body Memory Recall (BMR)
Jonathan Tripodi
Website: www.freedomfrombody
  memory.com

Emotional Freedom Technique
Website: www.eftuniverse.com

Evox
Website: zyto.com/products/EVOX

Eye Movement Dissociative Reprogramming (EMDR)
Website: www.emdr.com

Landmark Education Corporation
Website: www.landmarkworldwide
  .com

Madly in Love with Me
Christine Arylo
Website: www.madlyinlovewithme
  .com

New Realities
Website: www.newreality.com/aff/
  index.php?p=chorner&w=wcscnow

PAIRS
Website: www.pairs.com

Radical Forgiveness
Colin Tipping
Website: www.radicalforgiveness.com

TeleHealing with Gail Raborn, CHT
Transformational hypnosis and mind,
  body, spirit counselor
Phone: 707-937-2271
Website: www.telehealing.com

ENVIRONMENTAL TOXINS (INFORMATION)

Environmental Working Group
1436 U Street, NW, Suite 100
Washington, DC 20009
Phone: 202-667-6982
Website: www.ewg.org

Scorecard (Environmental Defense)
Website: www.scorecard.org

U.S. Environmental Protection Agency
Website: www.epa.gov

ESTRO-G 100

Websites: www.Femina-plus.com,
  www.estrog100.com, or
  www.nowfoods.com/Herbal-Pause-
  with-EstroG-100-60-Veg-
  Capsules.htm

FLAXSEEDS AND FLAX OIL

Barlean's Organic Oils
3660 Slater Road
Ferndale, WA 98248
Phone: 800-445-3529 or 360-384-0485
Fax: 360-384-1746
Websites: www.barleans.com or
  www.drchristinehorner.com

ORGANIC FOODS

Amy's Kitchen, Inc.
P.O. Box 449
Petaluma, CA 94953
Phone: 707-781-7535
E-mail: amy@amyskitchen.net
Website: www.amyskitchen.com

Small Planet Foods (makers of Cascadian Farms)
P.O. Box 9452
Minneapolis, MN 55440
Phone: 800-624-4123
Website: www.cascadianfarm.com
Organic foods, including frozen fruits and vegetables

Earthbound Farm
1721 San Juan Highway
San Juan Bautista, CA 95045
Phone: 800-690-3200
Website: www.ebfarm.com
Organic fruits and vegetables

Eden Foods
701 Tecumseh Road
Clinton, MI 49236
Phone: 517-456-7424, 888-424-EDEN
Fax: 517-456-7854
Website: www.edenfoods.com
Variety of organic foods

Horizon Organic
12002 Airport Way
Broomfield, CO 80021
Phone: 888-494-3020
Fax: 503-652-1371
Website: www.horizonorganic.com
Organic dairy

Lotus Foods
c/o WorldPantry.com, Inc.
1192 Illinois Street
San Francisco, CA 94107
Phone: 866-972-6879
Fax: 510-525-4226
Website: www.lotusfoods.com
Organic grains

Lundberg Family Farms
P.O. Box 369
Richvale, CA 95974
Phone: 530538-3500
Fax: 530-882-4500
Website: www.lundberg.com
Organic grains.

Melissa's/World Variety Produce Inc.
P.O. Box 21127
Los Angeles, CA 90021
Phone: 800-588-0151
Fax: 323-584-7385
E-mail: hotline@melissas.com
Website: www.melissas.com
Organic foods and many recipes

Organic Kingdom
192 West 1480 South
Orem, UT 84058
Phone: 866-699-4950
Fax: 801-426-7627
Website: www.organickingdom.com

Organic Valley Family of Farms/ CROPP Cooperative
One Organic Way
LaFarge, WI 54639
Phone: 888-444-6455
Fax: 608-625-3025
Website: www.organicvalley.com
Organic dairy

Purely Organic, Ltd.
P.O. Box 847
Fairfield, IA 52556
Phone: 877-201-0710
Fax: 641-472-1754
Website: www.purelyorganic.com
Imported organic condiments, grape juice from Italy

Seeds of Change
P.O. Box 4908
Rancho Dominguez, CA 90220
Phone: 888-762-7333
Website: www.seedsofchange.com

ShopOrganic
3450 S. Broadmont Drive, Suite 114
Tucson, AZ 85713
Phone: 520-792-0804
Website: www.shoporganic.com
Online organic food and products store

South Pacific Trading Company
15052 Ronnie Drive, Suite 100
Dade City, FL 33523
Phone: 888-505-4439 or 352-567-2200
Fax: 352-567-2257
Website: www.southpacifictrading
  .com

Sprouts Farmers Market
Corporate Office
11811 N. Tatum Blvd., Suite 2400
Phoenix, AZ 85028
Phone: 480-814-8016 or
  888-5-SPROUT (888-577-7688)
Fax: 480-814-8017
Website: sprouts.com

Stonyfield Farms
10 Burton Drive
Londonderry, NH 03053
Phone: 800-776-2697
Fax: 603-437-7594
Website: www.stonyfield.com
Organic dairy

SunOrganic Farm
411 S. Las Posas Road
San Marcos, CA 92078
Phone: 888-269-9888
Fax: 760-510-9996
Website: www.sunorganic.com
Online organic foods, free catalog

Whole Foods Market, Inc.
World Headquarters
550 Bowie Street
Austin, TX 78703
Phone: 512-477-4455
Fax: 512-482-7000
Website: www.wholefoodsmarket.com

FREQUENCY MEDICINE DEVICES & PRACTITIONERS

Computerized Devices
Asyra Pro
Website: www.asyra.com

Practitioners
Bach Flower Remedies: Alicia Sirkin
E-mail: info@sirkincreativeliving.com
Website: www.sirkincreativeliving
  .com

MVVT

Website: www.vedicvibration.com

GARLIC SUPPLEMENTS

Enzymatic Therapy
825 Challenger Drive
Green Bay, WI 54311
Phone: 800-783-2286
Fax: 920-469-4444
Website: www.eticonsumer.com

New Chapter
90 Technology Drive
Brattleboro, VT 05301
Phone: 800- 543-7279
Fax: 800-470-0247
E-mail: info@newchapter.com
Website: www.newchapter.com

Kyolic
23501 Madero
Mission Viejo, CA 92691
Phone: 949-855-2776, 800-421-2998
Fax: 949-458-2764
E-mail: info@wakunaga.com
Website: www.kyolic.com

GINKGO BILOBA

Nature's Way
Customer Service Department
3051 West Maple Loop Dr., Suite 125
Lehi, UT 84043
Phone: 800-962-8873
Website: www.naturesway.com

NOW Foods
Corporate Offices
244 Knollwood Drive, Suite 300
Bloomingdale, IL 60108
Phone: 888-669-3663
Website: www.nowfoods.com

Source Naturals
Customer Service Department
23 Janis Way
Scotts Valley, CA 95066
Phone: 800-815-2333
Website: www.sourcenaturals.com

GINSENG

Nature's Way
Customer Service Department
3051 West Maple Loop Dr. Suite 125
Lehi, UT 84043
Phone: 800-962-8873
Website: www.naturesway.com

NOW Foods
Corporate Offices
244 Knollwood Drive, Suite 300
Bloomingdale, IL 60108
Phone: 888-669-3663
Website: www.nowfoods.com

Source Naturals
Customer Service Department
23 Janis Way
Scotts Valley, CA 95066
Phone: 800-815-2333
Website: www.sourcenaturals.com

GRAPE SEED EXTRACT

Enzymatic Therapy
825 Challenger Drive
Green Bay, WI 54311
Phone: 800-783-2286
Fax: 920-469-4444
Websites: www.eticonsumer.com or
   www.drchristinehorner.com
Available in Protective Breast Formula

GREEN DRINKS

All Day Energy Greens
Institute for Vibrant Living
P.O. Box 3840
Camp Verda, AZ 86322
Phone: 800-218-1379
Website: www.IVLProducts.com

GREEN TEA

Blue Moon Tea
Website: www.bluemoontea.com

Celestial Seasonings
Website: www.celestialseasonings.com

Choice Organic Teas
Website: www.choiceorganicteas.com

Numi Teas and Teasans
Website: www.numitea.com

Stash Tea
Website: www.stashtea.com

Traditional Medicinals
Website: www.traditionalmedicinals
   .com/products

Yogi Tea
Website: www.yogiproducts.com

GREEN TEA SUPPLEMENTS

Enzymatic Therapy
825 Challenger Drive
Green Bay, WI 54311
Phone: 800-783-2286
Fax: 920-469-4444
Websites: www.eticonsumer.com or
   www.drchristinehorner.com
Available in Protective Breast Formula

New Chapter
90 Technology Drive
Brattleboro, VT 05301
Phone: 800-543-7279
Fax: 800-470-0247
E-mail: info@newchapter.com
Website: www.newchapter.com

GYMNEMA SYLVESTRE

Banyan Botanicals
6705 Eagle Rock Ave NE
Albuquerque, NM 87113
Phone: 800-953-6424
E-mail: info@banyanbotanicals.com
Website: www.banyanbotanicals.com

Nature's Way
Customer Service Department
3051 West Maple Loop Dr. Suite 125
Lehi, UT 84043
Phone: 800-962-8873
Website: www.naturesway.com

Source Naturals
Customer Service Department
23 Janis Way
Scotts Valley, CA 95066
Phone: 800-815-2333
Website: www.sourcenaturals.com

HERBAL ANTI-INFLAMMATORY (ZYFLAMEND)

New Chapter
90 Technology Drive
Brattleboro, VT 05301
Phone: 800-543-7279
Fax: 800-470-0247
E-mail: info@newchapter.com
Websites: www.newchapter.com or
   www.drchristinehorner.com

HERBAL SLEEP FORMULAS

Maharishi Ayurveda Products Int'l
1680 Highway 1 North, Suite 2200
Fairfield, IA 52556
Phone: 800-255-8332
Fax: 719-260-7400
E-mail: info@mapi.com
Website: www.mapi.com
Blissful Sleep and *Deep Rest*
**Use the code "radianthealth" for
   a 10% discount**

New Chapter
90 Technology Drive
Brattleboro, VT 05301
Phone: 800-543-7279
Fax: 800-470-0247
E-mail: info@newchapter.com
Website: www.newchapter.com
Tranquilnite™

HERBS

Frontier Natural Products Co-op
P.O. Box 299
3021 78th Street
Norway, IA 52318
Phone: 800-669-3275
Fax: 800-717-4372
Website: www.frontiercoop.com

World's largest supplier of organic herbs and spices—available in many stores including online stores.

HOME DETOX PROGRAMS

Enzymatic Therapy Natural Medicines
Website: www.eticonsumer.com
Whole Body Cleanse Kit

Maharishi Ayurveda
Website: www.mapi.com
Type in "home detox" into search engine to find several articles from past newsletters with instructions and recipes for home detox programs.

HOUSEHOLD CLEANING PRODUCTS

Country Save
19704 60th Avenue NE
Arlington, WA 98223
Phone: 360-435-9868
Fax: 360-435-0896
E-mail: info@countrysave.com
Website:
www.countrysave.com/prods.php

Earth Friendly Products
111 S. Rohlwing Road
Addison, IL 60101
Phone: 800-335-3267
Fax: 847-446-4437
Website: www.ecos.com

Ecover
P.O. Box 9111058
Commerce, CA 90091
Phone: 800-449-4925
Fax: 323-720-5732
Website: www.ecover.com

Planet, Inc.
2676 Wilfert Road, Suite 201
Victoria, BC V9B 5ZE
Canada
Phone: 250-478-8171 or
800-858-8449
Fax: 250-478-3238
Website: www.planetinc.com

INDOLE-3-CARBINOL SUPPLEMENTS

Enzymatic Therapy
825 Challenger Drive
Green Bay, WI 54311
Phone: 800-783-2286
Fax: 920-469-4444
Websites: www.eticonsumer.com or
www.drchristinehorner.com
Available in Protective Breast Formula

LIGNAN SUPPLEMENTS

Brevail
Barlean's Organic Oils
3660 Slater Road
Ferndale, WA 98248
Phone: 800-445-3529 or
360-384-0485
Fax: 360-384-1746
Websites:
www.barleans.com/brevail.asp or
www.drchristinehorner.com

LOW-EMF HAIR DRYER

CHI Pro Low-EMF Hairdryer
This hairdryer is sold on many different websites and retail stores. Search the Internet to find the best price.

MAGNESIUM SUPPLEMENTS

Natural Vitality
12200 Anderson Mill Road
Austin, TX 78726
Phone: 866-416-9216
Website:
  www.Naturalvitality.com/Natural-
  Calm/

MAITAKE MUSHROOM SUPPLEMENTS

Enzymatic Therapy
825 Challenger Drive
Green Bay, WI 54311
Phone: 800-783-2286
Fax: 920-469-4444
Websites: www.eticonsumer.com or
  www.drchristinehorner.com
Available in Protective Breast Formula

Mushroom Wisdom
1 Madison Street Blvd. F6
East Rutherford, NJ 07073
Phone: 800-747-7418
Email: customerservice@mushroom
  wisdom.com
Website: www.mushroomwisdom.com

MELATONIN SUPPLEMENTS

Integrative Therapeutics
825 Challenger Drive
Green Bay, WI 54311
Phone: 800-931-1709
Fax: 920-469-4444
Websites: www.integrativepro.com or
  www.drchristinehorner.com

MUSHROOMS, DRIED

Life Gourmet Shop, LLC
2814 Ashbury Heights Road
Decatur, GA 30030
Phone: 800-910-0849
E-mail: info@lifegourmetshop.com
Website:
  www.lifegourmetshop.com/dried-
  mushrooms.html

MycoLogical Natural Products, Ltd.
P.O. Box 24940
Eugene, OR 97402
Phone: 888-465-3247
Website: www.mycological.com

OILS, ORGANIC

Barlean's Organic Oils
3660 Slater Road
Ferndale, WA 98248
Phone: 800-445-3529 or
  360-384-0485
Fax: 360-384-1746
Website: www.barleans.com

New Chapter
90 Technology Drive
Brattleboro, VT 05301
Phone: 800-543-7279
Fax: 800-470-0247
E-mail: info@newchapter.com
Website: www.newchapter.com

OLIGONOL

Quality of Life Labs, Inc.
2975 Westchester Avenue, Suite G-01
Purchase, NY 10577
Phone: 877-937-2422
Website: www.qualityoflife.net

PERSONAL CARE PRODUCTS

Aubrey Organics
5046 W. Linebaugh Avenue
Tampa, FL 33624
Phone: 800-282-7394
Fax: 813-876-8166
Website: www.aubrey-organics.com

Burt's Bees
Attn: Consumer Care
P.O. Box 3900
Peoria, IL 61612
Phone: 800-849-7112
Fax: 800-429-7487
Website: www.burtsbees.com

Natracare, LLC
3620 West 10th Street, Unit B, #406
Greeley, CO 80634
Phone: 970-304-0076
Website: www.natracare.com
Chlorine-free feminine hygiene products

Tom's of Maine
P.O. Box 710
302 Lafayette Center
Kennebunk, ME 04043
Phone: 800-FOR-TOMS (800-367-8667)
Fax: 207-985-2196
Websites: www.tomsofmaine.com or www.drchristinehorner.com

PRANAYAMA

The Pranayama Institute
P.O. Box 660
Columbus, NM 88029
Website: www.pranayama.org

For instruction on how to perform *panchakarma,* **visit:**
www.yogajournal.com/practice/219

www.integralyogastudio.com/basic
pranayama.php
www.yogawiz.com/breathing-exercises.html

PRODUCTS FOR THE HOME

Gaiam
833 W. South Boulder Road
P.O. Box 3095
Boulder, CO 80307
Phone: 877-989-6321 or 800-254-8464 (in Canada)
Website: www.gaiam.com
Free catalog: Harmony

ShopOrganic
3450 S. Broadmont Drive, Suite 114
Tucson, AZ 85713
Phone: 520-792-0804
Website: www.shoporganic.com
Online organic food and products store

PROTECTIVE BREAST FORMULA

Enzymatic Therapy
825 Challenger Drive
Green Bay, WI 54311
Phone: 800-783-2286
Fax: 920-469-4444
Websites: www.eticonsumer.com or www.drchristinehorner.com

RAW-FOODS BLENDER

Vita-Mix Corporation
8615 Usher Road
Cleveland, OH 44138
Phone: 887-848-2649
Fax: 440-235-7155
Website: www.ultimateblender.com

RELAXATION DEVICES

Life Vessel Arizona
33747 North Scottsdale Road,
  Suite 115
Scottsdale, AZ 85266
Phone: 480-488-7780
Website: www.lifevesselarizona.com

Life Vessel Boulder
1625 Folsom Street
Boulder, CO 80302
Phone: 303-442-0122
Website: www.lifevesselboulder.com

Life Vessel California
31371 Rancho Viejo Road, Suite 102
San Juan Capistrano, CA 92660
Phone: 949-222-9991
Fax: 949-222-0630
E-mail: info@lifevessel.com
Website: www.lifevessel.com

Light Vessel Santa Fe
199 Paseo de Peralta, Suite D
Santa Fe, NM 87501
Phone: 505-473-1200
Website: www.lightvesselsantafe.com/
  about-light-vessel

New Realities
Transformational Guided Imagery
Website: www.drchristinehorner.com/
  transformationalguidedimagery.html

RESOURCE ORGANIZATIONS

National Green Pages
Co-op America Business Network
1612 K Street NW, Suite 600
Washington, DC 20006
Phone: 800-58-GREEN
Website: www.greenpages.org
Directory to socially and environmentally responsible businesses

Natural Products Association
2112 East 4th Street, Suite 200
Santa Ana, CA 92705
Phone: 800-966-6632
Fax: 714-460-7444
Website: www.npainfo.org

Organic Consumers Association
6771 South Silver Hill Drive
Finland, MN 55603
Phone: 218-226-4164
Website: www.organicconsumers.org

Organic Trade Association
28 Vernon Street, Suite 413
Brattleboro, VT 05301
Phone: 802-275-3800
Fax: 802-275-3801
Website: www.ota.com

U.S. Green Building Council
2101 L Street NW, Suite 500
Washington, DC 20037
Phone: 800-795-1747
E-mail: info@usgbc.org
Website: www.usgbc.org

Vegetarian Resource Group
P.O. Box 1463
Baltimore, MD 21203
Phone: 410-366-8343
Website: www.vrg.org

RESVERATROL SUPPLEMENT

Enzymatic Therapy
825 Challenger Drive
Green Bay, WI 54311
Phone: 800-783-2286
Fax: 920-469-4444
Websites: www.eticonsumer.com or
  www.drchristinehorner.com

ROSEMARY PRODUCTS

Frontier Natural Products Co-op
3021 78th Street
Norway, IA 52318
Phone: 800-669-3275
Website: www.frontiercoop.com

SAUNAS

Sunlighten Infrared Saunas
Website: www.drchristinehorner.com/
links.cfm

SELENIUM SUPPLEMENTS

New Chapter
90 Technology Drive
Brattleboro, VT 05301
Phone: 800-543-7279
Fax: 800-470-0247
E-mail: info@newchapter.com
Website: www.newchapter.com

SKIN CARE LOTIONS AND CREAMS

Aminocare Lotions: www.drchristine
horner.com/shop-oils.cfm
Makana: www.drchristinehorner.com/
shop-oils.cfm
NuSkin: email info@drchristine
horner.com for more information
Sarada Ayurvedic Remedies:
www.saradausa.com
Youthful Skin Cream: www.mapi.com.
Use the code: "radianthealth" for a
10% discount.

STEVIA PRODUCTS

Body Ecology/Stevia.Net
Website: www.stevia.net

HealthWorld Online
Website: www.healthy.net

Wisdom Natural Brands
1203 West San Pedro
Gilbert, AZ 85233
Phone: 800-899-9908
E-mail: wisdom@wisdomnatural
brands.com
Website: www.wisdomherbs.com

STHAPATYAVEDA (VEDIC ARCHITECTURE)

Maharishi Sthapatya Veda
Website: www.maharishivastu.org

SUPERFOODS

Longevity Warehouse
Phone: 805-870-5756
E-mail: support@longevitywarehouse
.com
Website: www.longevitywarehouse.com

Navitas Naturals
936 B Seventh St. Box # 141
Novato, California 94945
Phone: 888-645-4282
E-mail: info@navitasnaturals.com
Website: www.navitasnaturals.com/

TRANSCENDENTAL MEDITATION (TM)

Maharishi Foundation USA
1100 N. 4th Street, Suite 128
Fairfield, IA 52556
Phone: 888-LEARN TM (888-532-7686)
Website: www.TM.org

TURMERIC PRODUCTS

Enzymatic Therapy
825 Challenger Drive
Green Bay, WI 54311
Phone: 800-783-2286
Fax: 920-469-4444
Websites: www.eticonsumer.com or
www.drchristinehorner.com
Available in Protective Breast Formula

Frontier Natural Products Co-op
P.O. Box 299
3021 78th Street
Norway, IA 52318
Phone: 800-669-3275
Fax: 800-717-4372
Website: www.frontiercoop.com
*World's largest supplier of organic
herbs and spices—available in many
stores including online stores.*

New Chapter
90 Technology Drive
Brattleboro, VT 05301
Phone: 800-543-7279
Fax: 800-470-0247
E-mail: info@newchapter.com
Website: www.newchapter.com or
   www.drchristinehorner.com

VITAMIN SUPPLEMENTS

Enzymatic Therapy
825 Challenger Drive
Green Bay, WI 54311
Phone: 800-783-2286
Fax: 920-469-4444
Website: www.eticonsumer.com

New Chapter
90 Technology Drive
Brattleboro, VT 05301
Phone: 800-543-7279
Fax: 800-470-0247
E-mail: info@newchapter.com
Websites: www.newchapter.com or
   www.drchristinehorner.com

WAKAME & MEKABU SEAWEEDS

Eden Foods
701 Tecumseh Road
Clinton, MI 49236
Phone: 517-456-7424, 888-424-EDEN
Fax: 517-456-7854
Website: www.edenfoods.com

WATER-FILTRATION SYSTEMS

Building for Health Materials Center
Website: www.buildingforhealth.com

Nirvana Safe Haven
Website: www.nontoxic.com

WOMEN'S BREAST HEALTH FORMULAS

Institute for Vibrant Living (IVL)
661 E Howards Rd.
Camp Verde, Arizona 86322
Phone: 800-218-1378
Website: www.ivlproducts.com
ProShield

Integrative Therapeutics
825 Challenger Drive
Green Bay, WI 54311
Phone: 800-931-1709
Fax: 920-469-4444
Websites: www.integrativepro.com or
   www.drchristinehorner.com
Protective Breast Formula

WOMEN'S HORMONAL BALANCING FORMULAS

Institute for Vibrant Living (IVL)
661 E Howards Rd.
Camp Verde, Arizona 86322
Phone: 800-218-1378
Website: www.ivlproducts.com
Estro-Sync

ESTRO-G 100
Websites: www.Femina-plus.com,
   www.estrog100.com, or
   www.nowfoods.com/Herbal-Pause-
   with-EstroG-100-60-Veg-
   Capsules.htm

References

The references for all the studies included in this book can be found at **www.drchristinehorner.com**

Index

About the Author

Christine Horner, M.D., F.A.C.S., is a nationally known surgeon, author, and professional speaker residing in San Diego, California. She holds two board certifications: the National Board of Surgery and the National Board of Plastic Surgery. Dr. Horner was recognized as a leader in her field shortly after starting her plastic and reconstructive surgery practice because she successfully ran a national campaign to pass laws requiring insurance companies to pay for breast reconstruction following mastectomy. Her five-year crusade—the Breast Reconstruction Advocacy Project (BRA Project)—led to the passage of laws in thirty-five states and a federal bill, which was signed into law by President Clinton on October 21, 1998.

Dr. Horner has been featured in hundreds of national magazines, radio, and televisions shows, including *The Dr. Oz Show, Mercola.com Interviews, A Healthy You with Carol Alt, Flourish!* with Dr. Christiane Northrup, *CNN Live Saturday,* and *FOX & Friends.* In February 1999 *Glamour* magazine honored her as their "WOW—Woman of the Month." In 2000 Oprah recognized her as part of her "Angel Network" on her television program.

Dr. Horner is the author of the award-winning book, *Waking the Warrior Goddess: Dr. Christine Horner's Program to Protect Against and Fight Breast Cancer.* She has also contributed chapters to several books, including *The Fountain: 25 Experts Reveal Their Secrets of Health and Longevity* and *Chicken Soup for the Soul: Life Lessons for Loving the Way You Live.* A popular keynote speaker, Dr. Horner has traveled across the country and internationally for over twenty years and inspired thousands to achieve better health.

In 1999, Dr. Horner created and hosted the first-ever syndicated television news segment exclusively focused on complementary and alternative medicine and natural approaches to staying healthy. It aired on WCPO-TV and then WLW-TV in Cincinnati, and in 2001, the segment was syndicated on the WISDOM Television Network reaching 5.5 million households.

In June 2002, Dr. Horner left her plastic surgery practice so that she could dedicate herself full time to writing and teaching about her passion: prevention-oriented medicine and how to become and stay healthy naturally.

Dr. Horner stays in touch with her worldwide community through her Internet radio show *The Radiant Health Show with Dr. Christine Horner,* Facebook (www.facebook.com/drchristinehorner), Twitter @ https://twitter .com/DrHornerMD, YouTube channel (http://bit.ly/1KYnc6g), her free news-letter, and website: www.drchristinehorner.com.

CPSIA information can be obtained
at www.ICGtesting.com
Printed in the USA
FSOW02n0406291217
42465FS